HANNAH BARRETT

THE YOGA HAPPY YEAR

A MONTH-BY-MONTH GUIDE FOR A STRONGER AND CALMER YOU

Photography by Cecilia Cristolovean

Illustrations by Eleanor Hardiman

quadrille

MANAGING DIRECTOR Sarah Lavelle
EDITORIAL DIRECTOR Sophie Allen
ASSISTANT EDITOR Oreolu Grillo
COPY EDITOR Imogen Fortes
SENIOR DESIGNER Gemma Hayden
PHOTOGRAPHER Cecilia Cristolovean
ILLUSTRATOR Eleanor Hardiman
HAIR AND MAKE UP Danni Hooker
MODELS Giles Barrett, Geri East, Khala Ongdi, Maria Amparo Buaki-Sogo
VIDEOGRAPHER MikeGlide Photography
HEAD OF PRODUCTION Stephen Lang
SENIOR PRODUCTION CONTROLLER Gary Hayes

This book is not intended as a substitute for genuine medical advice. The reader should consult a medical professional in matters relating to their health.

The publisher would like to thank Liforme (liforme.com) for the generous loan of mats for the photoshoot.

Quadrille
Penguin Random House UK
One Embassy Gardens
8 Viaduct Gardens
London SW11 7BW

Quadrille Publishing Limited is part of the Penguin Random House group of companies whose addresses can be found at global.penguinrandomhouse.com

Penguin Random House UK

Penguin Random House values and supports copyright. Copyright fuels creativity, encourages diverse voices, promotes freedom of expression and supports a vibrant culture. Thank you for purchasing an authorized edition of this book and for respecting intellectual property laws by not reproducing, scanning or distributing any part of it by any means without permission. You are supporting authors and enabling Penguin Random House to continue to publish books for everyone. No part of this book may be used or reproduced in any manner for the purpose of training artificial intelligence technologies or systems. In accordance with Article 4(3) of the DSM Directive 2019/790, Penguin Random House expressly reserves this work from the text and data mining exception.

Published by Quadrille in 2024

www.penguin.co.uk

A CIP catalogue record for this book is available from the British Library

ISBN 978 1 83783 133 3
10 9 8 7 6 5 4 3 2 1

Copyright © Hannah Barrett 2024
Photography © Cecilia Cristolovean 2024
Illustrations © Eleanor Hardiman 2024
Videos © MikeGlide Photography 2024
Design © Quadrille 2024

Hannah Barrett has asserted her right to be identified as the author of this Work in accordance with the Copyright, Designs and Patents Act 1988

Colour reproduction by F1 Colour

Printed in China by C&C Offset Printing Co., Ltd.

The authorised representative in the EEA is Penguin Random House Ireland, Morrison Chambers, 32 Nassau Street, Dublin D02 YH68.

Penguin Random House is committed to a sustainable future for our business, our readers and our planet. This book is made from Forest Stewardship Council® certified paper.

FSC www.fsc.org MIX Paper | Supporting responsible forestry FSC® C018179

CONTENTS

START HERE

The Yoga Happy Year is designed to help you create a lasting and nourishing yoga habit in an *accessible* way. It isn't just a book of yoga sequences (also known as yoga flows); you will be encouraged to incorporate the other elements of a yoga practice, such as yogic breathing techniques, meditation, mindfulness and journaling, too. If this is all new to you, please don't worry – I break everything down into easy-to-digest chunks. And the best bit is, you will quickly start to see the benefits – not only gaining strength and flexibility but feeling less stressed and more connected, content and happier.

This section shares everything you need for the programme to make *sense* and to get *the most out of it* so please don't skip it.

WHAT DOES THE PROGRAMME INCLUDE?

More detail is given below but in summary, each month is based around a set theme and you will be incorporating the following four elements into a weekly routine:

1. A yoga flow (linked to the month's theme) to repeat three to four times per week.
2. A breathing exercise to practise at the start of each flow or whenever required.
3. A meditation or mindfulness exercise to practise daily.
4. A short daily – and a weekly – journaling exercise.

I am **not** expecting you to commit hours each day to your yoga routine; I fully appreciate that life can be hectic. The programme in this book can fit around you and your schedule. On days when you flow, the routine will take less than 30 minutes. On days when you don't get on your yoga mat, the routine can be less than 10 minutes. Commit to prioritising time each day for you and very quickly you will start to see the positive results.

Hannah xx

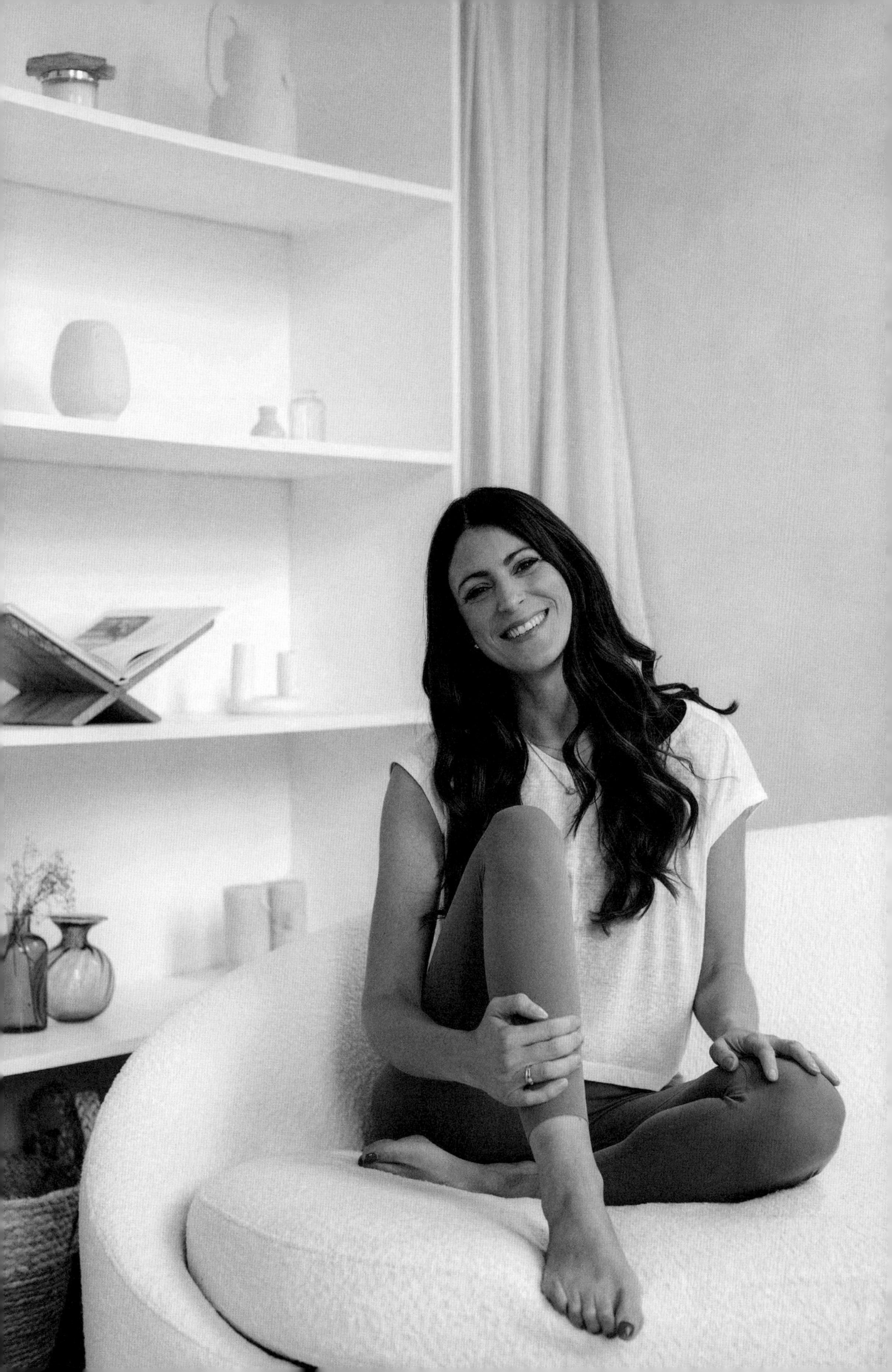

1. YOGA FLOW

Each month you are given a signature yoga flow that is based on the theme of the month and is designed to take around 20 minutes. I recommend that you aim to practise this flow three or four times per week. If on some days you have more time, feel free to repeat the flow or combine it with a flow from a previous month. All poses are broken down in detail in the appendix (see page 190), including ways to modify each pose.

In the later months, you may want to substitute two of your weekly practices with earlier signature flows instead of repeating the flow of the month throughout the week. Part of the practice of yoga is listening in to what your body needs, so this is the perfect opportunity to practise this concept of self-study.

In addition to the signature flows, I have included a warm-up seated flow (see page 10) that can be practised in isolation and/or before each signature flow. This sequence can also be completed in bed every morning as part of a revitalising morning routine, if you would like.

There is also a gentle bedtime flow (see page 13) designed to help calm the nervous system and prepare you for a restful night's sleep.

If you would like to practise all the yoga flows in this book with me, scan the QR code below, which will direct you to guided online classes that take you through versions of each of the flows.

2. BREATHING (*PRANAYAMA*) EXERCISES

The breath is at the heart of a yoga practice, and I will share more about why this is in later chapters. But beyond your breathing on a yoga mat, how we breathe is so important to our daily lives – it can directly impact our emotions. We breathe 24/7 and many of us do it *without* paying any attention to it. However, how we *breathe* is how we *feel*.

Each month I am going to share with you a breathing technique to add to your toolkit for life. Whether you're looking for energy, calm or anger relief, working with your breath can help you to find them. The monthly exercise or technique can be practised before you start the month's signature flow, or used whenever you need it. For example, I love practising the golden thread breath (see page 60) to keep me calm in the morning during the chaos of the school run.

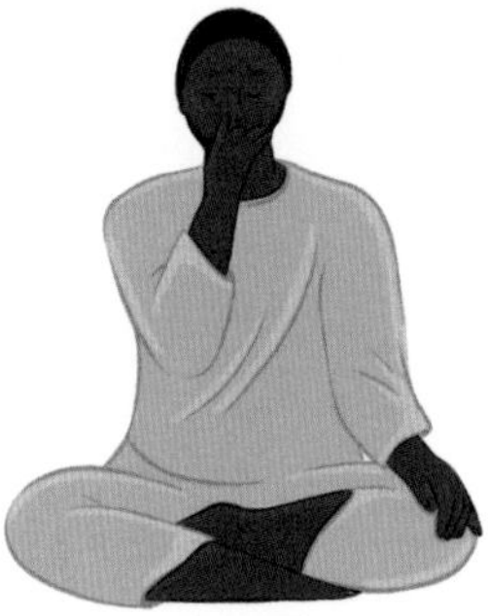

3. MEDITATION AND MINDFULNESS

MEDITATION

Meditation is a key component of yoga and, in fact, the physical practice of yoga (the *asana*) was designed to help prepare the body to be steady and comfortable when seated in meditation.

Perhaps you are sitting reading this thinking that meditation isn't for you. You're visualising meditation being something you do barefoot, in lotus pose, sitting on a hardwood floor for hours on end. But the reality is that you can practise meditation anywhere, on anything (comfy chairs allowed), wearing anything you wish and for as long as you want (a five-minute meditation can still provide great benefits!). Meditation, like all of yoga, is truly for everyone.

There are many interpretations of what meditation is and what it should be. There are also plenty of different techniques. Meditation is an accessible skill for everyone and if one of the practices in this book doesn't resonate with you, please don't worry, simply try another one.

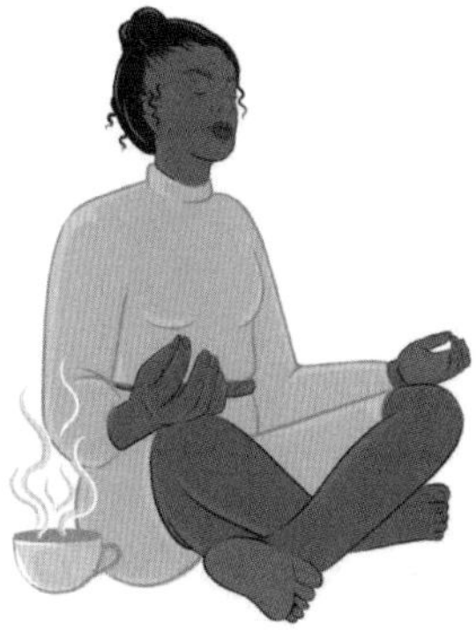

MINDFULNESS

People often get confused between mindfulness and meditation. Meditation is a form of mindfulness, but mindfulness isn't necessarily meditation. In a nutshell, mindfulness is about being fully present and aware of one's experiences, thoughts, emotions and sensations without judgement. It helps us avoid getting caught up in reactivity or automatic patterns of thinking. It also helps us forge a deeper connection to the world around us. A mindfulness exercise could be as simple as a walk in nature in which you take notice of the sights, smells and sounds around you, or a cold shower, during which you are conscious of the cold sensation and how it makes you feel.

Each month I will share a signature meditation or mindfulness exercise for you to practise daily. Prioritise at least five minutes for this or more time if you have it. The benefits of meditation and mindfulness can be huge, so I urge you to keep an open mind and notice the impact it has. As you get further through the book, simply pick the exercise that fits with what you need on that day.

THE REWARDS OF A REGULAR MEDITATION PRACTICE

- Reduced stress and anxiety.
- Enhanced self-awareness.
- Improved sleep quality.
- Encourages a healthy lifestyle.
- May slow ageing (both mind and body).
- Improved immunity.
- Encourages better control of unhelpful habits e.g. stress eating, nail biting.
- Improved self-efficacy (and self-esteem).
- Decreased blood pressure.
- Improved problem-solving abilities.
- Can help control pain.

4. JOURNALING

Journaling is a fantastic way to practise self-study and gain a deeper understanding of your thoughts, emotions and behaviours. I will explain how this links to yoga on page 142, but it is above all a way to recognise the abundance of joy you have in your life already and to reflect on the events of each day: what went well, what didn't and what you can work on. Both yoga and journaling have been shown to improve happiness.

You don't need to have done it before or have a fancy journal. Just grab a plain notebook and follow the structure set out opposite. It's divided into two parts: daily journaling (which will take five to ten minutes) and a weekly reflection.

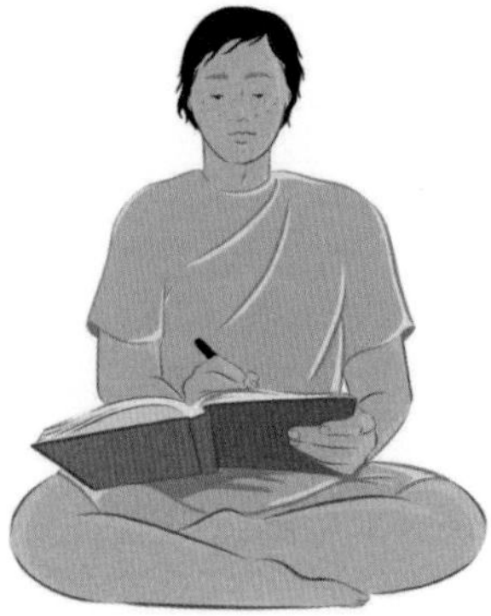

DAILY JOURNALING

Morning: Gratitude

Start every day with gratitude and set a positive tone for the rest of your day. Each morning, write down five things you are grateful for. Be as detailed as you can and try to avoid repeating the same things each day as much as possible. When times are hard, this can feel difficult; I find it helps to think of the things we label as 'small'. For example, a warm place to sleep or the food on the table. The things we might consider minor, but when you properly think about them, are actually so important.

I could write a whole book on why gratitude will change your life but in short, research has shown that gratitude:

- is strongly and consistently associated with greater happiness;
- has shown to help people feel better and more positive about their lives;
- increases exercise frequency and improves physical health;
- facilitates positive emotions and improves resilience;
- increases self-esteem;
- improves relationships and friendships;
- reduces materialism and improves life satisfaction;
- improves decision-making and patience;
- reduces blood pressure;
- improves sleep quality.

Evening: Learning Point

Each evening, reflect on what you can learn from the day. Maybe something didn't go well but instead of ruminating on that fact, think, 'What could I do differently tomorrow?' For example, maybe you spent too long getting lost down a social media rabbit hole. Your reflection could be to be more mindful when you pick up your phone, set time limit boundaries, and each time you pick it up ask yourself if you want to look at it or whether it is habit. That pause will allow you a moment of mindfulness and is surprisingly helpful.

This learning point gives you something to work with; it can help identify patterns that aren't serving you and allow you to change your routine or add more positive habits to it instead.

Evening: Wins

Each evening, write down three wins of the day: what went well or what you enjoyed. A positive reflection before bed is a powerful way to clear your brain of negativity, help you relax and prepare for a restful night's sleep. In fact, there's evidence to suggest that positive thinking can change your brain structure and the way you respond to the world around you.

WEEKLY JOURNALING

Reflection

Alongside the daily journal prompts, each month I provide a set of signature self-study questions. These are based on the theme of the month and should be included in your weekly routine. I find it helpful to set aside time every Sunday to reflect on the week just gone and prepare for the week ahead.

PLANNING AND STRUCTURING YOUR YOGA HAPPY PRACTICE

To give yourself the biggest chance of success with this programme and create a lasting yoga habit, I recommend two things:

1. Each week, plan when you are going to fit in the three or four yoga flow sessions. If you physically pencil them into your diary or mark them in your digital calendar, you are making your wellness a priority and you are more likely to find time to do them.
2. Get up 10–15 minutes early to complete the meditation, breathwork and journaling. This allows you to start your day on the best foot possible and bring your focus inwards (rather than reaching for your phone and immediately connecting to potential external stressors).

'THE BEGINNING IS THE MOST IMPORTANT PART OF THE WORK.'

PLATO

SEATED WARM-UP FLOW

This flow can be practised in isolation or before each monthly signature flow. It's a perfect mindful flow for first thing in the morning; you could even do this in your bed. Focus on breathing in and out through the nose with the inhale and exhale being fairly equal in length.

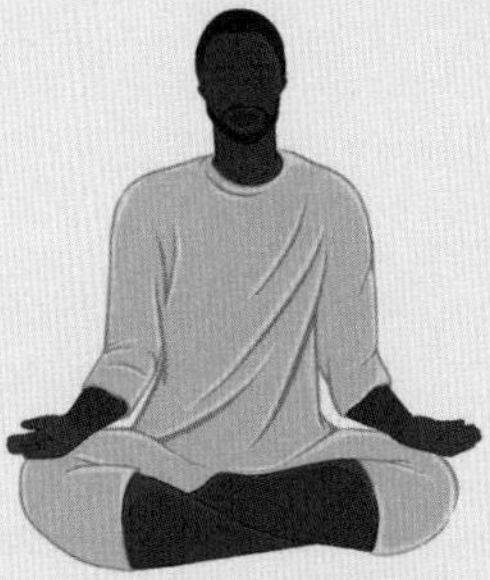

1. EASY POSE

Begin seated and take 5 slow and mindful breaths through the nose for grounding.

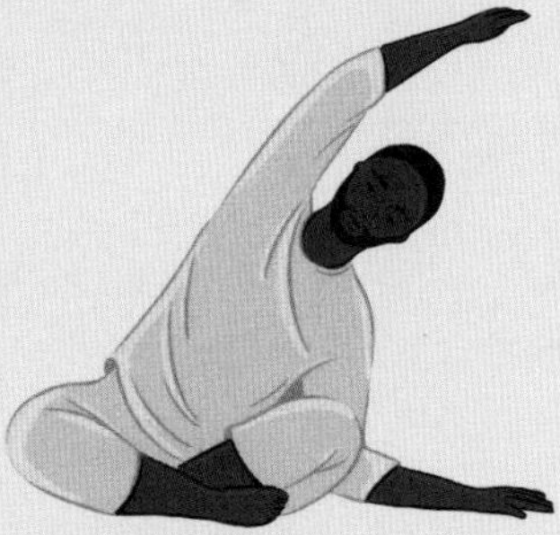

2. SEATED SIDE STRETCH

Repeat 5 times on both sides.

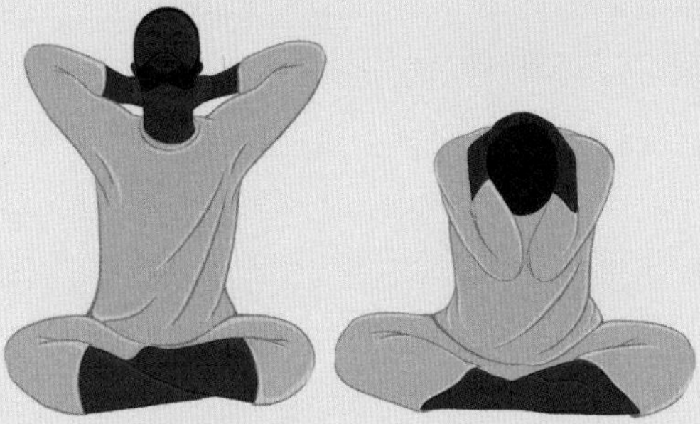

3. HEART OPENER

Inhale to open the heart, exhale to round in. Repeat 5 times.

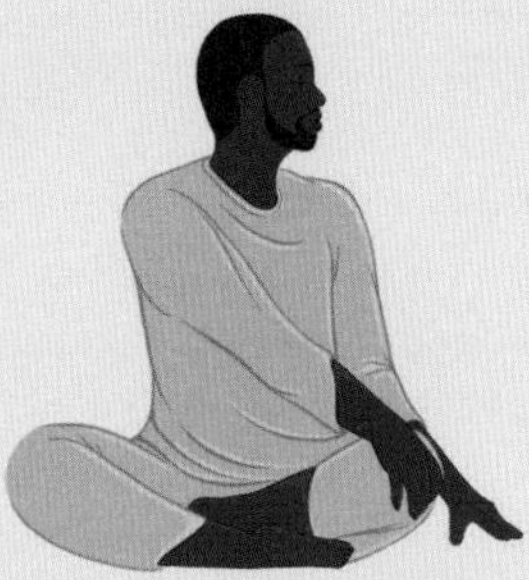

4. SEATED TWIST

Hold for 5 breaths on each side.

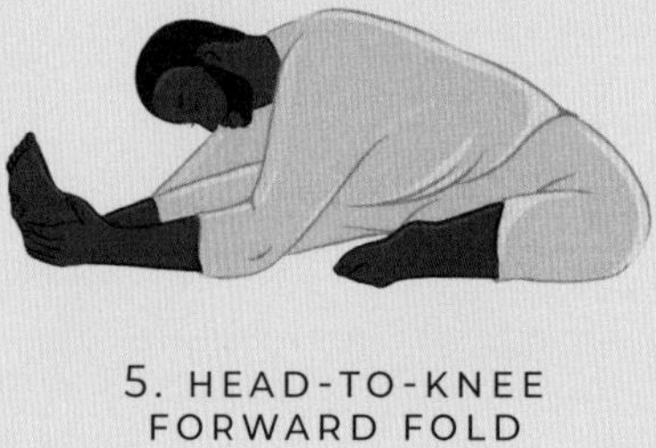

5. HEAD-TO-KNEE FORWARD FOLD

Bend the knee of the extended leg as much as you need. Hold for 5 breaths on each side.

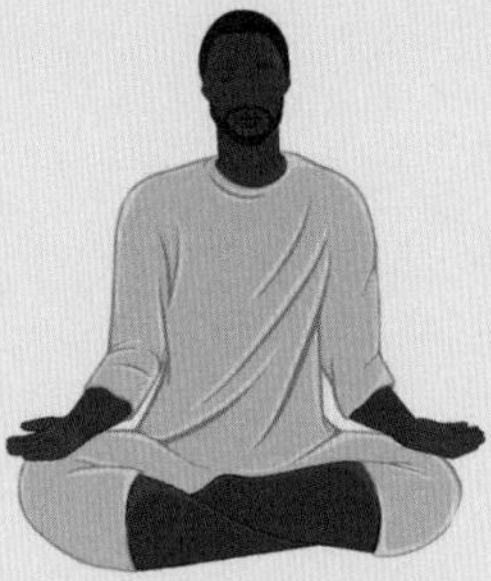

6. EASY POSE

Return to easy pose for 3 final grounding breaths.

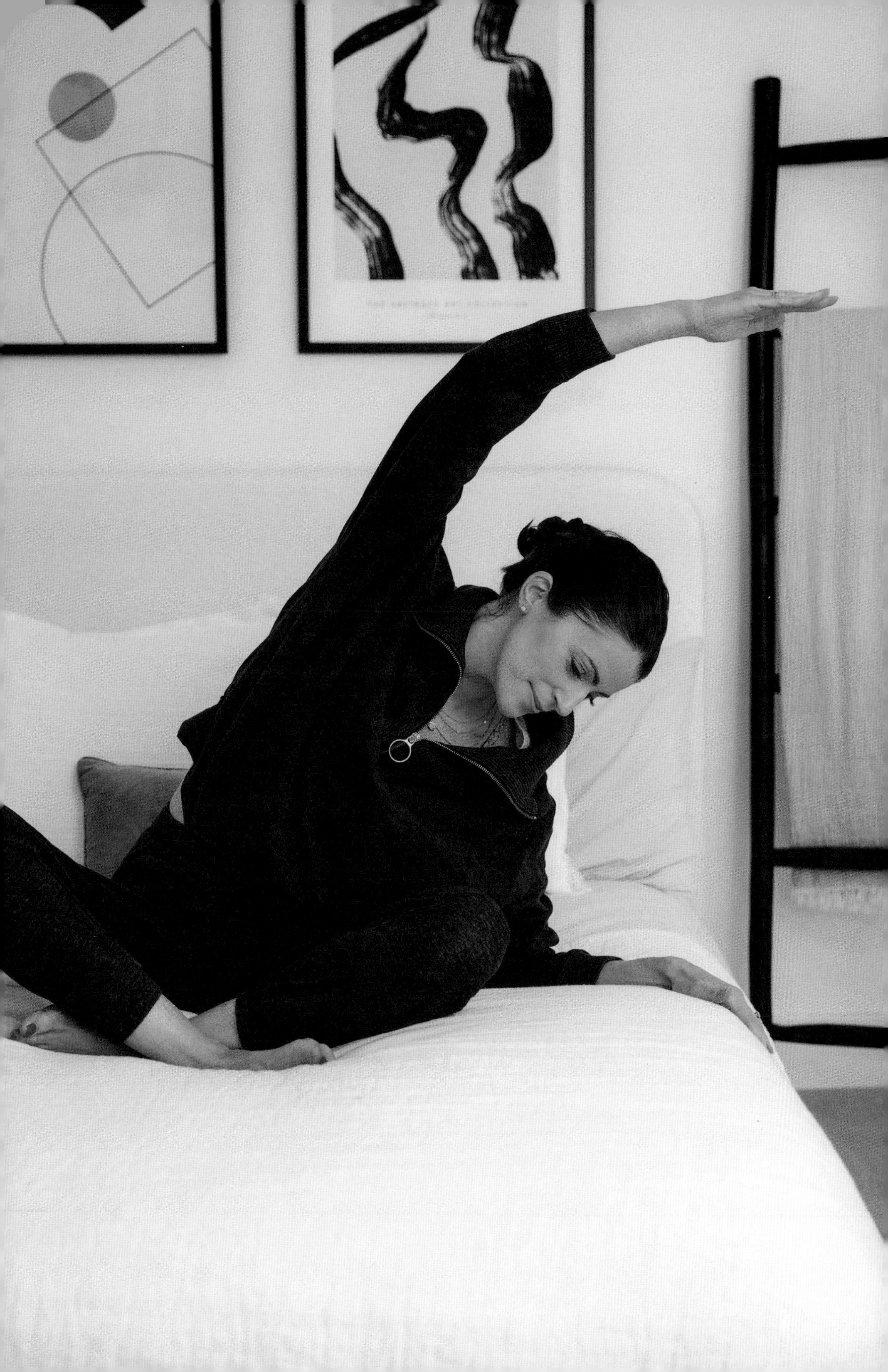

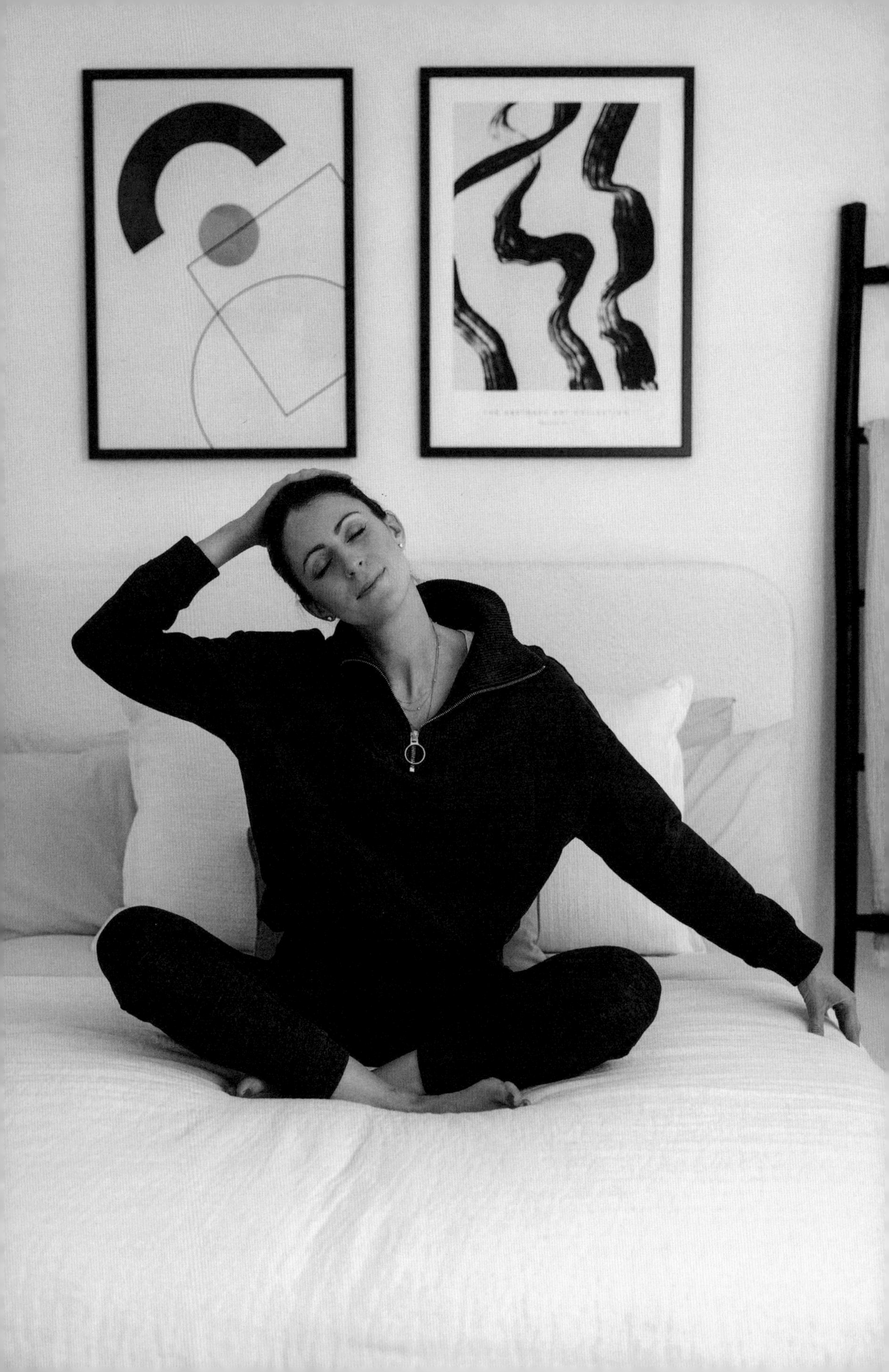

GENTLE BEDTIME FLOW

This flow can be done from a yoga mat or from the comfort of your bed. It's designed to be used as a nourishing bedtime routine to help calm the nervous system, release the tension of the day and prepare you for a restful night's sleep.

Focus on slowing and lengthening the exhales and releasing anything that isn't serving you.

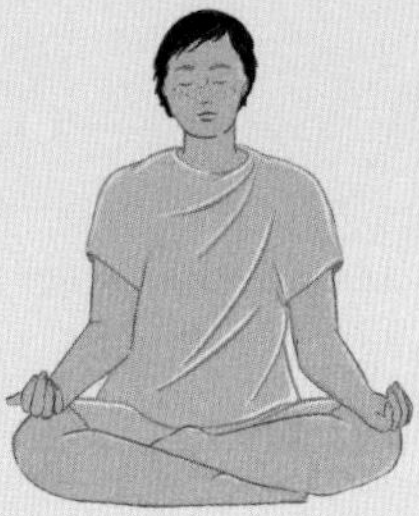

1. EASY POSE

Begin seated and take 5 slow and mindful breaths through the nose for grounding.

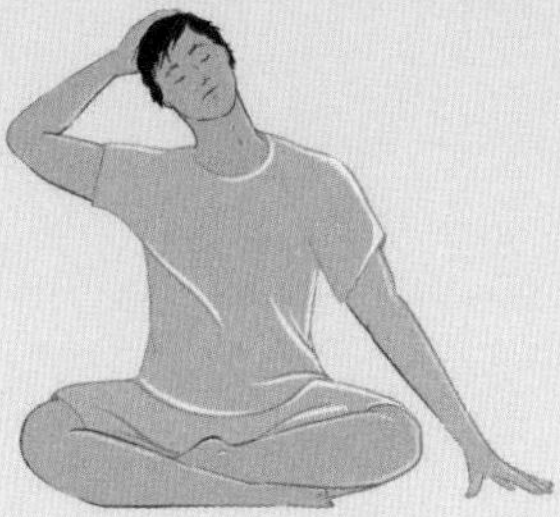

2. SEATED NECK STRETCH

Hold for 5 breaths each side.

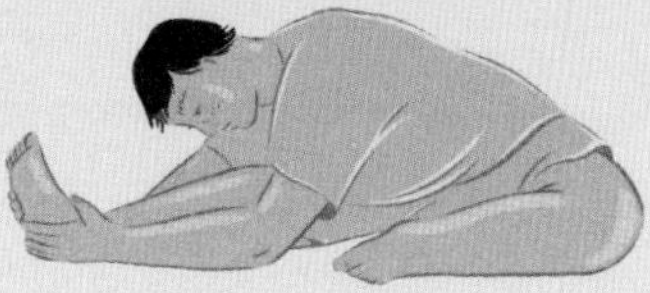

3. HEAD-TO-KNEE FORWARD FOLD

Bend the knee of the extended leg to make the pose more restorative. Hold for 5 breaths on each side.

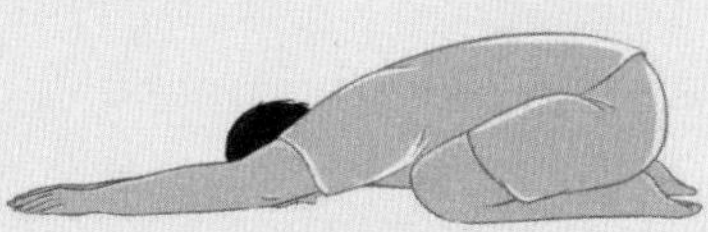

4. CHILD'S POSE

Melt back into child's pose for 5 slow breaths.

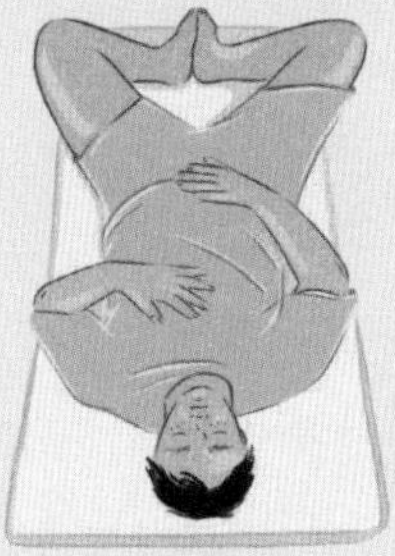

5. RECLINED BOUND ANGLE POSE

Release back and hold for 10 breaths or more.

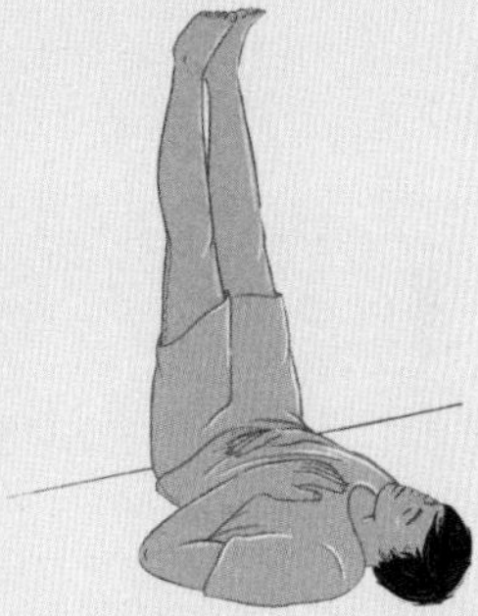

6. LEGS UP THE WALL

Extend the legs and hold for 10 breaths or more. Option to skip this pose if in bed.

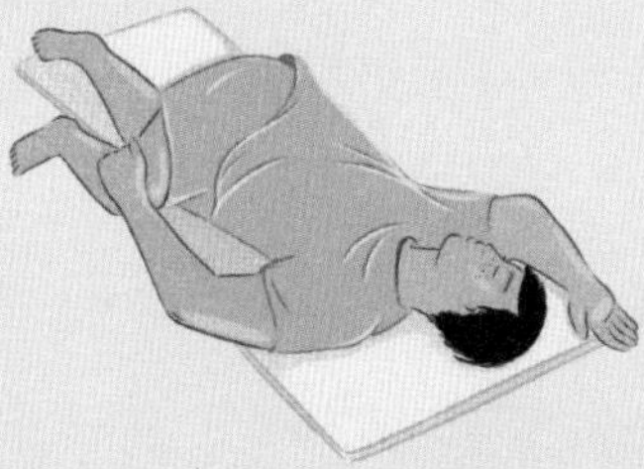

7. SUPINE TWIST

Hug the right knee in and come into a supine twist. Hold for 5 breaths before repeating on the opposite side.

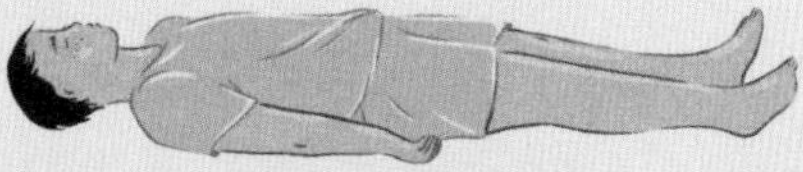

8. SAVASANA

Release into savasana and take 10 rounds or more of 2:1 breathing (see page 143).

SUN SALUTATIONS *(SURYA NAMASKAR)*

Sun salutations, or *surya namaskar,* have been practised for centuries and are deeply rooted in traditional yogic philosophy. They are believed to have been a Vedic ritual and originated as a way to worship the sun, a valued symbol of energy and enlightenment in many cultures, but also an awakening of the inner sun, the inner source of light, wisdom and vitality within each individual. There are different versions of the sun salutation and whilst the basic structure of the sequence typically involves a series of movements that flow and coordinate with the breath, specific variations may differ based on factors such as the tradition, lineage and teacher's preference.

For our Yoga Happy year I am sharing *surya namaskar* A and B which set the foundation of Ashtanga yoga. This is a style of yoga that was developed by Sri Krisha Pattabhi Jois and Tirumalai Krishnamacharya in the 20th century and its sun salutation sequences are the ones I teach in my classes. As well as being rich in physical benefits, such as increased strength, flexibility and endurance, the repetitive and flowing nature of the sun salutations also provides mindful awareness and a moving meditation. The sequences can reduce stress, improve concentration, deepen the mind–body connection and elevate energy levels.

If you are new to the sun salutations, you can always drop the knees in yoga push-up (*chaturanga*); please listen to what your body needs and how the posture feels. For sun salutation B (see pages 18–20), when you transition out of warrior I, over time it will become easier to exhale through plank straight into yoga push-up. However, feel free to take an extra breath in plank, if helpful, before exhaling through yoga push-up.

BEGIN SUN SALUTATIONS WHEN YOU SEE THESE SYMBOLS:

SUN SALUTATION A

See page 16

SUN SALUTATION B

See page 18

PLEASE NOTE
The appendix on page 190 includes a detailed breakdown of each pose, plus variations and modifications. Remember to listen to your body; yoga should never be painful and you can chose to skip any pose that doesn't feel right for you.

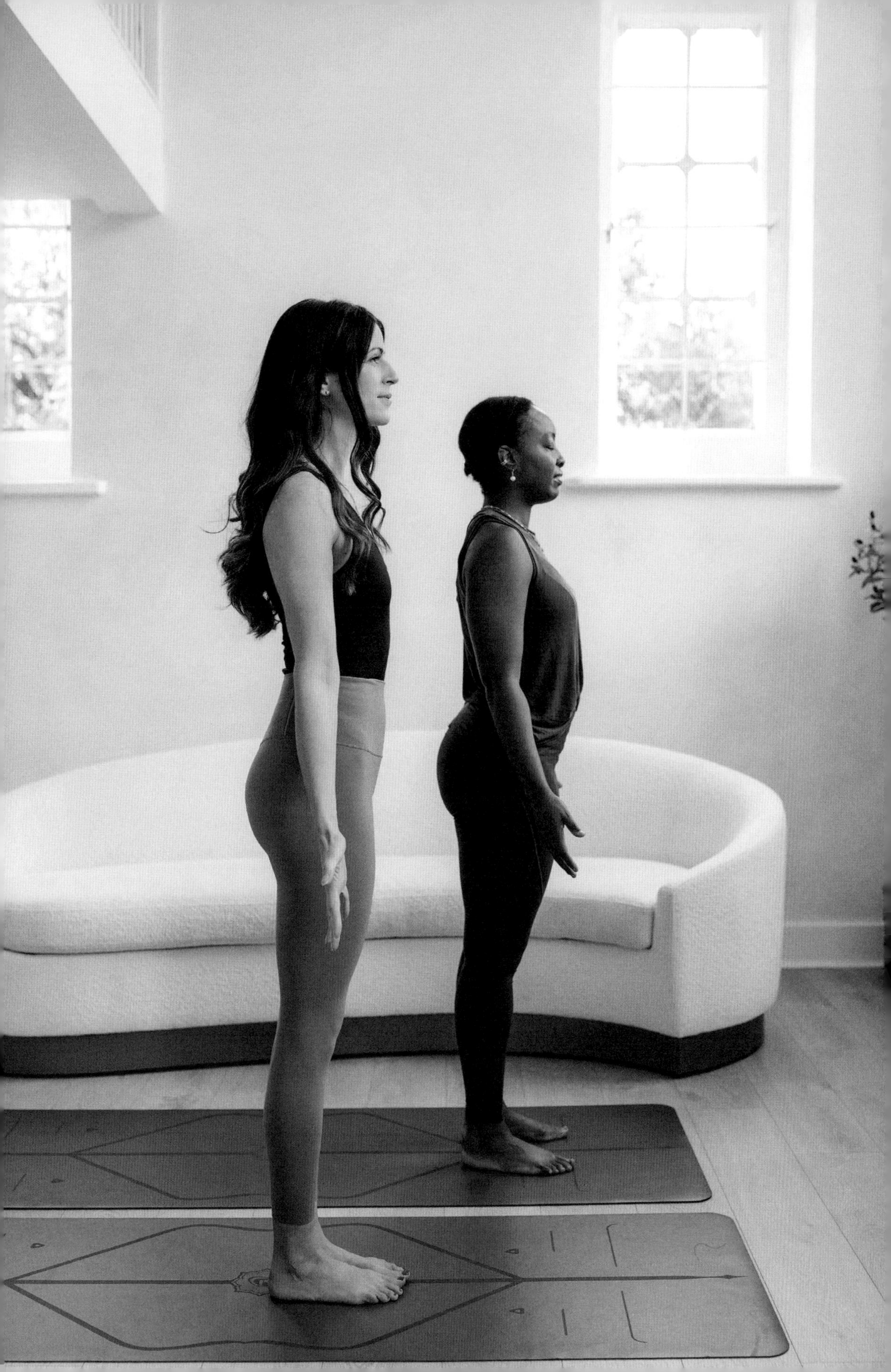

SUN SALUTATION A

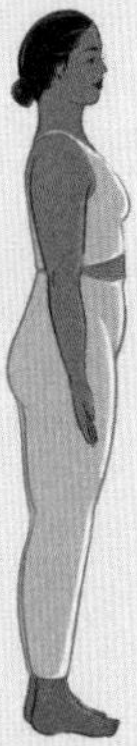

1. MOUNTAIN POSE

Start at the top of your mat in mountain pose.

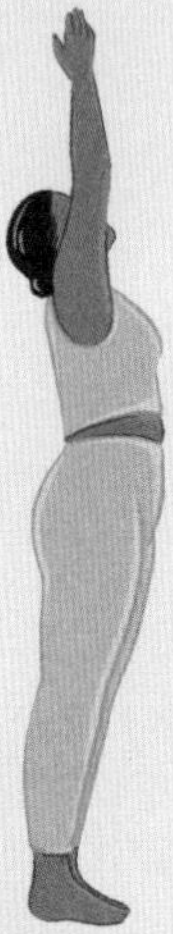

2. UPWARD SALUTE

Inhale, as you root down through the feet. Lift the fingertips to the sky.

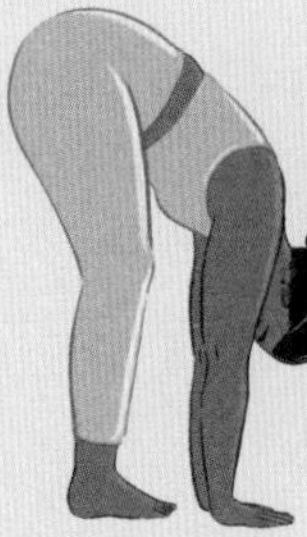

3. STANDING FORWARD BEND

Exhale as you hinge from the hips and fold to the floor. Use blocks if helpful.

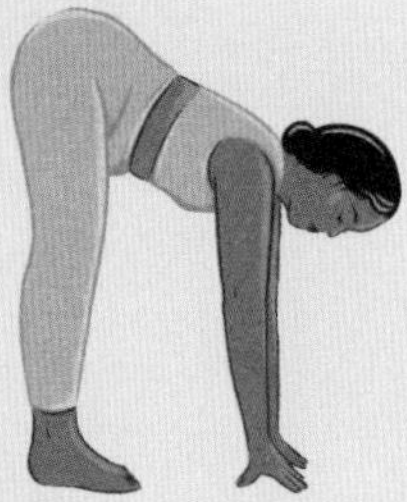

4. STANDING HALF FORWARD BEND

Inhale, lifting the torso halfway and lengthening the spine. Use blocks if helpful.

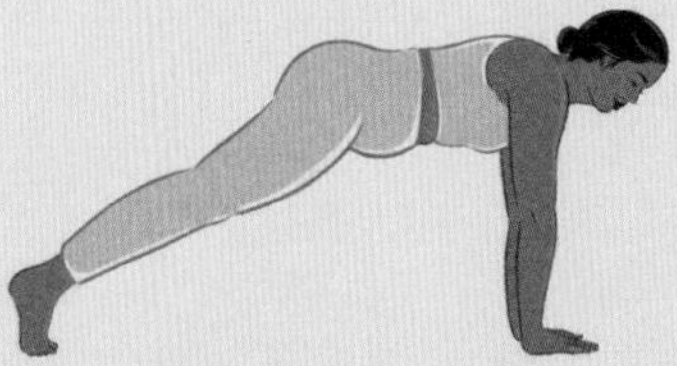

5. PLANK

Exhale, planting the hands firmly and stepping back into plank.

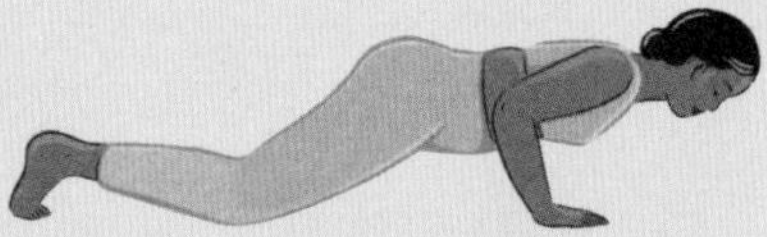

6. YOGA PUSH-UP

Continue to exhale as you lower through yoga push-up all the way to the floor.

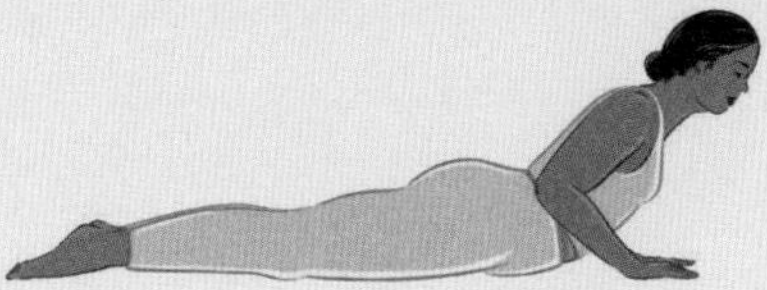

7. COBRA

Inhale, opening the chest into cobra or upward-facing dog.

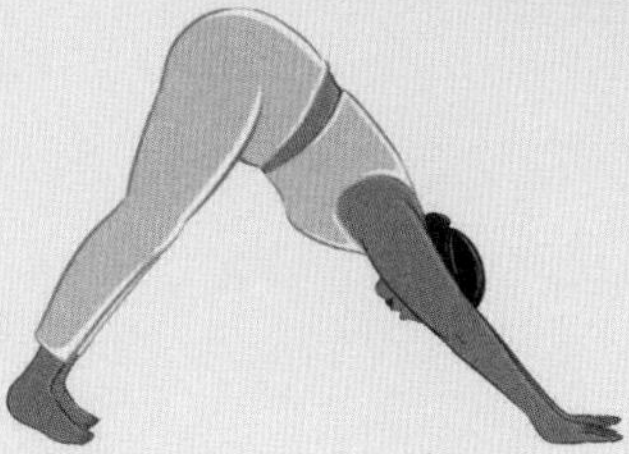

8. DOWNWARD-FACING DOG

Exhale, lifting the hips to the sky to find downward-facing dog. Hold for 5 breaths.

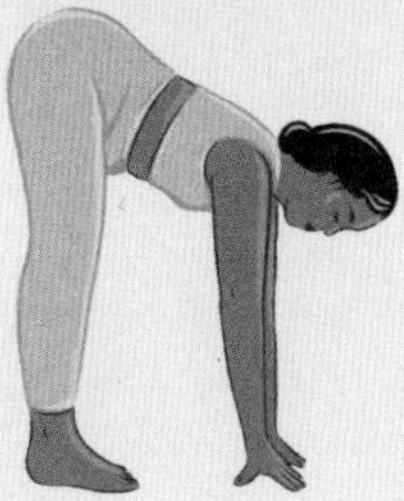

9. STANDING HALF FORWARD BEND

Inhale, stepping forward and lifting the torso halfway.

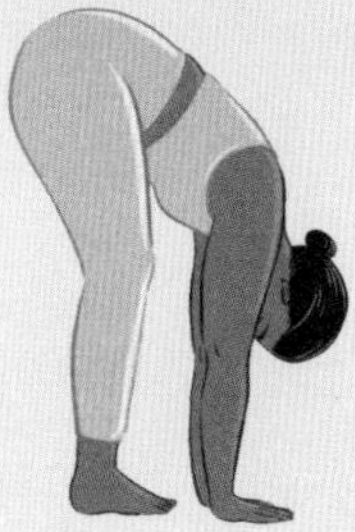

10. STANDING FORWARD BEND

Exhale as you fold down to the floor.

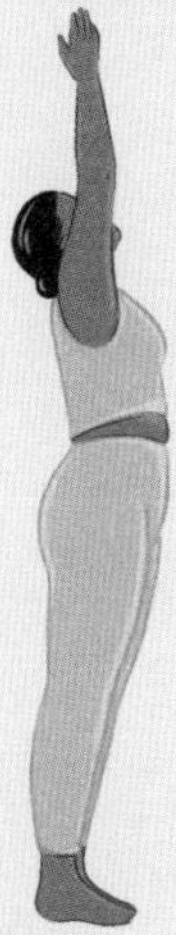

11. UPWARD SALUTE

Inhale, rooting down through the feet, coming up to standing and lifting the fingertips to the sky.

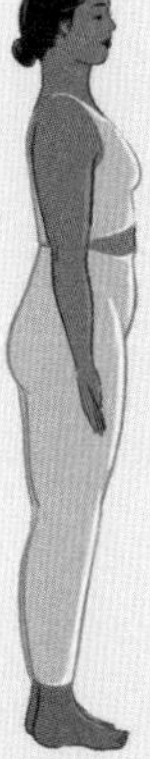

12. MOUNTAIN POSE

Exhale, releasing the hands and finding mountain pose. Repeat the sequence 1–5 times.

SUN SALUTATION B

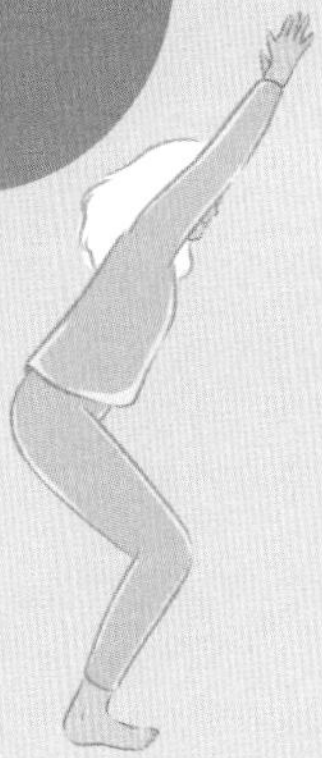

1. CHAIR

From the top of your mat, inhale, sweeping into chair pose.

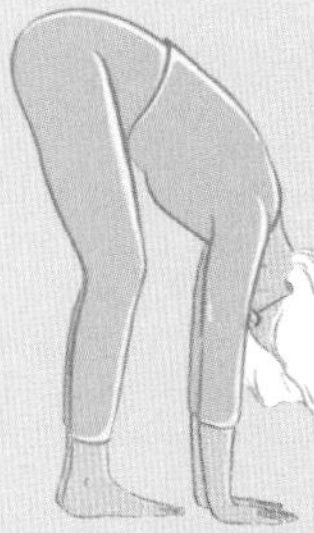

2. STANDING FORWARD BEND

Exhale as you hinge from the hips and fold to the floor.

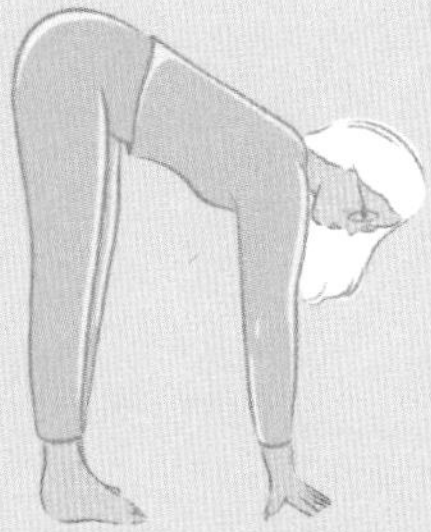

3. STANDING HALF FORWARD BEND

Inhale, lifting the torso halfway and lengthening the spine.

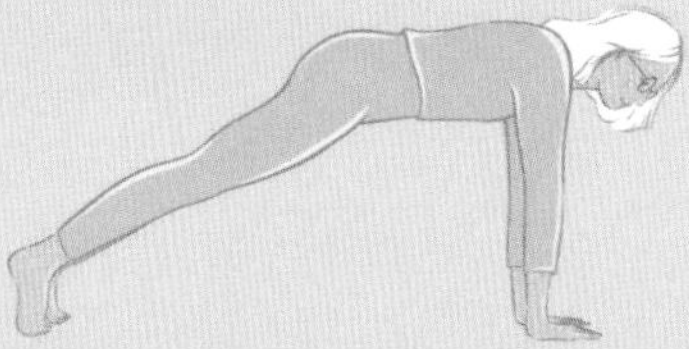

4. PLANK

Exhale planting the hands firmly and stepping back into plank.

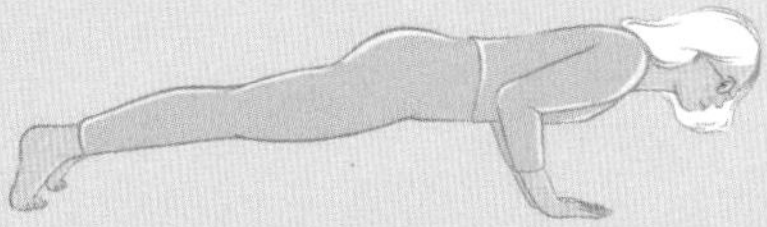

5. YOGA PUSH-UP

Continue to exhale as you lower through yoga push-up.

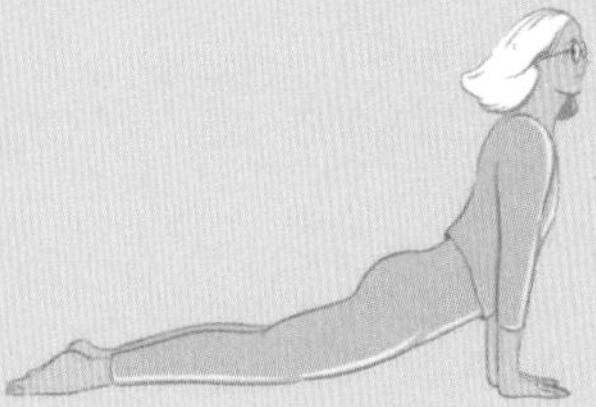

6. UPWARD-FACING DOG

Inhale, opening the chest into cobra or upward-facing dog.

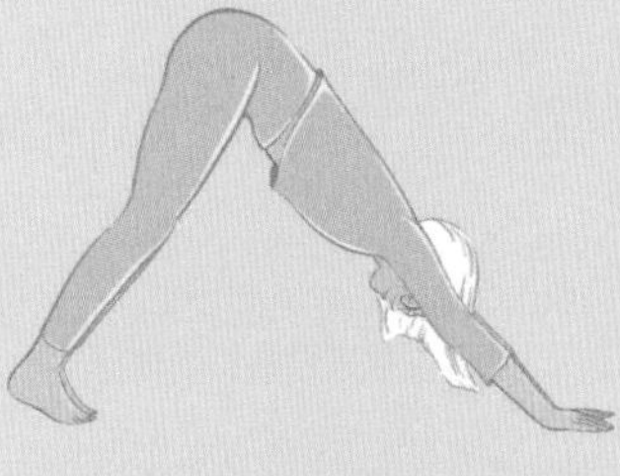

7. DOWNWARD-FACING DOG

Exhale, lifting the hips to the sky to find downward-facing dog.

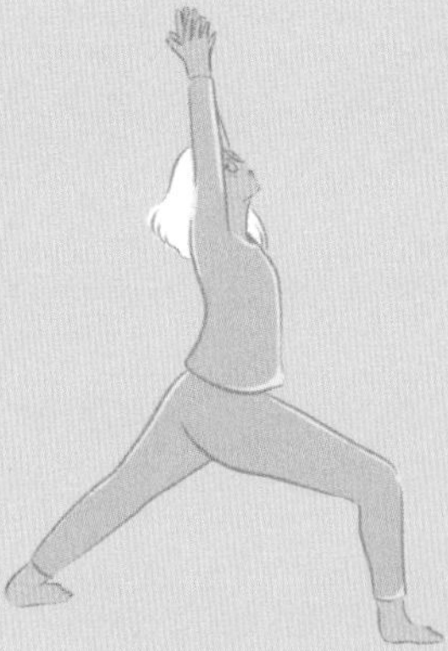

8. WARRIOR I

Inhale, stepping the right foot forward to the front of the mat and lifting into warrior I.

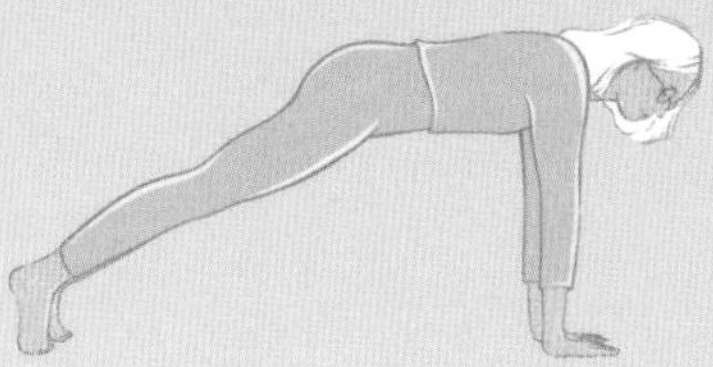

9. PLANK

Exhale, framing the front foot and stepping back into plank pose.

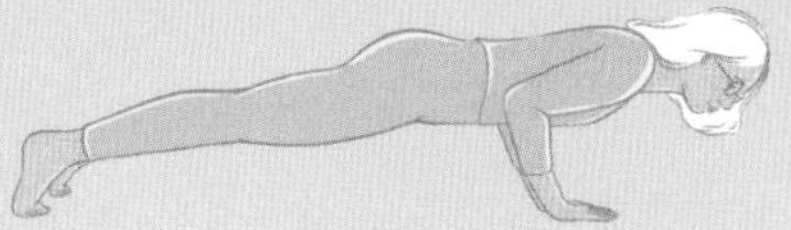

10. YOGA PUSH-UP

Continue to exhale as you lower through yoga push-up.

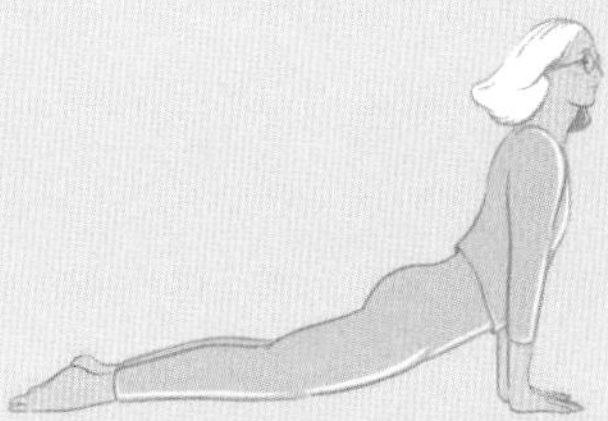

11. UPWARD-FACING DOG

Inhale, opening the chest into cobra or upward-facing dog.

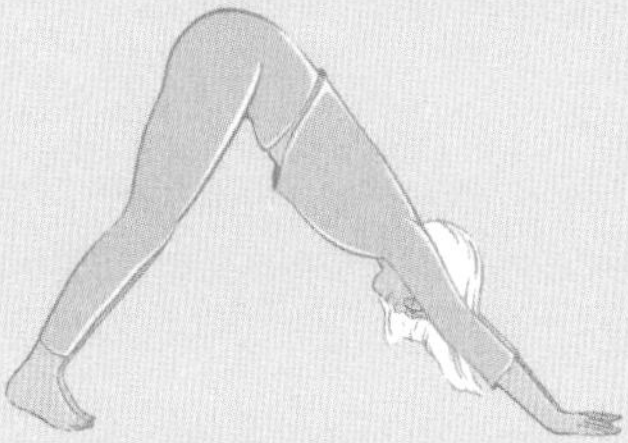

12. DOWNWARD-FACING DOG

Exhale, lifting the hips to the sky to find downward-facing dog.

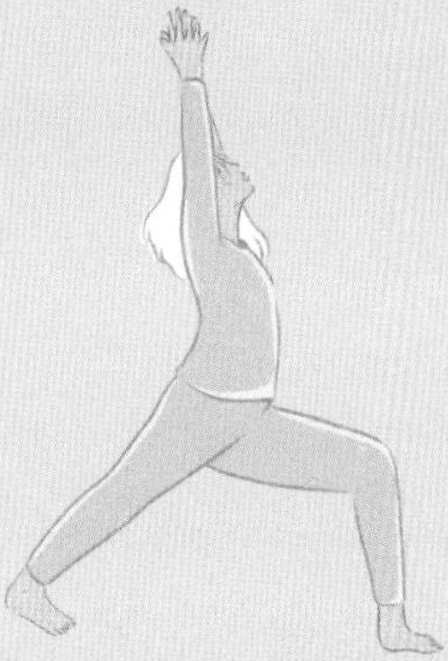

13. WARRIOR I

Inhale, stepping the left foot forward to the front of the mat and lifting into warrior I.

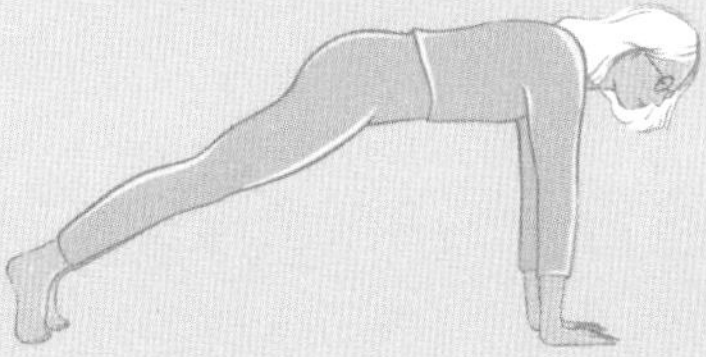

14. PLANK

Exhale, framing the front foot and stepping back into plank pose.

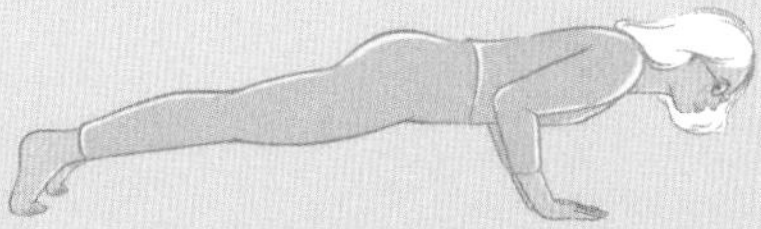

15. YOGA PUSH-UP

Continue to exhale as you lower through yoga push-up.

SUN SALUTATION B

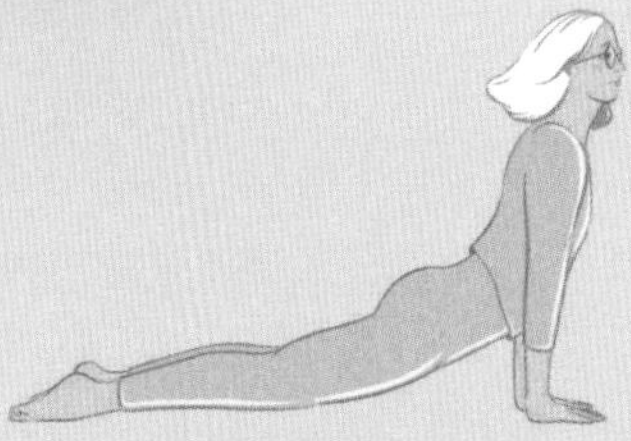

16. UPWARD-FACING DOG

Inhale, opening the chest into cobra or upward-facing dog.

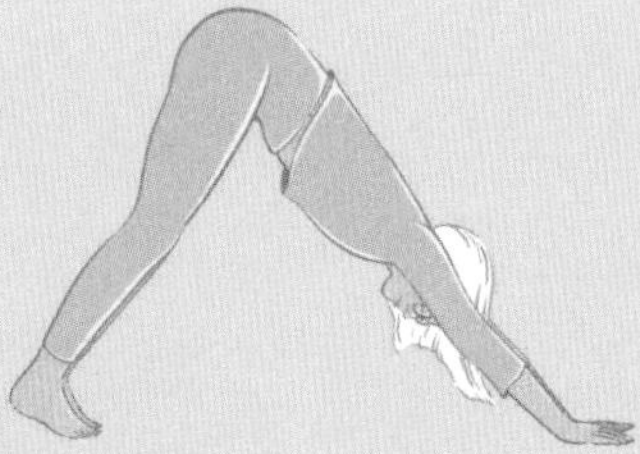

17. DOWNWARD-FACING DOG

Exhale, lifting the hips to the sky to find downward-facing dog. Hold for 5 breaths.

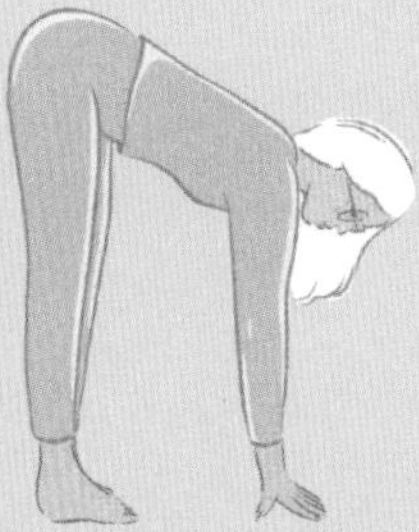

18. STANDING HALF FORWARD BEND

Inhale, stepping forward and lifting the torso halfway.

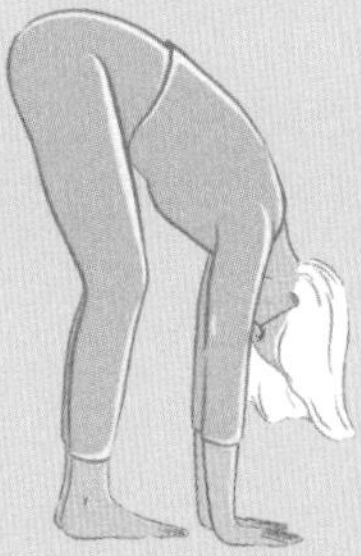

19. STANDING FORWARD BEND

Exhale as you fold down.

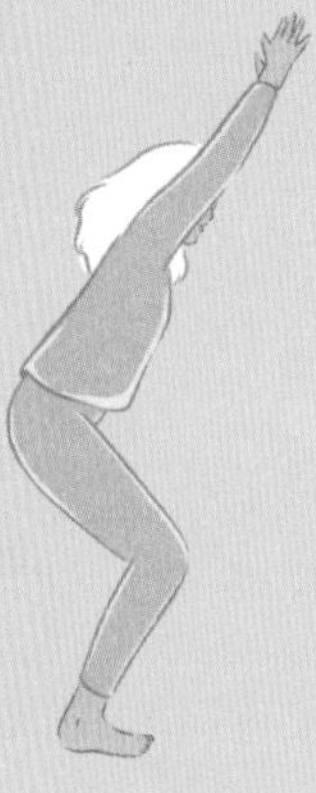

20. CHAIR

Inhale, rooting down through the feet as you sweep up into chair pose.

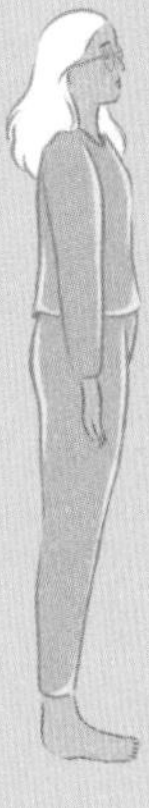

21. MOUNTAIN POSE

Exhale, releasing the hands and finding mountain pose. Repeat the sequence 1–5 times.

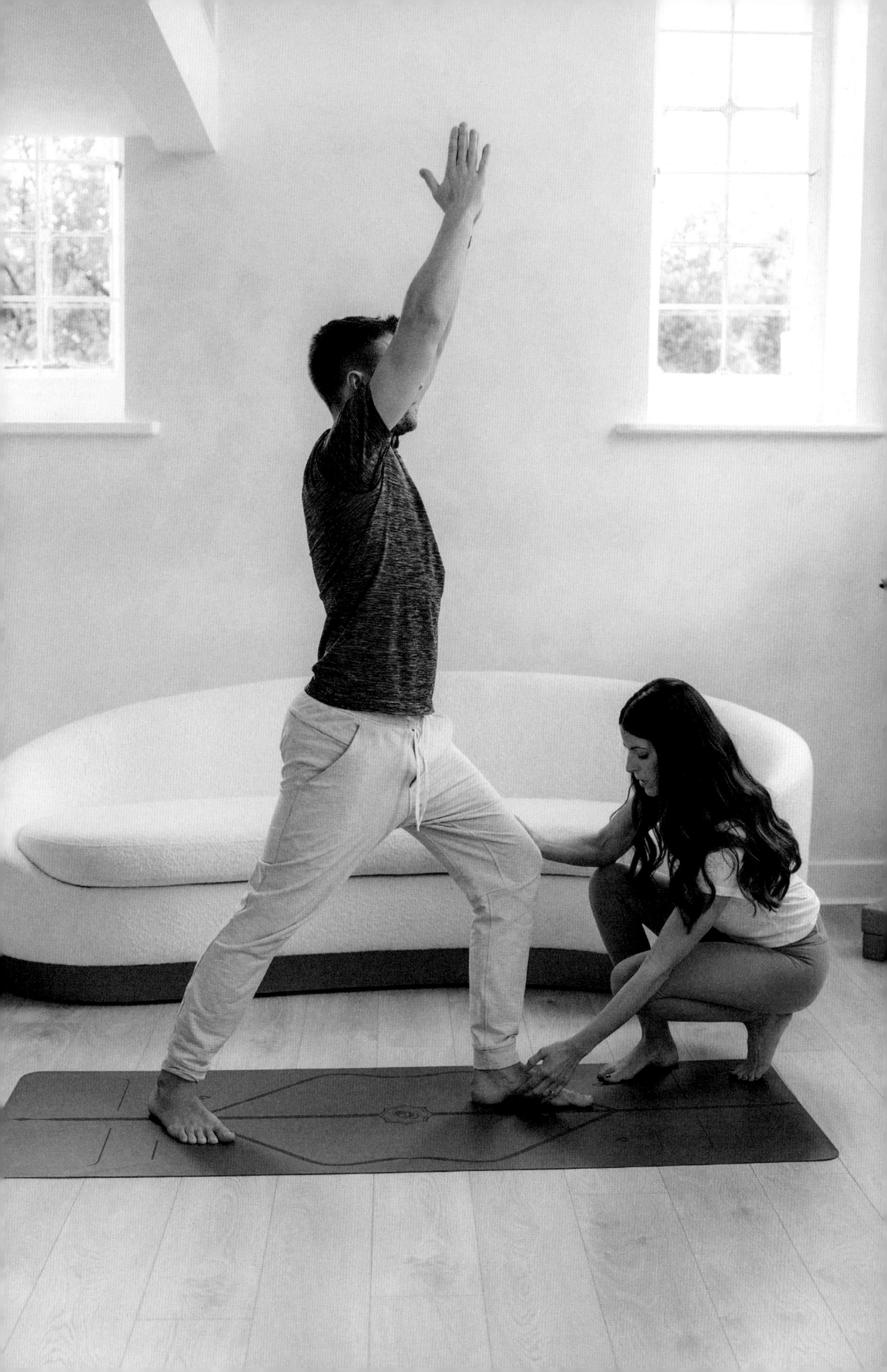

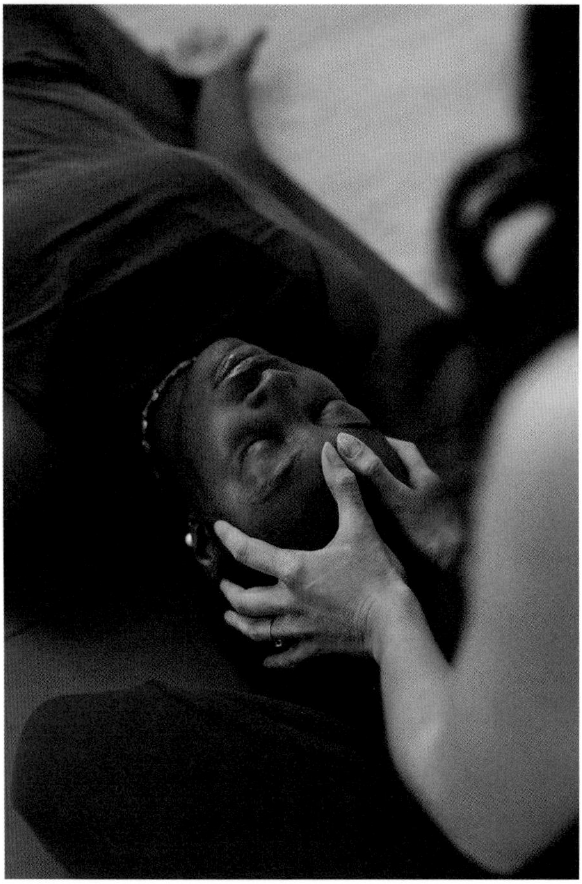
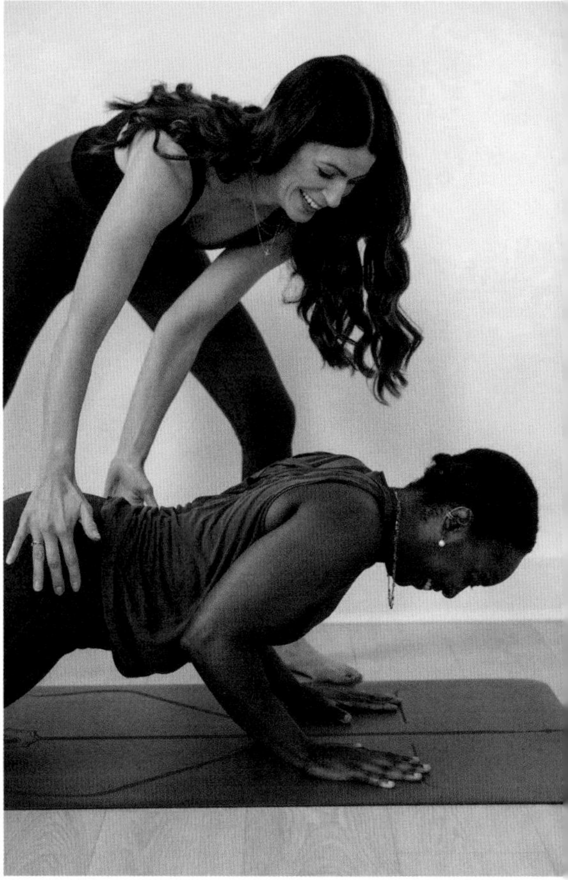
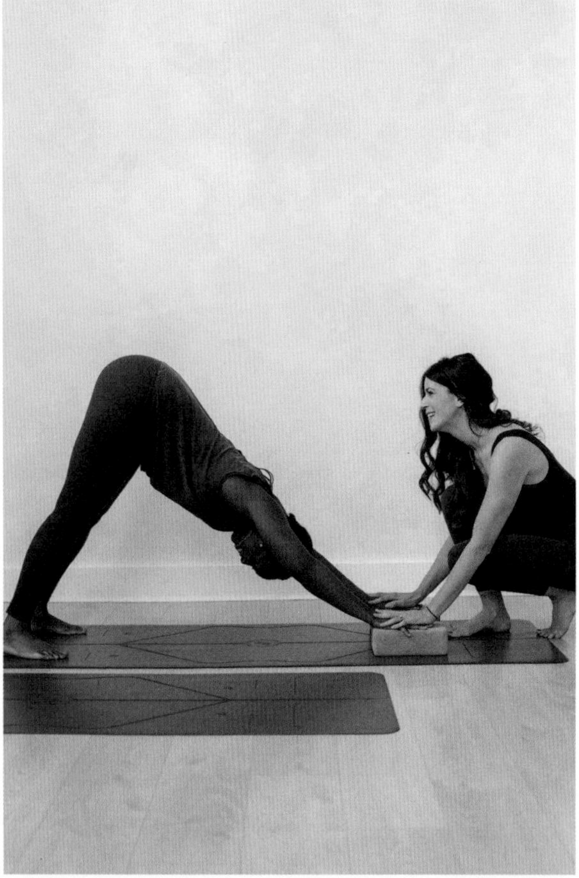
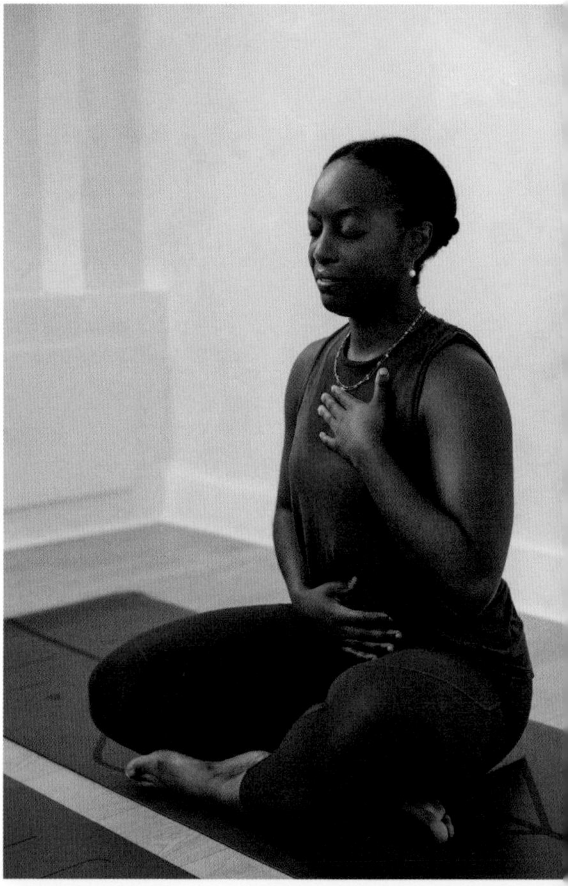

MONTH 1
MOUNTAIN

'THE JOURNEY OF A THOUSAND MILES BEGINS WITH ONE STEP.'

LAO TZU

MOUNTAIN

We start our Yoga Happy year with a mountain theme. 'Mountain month' is going to help you launch your practice in a strong and committed way. When we think of mountains, we tend to think of strength, stability and resilience – all traits yoga helps us with. We might also think of 'peaks' and 'valleys'. I wish I could say that starting yoga is an effortless process with only peaks in sight. But, like anything, there will be highs and lows, steps forwards and some steps back. What I can promise, though, is that it is worth the process.

The start of a yoga practice is often the hardest part, particularly if you struggle with flexibility, strength or have never practised yoga before. Don't think of this programme as if you are staring up at a huge mountain wondering how on earth you will reach the top. I am going to break down your yoga practice into simple steps to help make your journey as manageable and successful as possible. Visualise each step forward and remember there will be steps back too, but don't let this put you off.

Mountain pose, or *tadasana*, is a foundational yoga pose that looks so simple, yet done consciously it will light up your body and make you feel powerful. The principles behind this pose will also help with a number of other poses too. For some, mountain pose purely looks like standing at the top of a yoga mat. How hard can standing be, right? Well, jump up onto your feet now, spread your toes and push down strongly into the floor. At the same time lift up through the crown of your head like you're growing into the ceiling. Notice how these cues help you gently engage the core, glutes (butt muscles) and legs, and bring your body into alignment. Bring your arms by your sides, palms facing forward and reach downwards through your fingers like you're trying to touch something just out of reach. There's a lot going on isn't there? It's definitely not easy to hold this pose with conscious engagement and alignment.

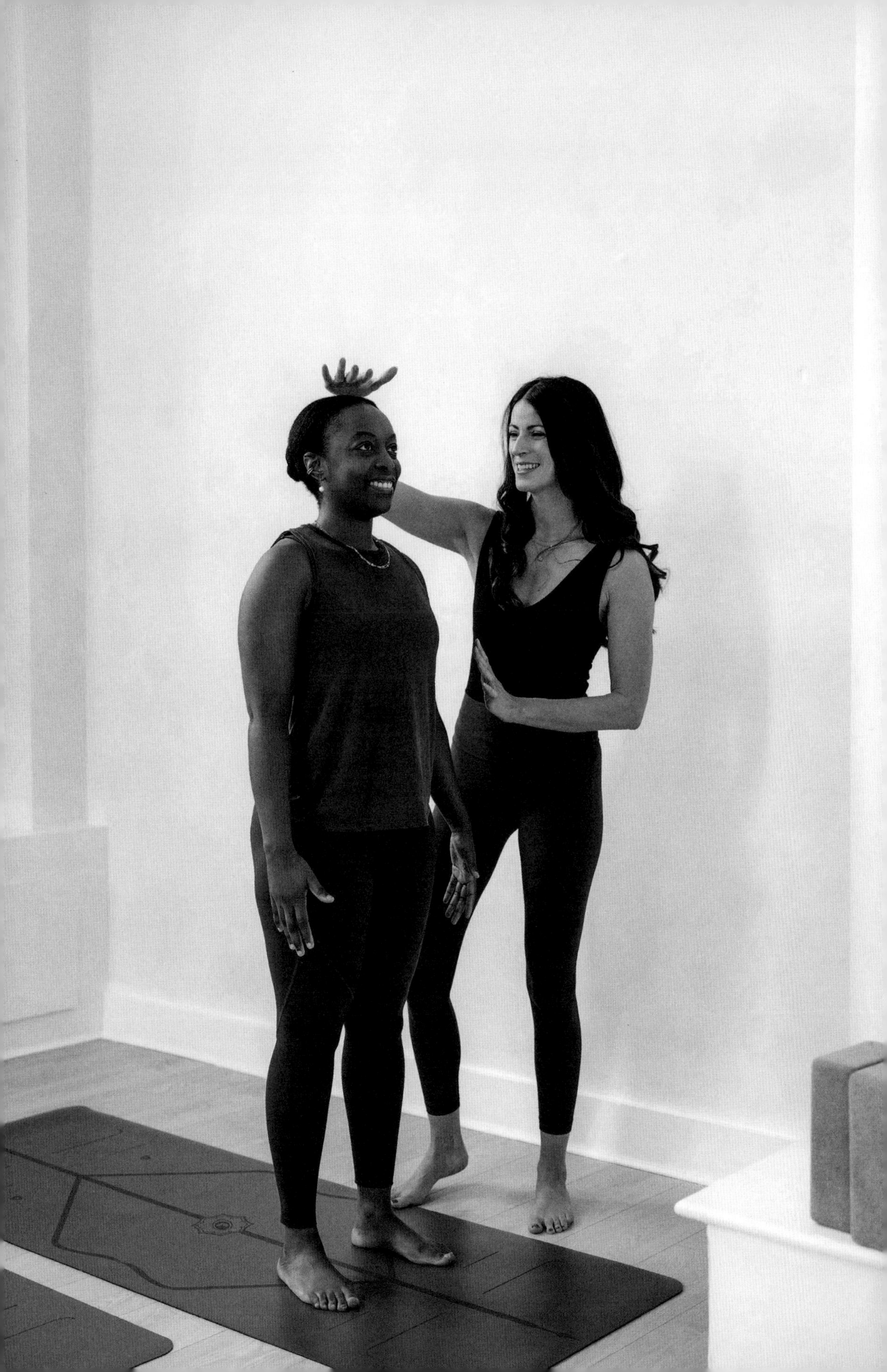

PATAÑJALI'S EIGHT-FOLD PATH OF YOGA

Yogic philosophy, like climbing a mountain, can seem overwhelming at the start. There is a lot to learn and it can often feel quite heavy. It doesn't need to be overwhelming though and if you want to practise yoga, it can't be skipped. With my students I like to break it down into bite-sized chunks and the starting point is often the ten *yamas* and *niyamas*, which are ethical principles from *The Yoga Sutras of Patañjali*, arguably one of the most influential yoga books of all time.

The book is a collection of 196 observations (sutras, or threads) written by the ancient sage Patañjali. They provide guidance on yoga's aims, practices, obstacles and the results that can be obtained. The observations outline a path towards the goal of yoga – freedom or liberation from the binds of the material world. It isn't a book of yoga poses, but rather a path of liberation through meditation and connection to our true Self. *The Yoga Sutras of Patañjali* is a comprehensive guide to understanding the nature of the mind and the suffering caused by material bondage. While Patañjali's teachings were originally intended for students who actively disengaged from activity in the world, for us, these teachings offer a way to live life with more meaning, purpose and freedom.

In this book I share an adapted interpretation of Patañjali's teachings to demonstrate how they are relevant and useful to us in the light of today's challenges. They help us to better navigate our relationships with ourself, others and the world.

Interestingly, Patañjali only mentions *asana* (the physical postures) a few times. He mentions the postures in relation to them being 'steady and comfortable' (*sutra 2.46 sthira sukham asanam*) and as a means to help the body be at ease in seated meditation. But what Patañjali is really telling us is that yoga isn't the postures; the postures are a means of helping us find comfort in meditation, which in turn helps get us closer to yoga's wider philosophy.

Patañjali sets out an eight-limbed path that supports us in transforming how we think, communicate and act by directing our attention inwards and stilling the mind – something that is surprisingly hard to do in this current world full of technology and noise. One of the limbs is the physical postures and the others are a collection of methods and tools that can help us live life with more compassion and intention.

1. ***Yamas*** – moral disciplines or restraints
2. ***Niyamas*** – observances
3. ***Asana*** – physical postures
4. ***Pranayama*** – breathing techniques or the expansion of life force
5. ***Pratyahara*** – sense withdrawal
6. ***Dharana*** – concentration
7. ***Dhyana*** – meditation
8. ***Samadhi*** – enlightenment

So, now you see why *The Yoga Happy Year* can't just be a collection of poses and sequences. We must look at the other limbs and also incorporate them into the daily practice to deliver all the incredible benefits of yoga. Each month I will delve into a yogic concept and share ways you can practise it off the yoga mat. I want to help you realise we have the opportunity to practise the philosophy that yoga teaches us through every interaction we have.

AHIMSA (KINDNESS)

I ALONE AM RESPONSIBLE FOR MY THOUGHTS, WORDS AND ACTIONS.

The first of Patañjali's limbs are the five *yamas*, set out below. The *yamas* can be thought of like our moral backbone. They are ethical considerations on how to avoid harming ourselves, others or the world we live in. The beauty of the *yamas* (and *niyamas*, see page 100) is that the more we practise them, the greater the ripple effect they will have. By bringing them into our lives, we are planting positive seeds of change that others can follow.

1. ***Ahimsa*** – non-violence in thought, word and deed
2. ***Satya*** – truthfulness
3. ***Asteya*** – non-stealing
4. ***Brahmacharya*** – celibacy or the 'right use of energy'
5. ***Aparigraha*** – non-attachment

At the heart of yoga is love. The first *yama* is *ahimsa* and it translates as 'non-violence' or 'absence of injury'. Think of it as a reminder of love. To act with love through all words, thoughts and actions: towards ourselves, as much as towards humanity and the planet. This allows us to live a more conscious and balanced life of harmony. *Ahimsa* is the foundational *yama* and the rest of the *yamas* build on it.

How *ahimsa* can be applied to everyday life

▸ **On the yoga mat:** Cultivate a compassionate and non-harming approach to your practice. Listen to your body's needs and know that these can change day to day, minute to minute. Avoid criticism or self-judgement and avoid pushing yourself into poses that feel painful or unsafe – always modify or pick a different pose that feels right for you.

▸ **Self-compassion:** Avoid limiting beliefs that hold you back from your full potential and cause you to engage in self-destructive behaviours, negative self-talk and criticism. We have to treat ourselves with the kindness, love and compassion we would show others – *ahimsa* begins with us.

▸ **Compassion towards others:** Show others empathy, offer to help those in need and treat others with the respect and dignity they deserve to embody the lessons of *ahimsa*.

▸ **Communication:** Avoid gossiping about or judging others and instead foster understanding, compassion and full communication, asking questions where necessary and without using harsh or hurtful language.

▸ **What you consume:** Think about what food you eat and the things you buy and be conscious in your choices, paying attention to where the food has come from, its impact on the planet and other people, and be mindful about waste.

▸ **Environmental consciousness:** *Ahimsa* includes taking care of the earth and we can all contribute to the well-being of the planet and minimise harm to the ecosystem and its inhabitants. Be mindful of sustainability, conserving resources and reducing waste.

▸ **Social activism:** Stand up to injustice, inequality and violence (*ahimsa* helps us contribute to a more compassionate and peaceful society).

FIRM FOUNDATIONS

This month's flow (see page 32) introduces some foundational yoga poses – the building blocks that will help you advance your yoga practice. All of the poses can be modified to suit you and your body and nothing in this book should cause pain. For example, in plank you could drop your knees to lower the intensity, come on to your forearms if you have wrist pain or even lift a leg or arm if you want to ramp up the intensity. There is a huge misconception that yoga is only for a certain type of person. This couldn't be further from the truth; it is a practice for all and we can adjust any sequence to make it appropriate for our body. Remember, the appendix on page 190 can help you with modifications and includes a detailed breakdown of each pose.

Another way of thinking about the foundations is by looking at the body's foundations in each pose, i.e. the parts of the body touching the mat. Being aware of and using the body's foundations gives us a way to find strength and stability in the postures. Some examples include:

▸ **Downward-facing dog** Spreading the fingers, push firmly through the hands and energetically dial them outwards (imagining you are screwing jam jar lids in opposite directions but your hands aren't actually moving). Notice the muscular engagement throughout the arms and shoulders as you do this.

▸ **Mountain pose** Spread the toes, imagining your feet have four corners and push them firmly into the mat as you lift the arches of the feet. Notice the energy that runs up the legs and ignites the core with this cue.

The body's foundations matter as they help us establish strength, stability and balance in our yoga poses. By consciously aligning the body's base, whether through the feet, hands or sitting bones, you can create a solid pedestal to better advance your strength and practice. It also helps you avoid stretching beyond what your body can handle or putting unnecessary stress on the joints and muscles.

Foundations can help in other ways, too. The yogic concept of *prana* is the 'energy' or 'vital life force' that flows through the body. It is the subtle energy that animates us and sustains our physical, mental and spiritual well-being. Just as we have channels for the flow of blood through the body, we have *nadis* for the flow of *prana*. In yoga, *prana* is believed to be influenced and enhanced through practices such as breath work, *asana* and meditation. When the foundations of the body are aligned and engaged, it is thought that the energy can flow more freely.

Having strong foundations allows us to be more mindful, present and connected in our yoga practice. The transitions between poses are done consciously, with thought, and they allow us to become more aware of the physical sensations within the body and the breath.

HOW TO CREATE A LASTING YOGA HABIT

1. **BELIEVE IN YOURSELF**
   Believe that you practising yoga is possible and embrace the change – this is an essential step!

2. **START SMALL**
   A 20-minute flow, like the ones in this book, is not only going to feel amazing, it will reap huge benefits when practised regularly. Think about consistency over quantity and aim to get on your yoga mat every one or two days. I have found that my students are much more likely to stick to their practice if they commit to it regularly rather than simply doing a 60-minute class once a week.

3. **KNOW IT'S GOING TO BE HARD**
   It is hard at first, particularly for beginners, but dedication is a big part of the practice and quickly you will start to see things become easier and the benefits flow into your life on and off the mat.

4. **MAKE IT ENJOYABLE**
   Perhaps this is by listening to your favourite playlist, burning a scented candle or being outside. Make each practice a small ritual to look forward to.

5. **BE PATIENT**
   It will take longer to feel comfortable in certain poses than others (it took me years to feel comfortable in some) but try not to feel frustrated with the journey. Each step is going to teach you something if you tune in and listen – even the fails.

6. **SET SMALL, REALISTIC GOALS**
   For most people, the goal of nailing a handstand in a few weeks is not going to be achievable. Instead set something motivating but realistic. Perhaps it's to practise for 20 minutes five times a week. Or to work on arm strength for *chaturanga* (yoga push-up) three times every week.

7. **COMMUNITY SUPPORT**
   Bring someone else on this journey with you. Practise with them online, in person or keep yourselves accountable over messages. Your odds of success in building new habits increase drastically when you are part of a group.

8. **BE SPECIFIC**
   At the start of each week, think about what you want to practise and when you're going to do it. The beauty of this book means that the 'what' is taken care of for you!

9. **BE PREPARED FOR SETBACKS**
   Think about what could hold back your new habit. For example, if you want a morning practice but have a tendency to hit snooze on your alarm. Identify these setbacks in advance and try and come up with solutions to avoid them; for example, you could place your alarm clock on the other side of the room.

10. **BE OKAY WITH SETBACKS**
    Setbacks will happen. Maybe you go a week without practising for whatever reason. But remember that you need to be consistent, not perfect. We are human, life happens. Jump right back into the habit as soon as you can and don't beat yourself up about it.

A NOTE ON POSTURE

Maintaining good posture when you move around the yoga mat promotes efficient movement patterns and helps to distribute the body's load and muscle forces evenly throughout the body. Focusing on posture can also enhance body awareness and mindfulness. However, it would be completely unrealistic for me to tell you to keep perfect posture throughout your whole day.

We are human and in fact, we should be training to have strength and control in lots of positions and ranges of motion. The issue is that most people tend to live in one fixed posture for long periods of time, for example, hunched over at a desk at work. What is really important is to regularly move the body in all different ways and directions – even if it's for one minute – as you will be doing with this programme. Regular movement is crucial for overall health and well-being. If you spend lots of the day in one position, I recommend setting an alarm every half-hour or hour to get up and move.

A final point to mention on posture is in relation to the breath. Posture matters with the breath because it directly impacts the mechanics of respiration. Good posture allows for optimal lung expansion and the diaphragm to move freely, which enables deeper and fuller breaths. Deep abdominal breathing encourages full oxygen exchange and optimal use of the lungs, meaning our body can function more efficiently. The diaphragm is also one of our deep core muscles and proper activation of the diaphragm during breathing promotes optimal engagement of the core muscles and supports core stability.

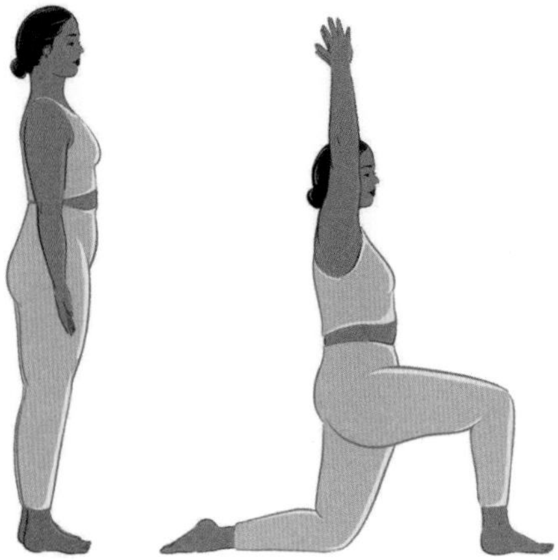

THE BREATH

THE THREE-PART BREATH

When I visualise a mountain, I first think of its solid and unwavering presence. Stability and feeling grounded are qualities that we look for as humans and breathwork can provide them. I mentioned on page 6 that we can change the way we feel by changing the way we breathe. Conscious, deep breathing techniques (like this three-part breath) can anchor us in the present moment and offer us a sense of stability when life becomes chaotic.

And just as a mountain provides an expansive view of its surroundings, breathwork can also heighten our awareness. When we focus on the breath, it allows us to tune in to our internal experiences, emotions and sensations. It allows us to expand our conscious awareness and helps us to feel more connected to the world around us.

This month's breathing technique is a foundational technique called the three-part breath. It is one of my favourite breathing techniques and for those who shallow chest-breathe (there will be many of you!), this breath is going to be transformational.

Use this technique anywhere to help you find calm and inner strength, to reduce anxiety, help fight insomnia and to anchor you to the present.

Directions:

1. Come into a comfortable seated position, growing tall through the crown of the head and allowing the spine to be neutral and long.
2. Option to place one hand over the belly and one onto the heart to channel awareness to the movement of the breath.
3. Take a slow, deep inhale through the nose from the base of your stomach, feeling the stomach expand like you're gently blowing up a balloon. Keep inhaling, sending the breath upwards through the mid-chest, feeling the ribs moving outwards, sideways and backwards. Finally, send the breath all the way to the upper chest, keeping the shoulders and collarbones neutral and soft.
4. Exhale slowly through the nose, feeling the body release all the way down to the base of the stomach.
5. Aim for each inhale and exhale to be as slow as possible (4–8 counts or longer).
6. Repeat for 10–20 rounds, 2–3 minutes, or for as long as desired.

THE MOUNTAIN FLOW

The mountain month's signature flow is a slow and energising flow with a focus on a number of yoga's foundational poses. Each time you step onto your yoga mat, bring with you the concept of *ahimsa*. Focus on being kind to yourself and if you're finding it tough, remember that each pose can be modified in a number of different ways to suit your body and your practice (see the appendix on page 190). Aim to practise this flow three or four times per week and if you have longer, feel free to include the seated warm-up flow on page 10 at the start or repeat the flow multiple times.

I recommend that as you move through the postures you breathe in and out through the nose as much as possible. Don't feel disheartened if you find this hard; over time it will get much easier. As long as you continue to breathe consciously and avoid holding your breath, you are practising yoga.

As you move around your yoga mat, bring some mountain qualities with you:

▸ **Strength and stability**: Just as a mountain embodies strength and stability, cultivate a strong foundation, move slowly and mindfully and harness your inner and outer strength.

▸ **Grounding**: Mountains are firmly rooted in the earth and connected to the present moment. Feel connected as you flow around the mat by focusing on the breath and sensations within the body. Come back to those solid foundations to find balance and stability.

▸ **Perspective**: The vastness of a mountain provides a higher vantage point and broader perspective. On the mat notice how over time the tools of yoga and the breath married with movement helps us broaden our awareness and cultivate a sense of connection not only to ourselves but to the world as a whole.

If you would like to practise all the yoga flows in this book with me, scan the QR code below, which will direct you to guided online classes that take you through versions of each of the flows.

PRIVACY.FLOWCODE.COM

PLEASE NOTE

The appendix on page 190 includes a detailed breakdown of each pose, plus variations and modifications. Remember to listen to your body; yoga should never be painful and you can chose to skip any pose that doesn't feel right for you.

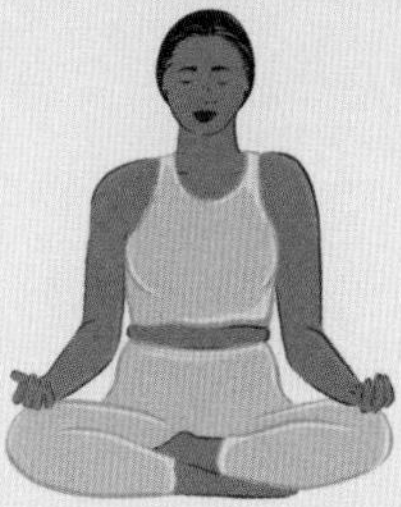

1. SEATED THREE-PART BREATH

In a seated position, take 10 rounds of the three-part breath (see page 31).

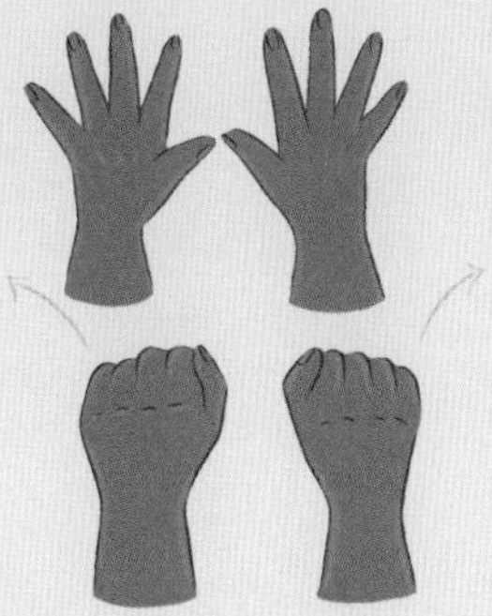

2A. WRIST WARM-UP SEQUENCE

From seated, reach the arms out straight in front of you and make 30 fists then stars with your hands.

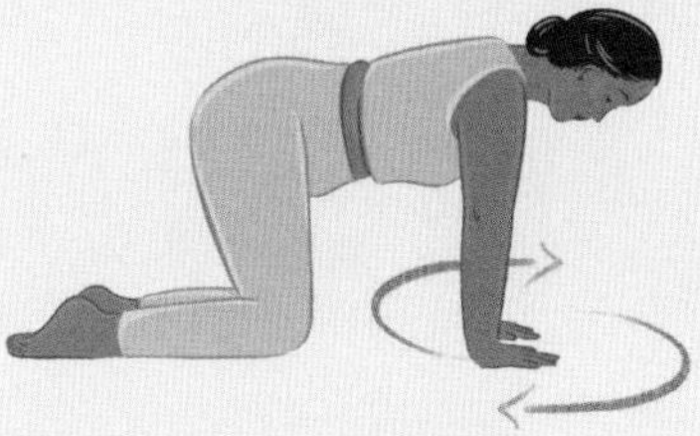

2B. WRIST WARM-UP SEQUENCE

Coming onto all fours, inhale forwards circling the shoulders over the wrists, exhale and circle the hips back towards the heels. Repeat 5 times in each direction.

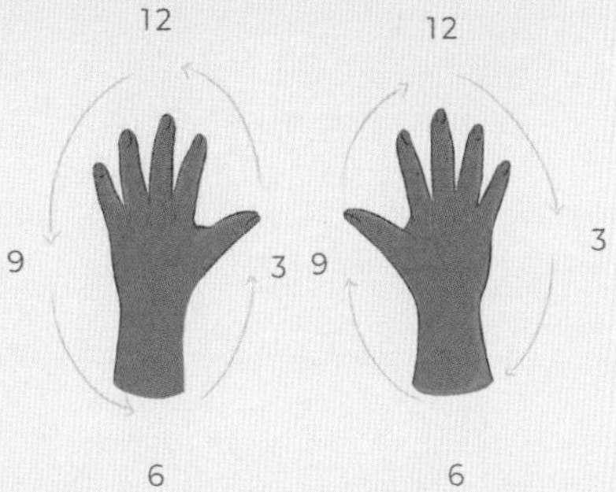

2C. WRIST WARM-UP SEQUENCE

From all fours, move your right hand clockwise to 3 o'clock, then 6 o'clock, and back to 3, 12, and 9 o'clock. At the same time, move your left hand anticlockwise to 9 o'clock, then 6 o'clock, and back to 9, 12, and 3 o'clock. Return both hands to 12 o'clock. (See page 221.) Repeat 5 times.

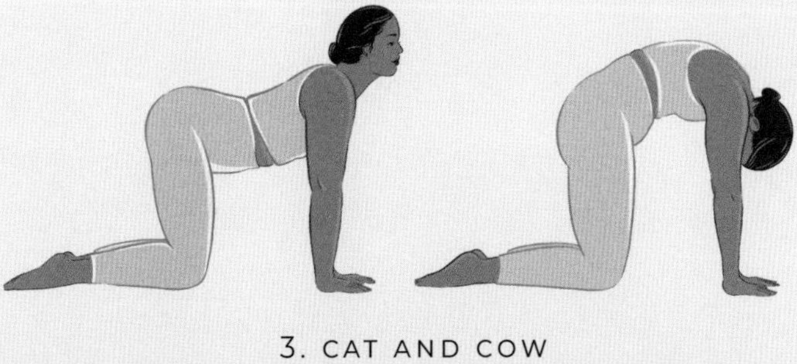

3. CAT AND COW

Inhale into cow pose and exhale into cat pose. Repeat 5 times.

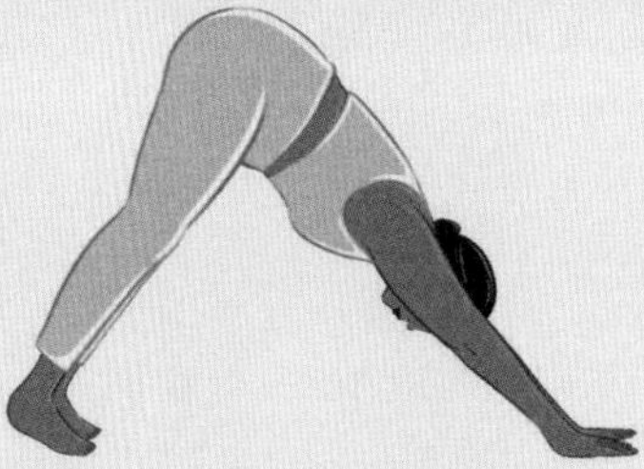

4. DOWNWARD-FACING DOG

Exhale, lifting the hips into downward-facing dog and hold for 5 breaths.

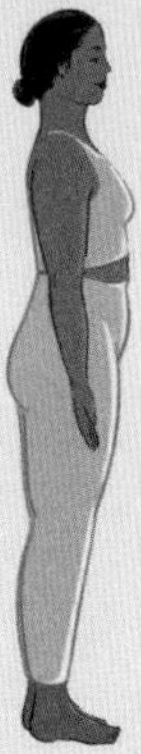

5. MOUNTAIN POSE

Step the feet forward and inhale, lifting into mountain pose for 5 breaths.

SUN SALUTATION A

Complete 1–5 rounds of sun salutation A (see page 16 for details).

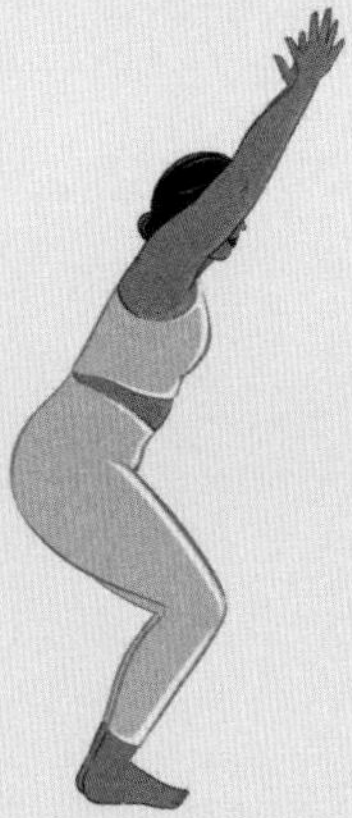

6. CHAIR POSE

Inhale, reaching the fingers high and bending the knees finding chair pose. Hold for 5 breaths.

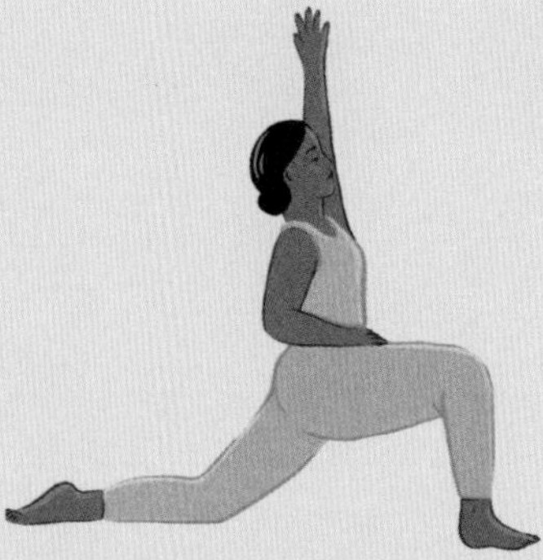

7. LOW LUNGE SIDE STRETCH

Exhale and step the left foot back into low lunge. Take a side bend to the right and hold for 5 breaths.

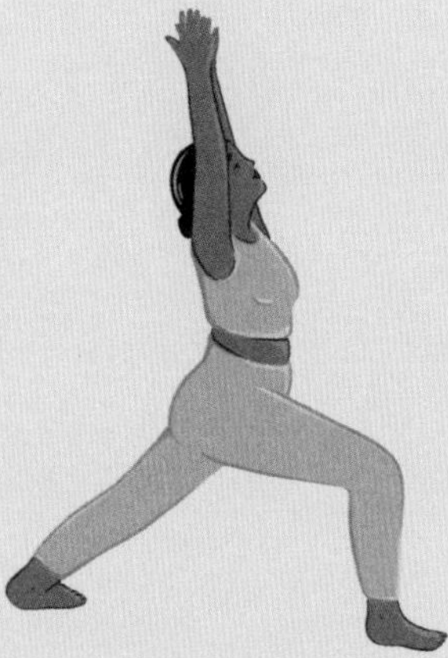

8. WARRIOR I

Exhale tucking the back toes and lifting up into warrior I or high lunge. Hold for 5 breaths.

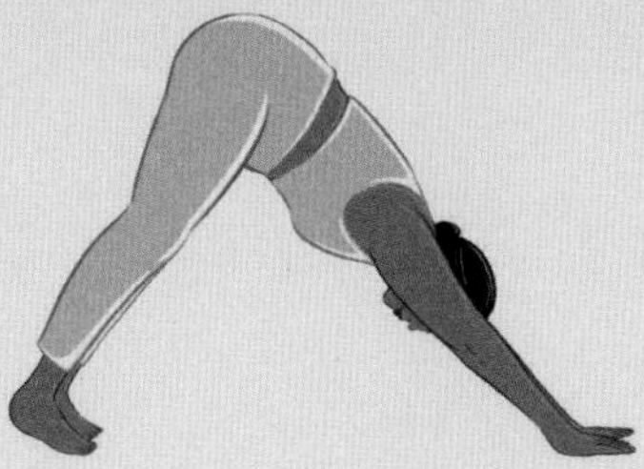

9. DOWNWARD-FACING DOG

Plant the hands and step back, lifting the hips high finding downward-facing dog. Hold for 5 breaths.

REPEAT ON THE LEFT SIDE

STEPS 7–9

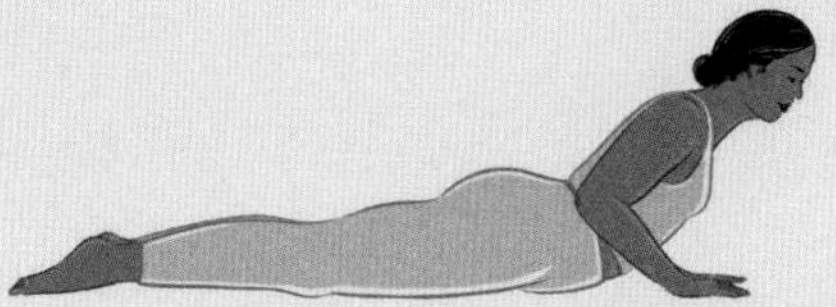

10. COBRA ROLLS

Exhale as you shift forward releasing all the way to the belly. Inhale into cobra, exhale back to belly. Repeat 5 times.

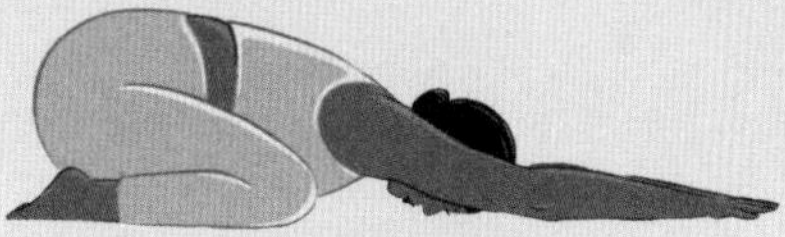

11. CHILD'S POSE

Exhale and push back into child's pose. Hold for 5 breaths.

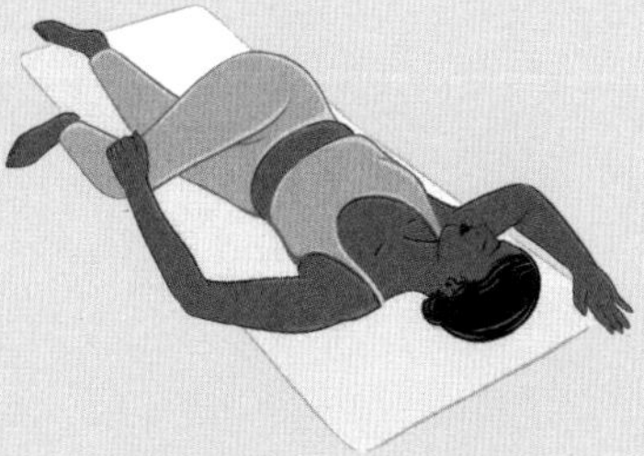

12. SUPINE TWIST

Coming onto your back, hug the right knee in and come into a supine twist. Hold for 5 breaths before repeating on the opposite side.

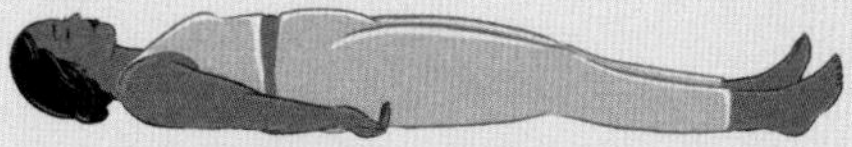

13. SAVASANA

Lie back and melt into savasana for 2 minutes or more.

MEDITATION

BREATHING MEDITATION

When you're just starting, meditation itself is like climbing a mountain.

Many people give up immediately, thinking, 'this isn't for me'. But *everything* requires practice. If you want to learn French, you don't expect to be fluent after the first lesson. One of the myths of meditation is that it's easy and another is that we need not think. Mahatma Gandhi explained meditation beautifully when he said, 'Meditation is a dance between the thoughts that come in and your anchor back to the present moment'.

As human beings, thoughts are going to be there. A meditation practice involves letting the thoughts drift away like clouds overhead. When you realise that your attention has been lost thinking about your to-do list, you gently, with compassion, bring your focus back to the now. The important thing is to think about the why, to have an *intention* for your practice. This intention will make creating a meditation habit easier. Your intention could be linked to one of the benefits on page 7. You might want to meditate daily to help improve your sleep quality and lower your stress levels, or your motivation could be as simple as wanting to prioritise time daily to pause and give your body and mind the rest it deserves.

The first meditation I am sharing with you is very simple, and you can do it anywhere. The breath in this meditation acts as the anchor to the present moment, allowing the mind to settle. Whenever your mind runs away during this meditation, simply bring your awareness back to your breath.

Directions:

1. Come into a comfortable seated position on a chair with an upright spine, somewhere you can be free of distractions.
2. Set a timer for 5 minutes or as long as you have.
3. Gently close your eyes; if you don't like to close your eyes, you can have the eyes slightly open with the gaze lowered to the floor in front of you to keep your forehead soft.
4. Softly close your lips and let your breath come in through the nose and out through the nose or mouth in its natural rhythm.
5. Before each meditation begins, feel your sitting bones on the chair and your feet on the floor. Imagine roots winding down from these areas, helping you feel secure and grounded.
6. Release control of the breath and simply start to observe it. Notice how each breath looks different, how various parts of your body move as you breathe. Notice the slight pause between each inhale and exhale, exhale and inhale. Notice any sounds the breath makes and every sensation that each breath brings.
7. Each time your mind starts to wander, gently bring your awareness back to your breath and the present moment.
8. When the timer finishes, take a moment with your eyes still closed to sit and notice how you feel and any thoughts or feelings that arose.

JOURNAL PROMPTS

Below I have given you eight self-reflection questions linked to this month's theme and the yogic concept of *ahimsa*. Try answering two questions weekly alongside the daily journal prompts set out on pages 8–9.

▸ Imagine yourself as a mountain. What strengths and stability do you possess? How can you draw upon those qualities during challenging times?

▸ Does the voice within you align with the principle of *ahimsa*? Are you practising self-compassion and empathy? Can you cultivate a more loving internal dialogue?

▸ Consider the metaphorical 'peaks' and 'valleys' in your life, i.e. the high points of success and the challenging low points. What lessons have you learnt from these experiences? How have they shaped you?

▸ Consider how you can practise *ahimsa* towards the world we live in. What changes can you make to be more conscious in the way you live your life to minimise harm and contribute to the well-being of the planet?

▸ Mountains are part of a huge, interconnected ecosystem, much like us. What can you do to nurture and contribute to the well-being of the community around you?

▸ Consider the last time you gossiped or passed judgement on another human. How did it truly make you feel? How can you extend the concept of *ahimsa* more towards others in your daily interactions?

▸ Mountains are known for their resilience and ability to weather the storm and treacherous conditions. Think of a time you demonstrated resilience in your life. How could you further develop this quality and can anything you've learned this month through your practice help you?

▸ Are there behavioural patterns that contribute to stress, harm or conflict in your life? This could even be the things you watch on television or where you buy your vegetables from. How can you challenge these patterns, practising *ahimsa* and creating more positive change?

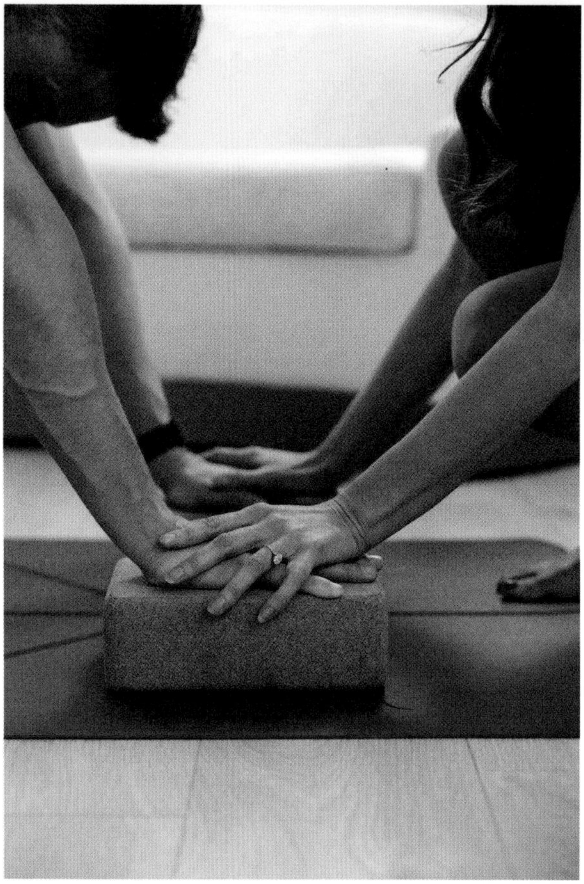
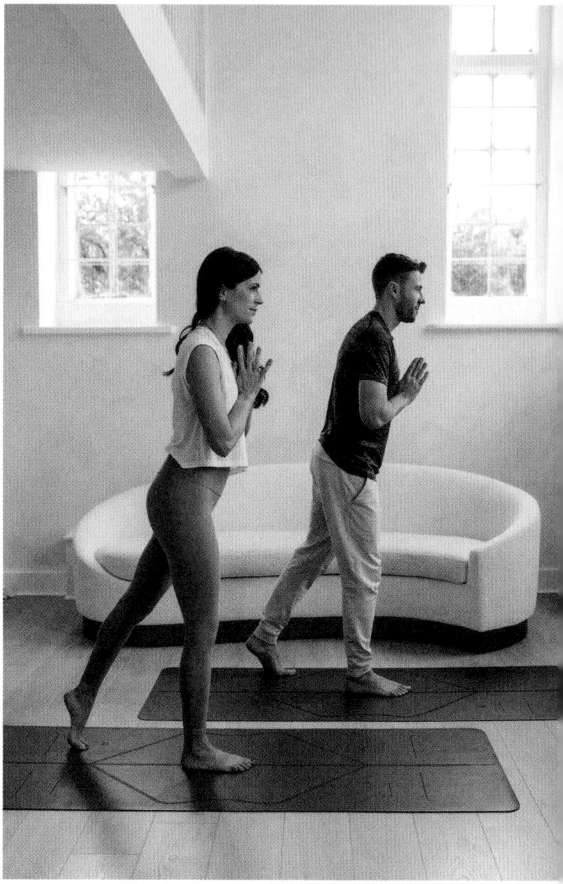
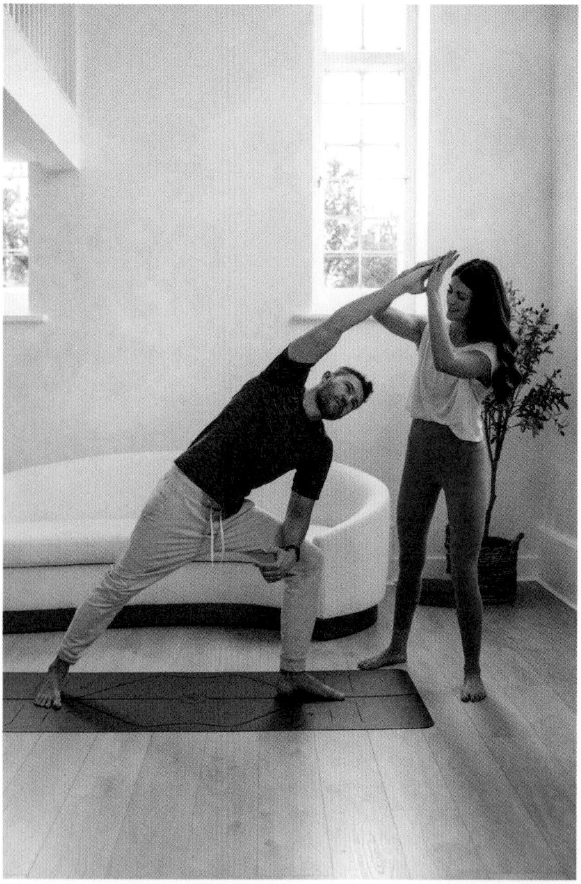
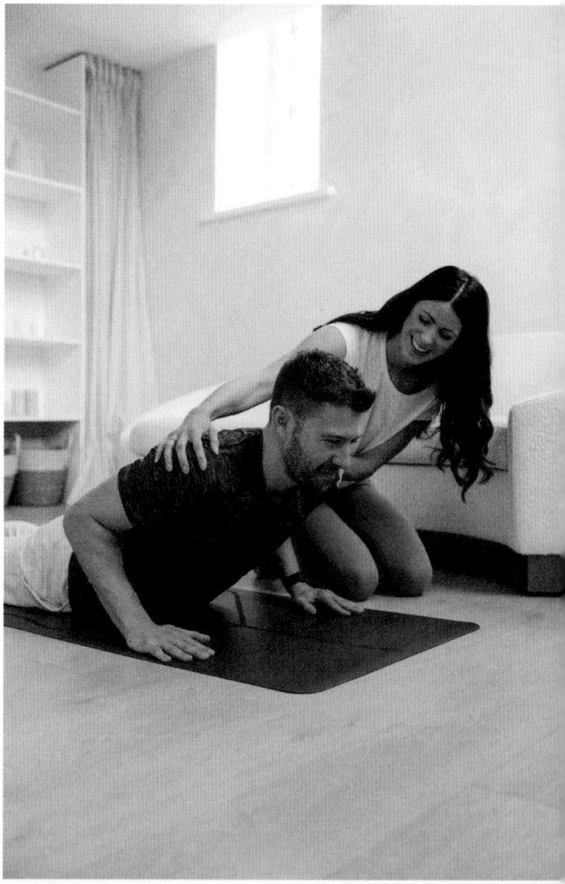

MONTH 2
WARRIOR

'THE TRUE WARRIOR IS GOOD, GENTLE AND HONEST. HIS BRAVERY COMES FROM WITHIN HIMSELF; HE LEARNS TO CONQUER HIS OWN FEARS AND MISDEEDS.'

BRIAN JACQUES

WARRIOR

'Warrior month' is going to help you harness strength, discipline and mindfulness. Warriors require resilience and physical and mental strength to endure and overcome difficulties. Over time, yoga can help you attain all these qualities and more. It gives you the ability to face challenges with a balanced and grounded approach.

As we start the second month of creating a yoga habit, continued discipline is key. Keep showing up to these practices and yoga *will* get easier. Some days it's going to feel hard and some poses might feel impossible, but remember that every pose can be adjusted for you and your body (the appendix on page 190 can help show you how). As you'll learn in this chapter, truthfulness is an essential foundation in building our ethical backbone and therefore of working towards yoga's aim of living with meaning and purpose. If something doesn't yet feel right for your body, that's okay, come back to it in a week or two, but whatever you do, don't give up.

The signature flow this month plays with the warrior poses, which epitomise the essence of the practice. They are seemingly simple but held for time, with truth and in alignment, they will challenge your strength and endurance.

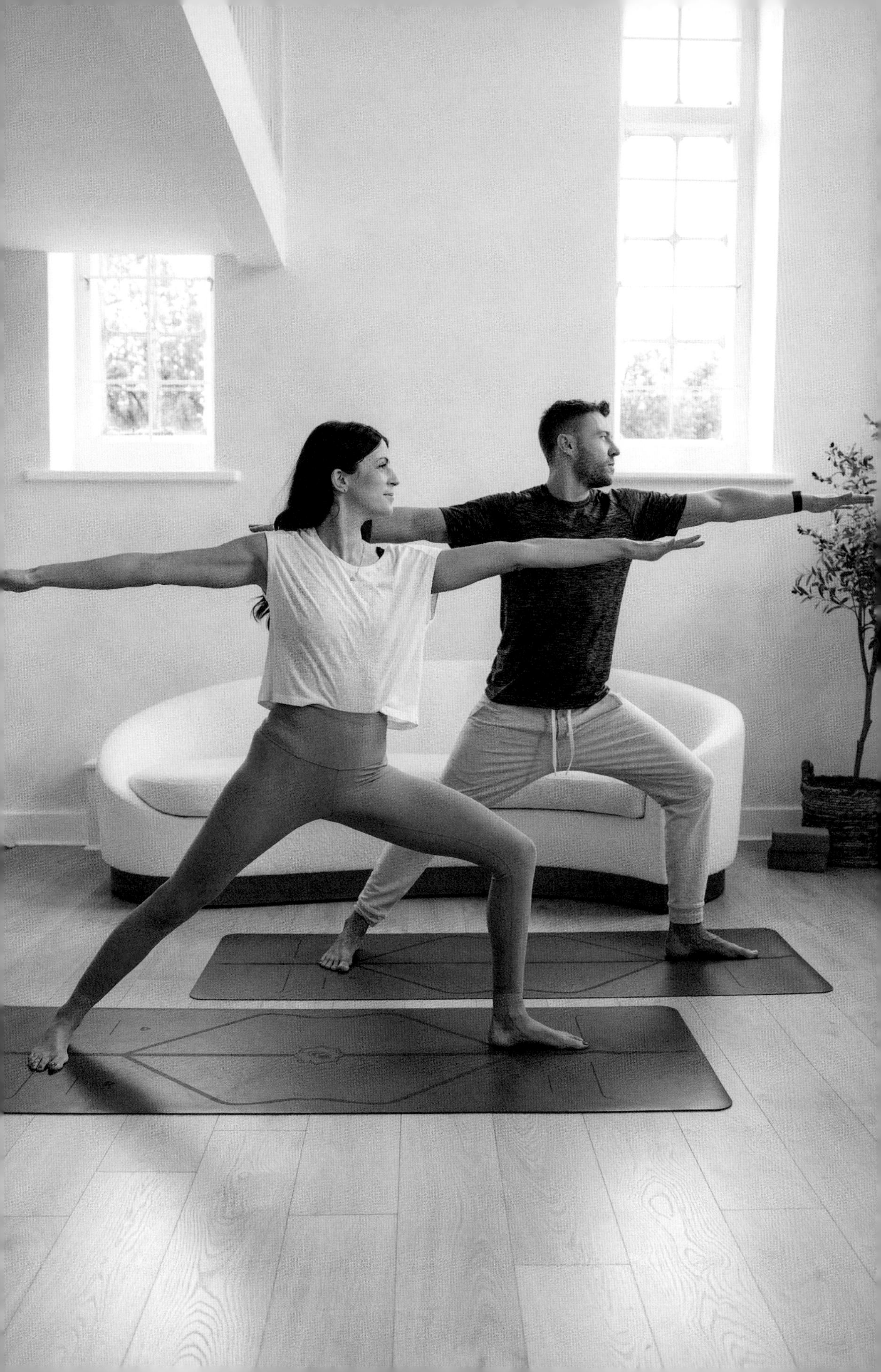

SATYA (TRUTH)

MY THOUGHTS, WORDS AND ACTIONS WILL BE CONSISTENT, HONEST AND FILLED WITH LOVE.

Satya is the second of the *yamas* and it translates as 'truthfulness'. Truthfulness is present when our words, thoughts and actions are aligned and honest. This authenticity requires inner strength and self-awareness, much like the qualities exhibited by a warrior in battle. *Satya* goes side-by-side with *ahimsa* (kindness, see page 27), as when we communicate with ourselves and others clearly and honestly, it prevents harm and suffering.

There's an ancient philosophy that helps explain the marriage of *satya* and *ahimsa*:

Is it kind?
Is it true?
Is it necessary?

Let me give you an example: imagine a child who doesn't find writing or spelling easy. They come to you with a handwritten note that is so sweet and beautiful and riddled with spelling mistakes. If, in response, you speak the full truth without kindness, saying, 'You've spelt almost every word incorrectly,' you would cause them pain and potentially risk them not wanting to try writing impromptu notes in future. In this case, is it not more appropriate to remember the concept of *ahimsa* and use a softer approach to the truth?

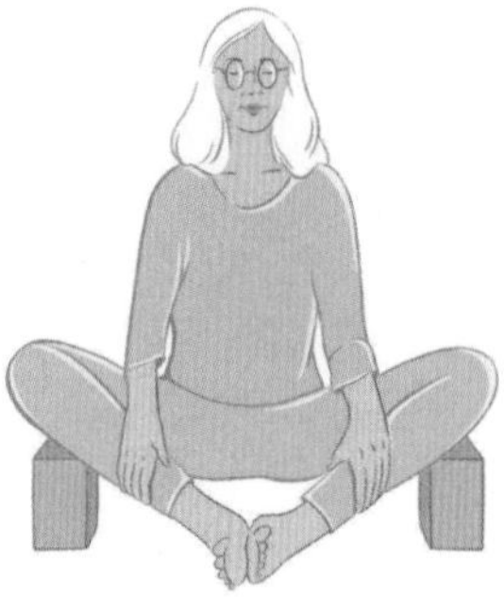

So, how can we incorporate *satya* into our daily lives:

▸ **On the yoga mat:** Start each practice with an intention – this is the truth behind why you are practising today. Cultivate a truthful approach to your movement and ask yourself, are you pushing yourself too much or too little? Is there an area of pain, tightness or weakness that you're ignoring? Are you modifying poses according to what your body needs? *Satya* teaches us to tune in and really listen to the answers.

▸ **Nice or real?:** As human beings we can be predisposed to want people to like us. However, this can mean that we end up modelling ourselves into different things for different people, striving for 'nice' rather than 'real'. The truth is, it is impossible for everyone to like us and isn't it better to aim for being real as this is in fact being truly known?

▸ **Avoiding gossip:** Have you noticed how speaking badly of others leaves a bad aftertaste that lingers and doesn't feel good? *Satya* teaches us to be aware of and distance ourselves from gossip. It's addictive and it's everywhere. Can you instead ask questions, have compassion and an open mind and seek out other sides of the story before jumping to judgement?

▸ **Inner dialogue check:** Pay attention to the voice within your head – your inner dialogue. Notice if it is speaking opinion or truth. If it's opinion, can you take time to explore the truth of the situation? Notice how often you let the words or emotions from within or the words from others cloud what is true for you.

▸ **Time truthfulness:** Time is precious and we lie to ourselves about it often, both by overestimating how many tasks we set ourselves to complete in one day, or by planning a day with back-to-back meetings or assignments. This gives us no wiggle room for things to go wrong or to take longer than we allowed, or even for rest breaks. Perhaps you've lied to yourself about how long you have spent mindlessly scrolling social media? Appreciate the value of time and commit to being truthful about how much you have and what you choose to do with it.

▸ **Sitting with discomfort:** Practising truthfulness means acknowledging and accepting the reality of situations, even when it's uncomfortable. *Satya* encourages us to confront our limitations, fears and shortcomings without evasion.

PROPS HELP US STAY TRUTHFUL

Please listen when I say that yoga props are your friends. A prop is an object that is used to aid the practice of *asana*. Some common props are set out below.

- **Blocks and bricks** can be used to modify poses, provide support, assist with alignment, bring the floor closer to the hands and add height to seated poses.
- **Yoga straps** extend our reach and can be used in assisting, attaining and holding positions.
- **Blankets** are useful as padding and support for sensitive knees. They can be rolled up to add height to seated poses and used as a cover for relaxation during *savasana*.
- **Bolsters and cushions** can provide support in restorative poses, aid in alignment (for example, sitting on a cushion in easy pose or *sukasana*) and help us be more mindful in our practice by allowing us to relax into the pose, and focus on the breath and sensations.

There is a misconception that props are purely for beginners and make things easier. People shy away from using them as they think it means they are 'not good at yoga'. Firstly, yoga props have the capacity to completely transform the way your yoga practice feels. All bodies are built differently – my anatomy and biomechanics will be very different to yours. It may be easier for me to reach the ground in triangle pose as a result of my anatomy, but not needing to use a block under my hand does not make me 'better at yoga'. You will often hear me say that the poses aren't the goal of yoga. The art of developing a strong and truthful practice is in tuning in and being *truthful* with how the poses feel for you. Ask yourself if a prop could make it feel better or make another variation more accessible. Don't let your ego take over and tell you not to take up the wonderful prop. In the appendix of postures (see page 190) I have included many examples of how props can make the poses more accessible.

Secondly, I also want to flag that props can also make a practice HARDER! Balance on a block in warrior III and see the added concentration and focus it takes. Or squeeze a block between the thighs in chair pose and feel the inner thighs and core light up.

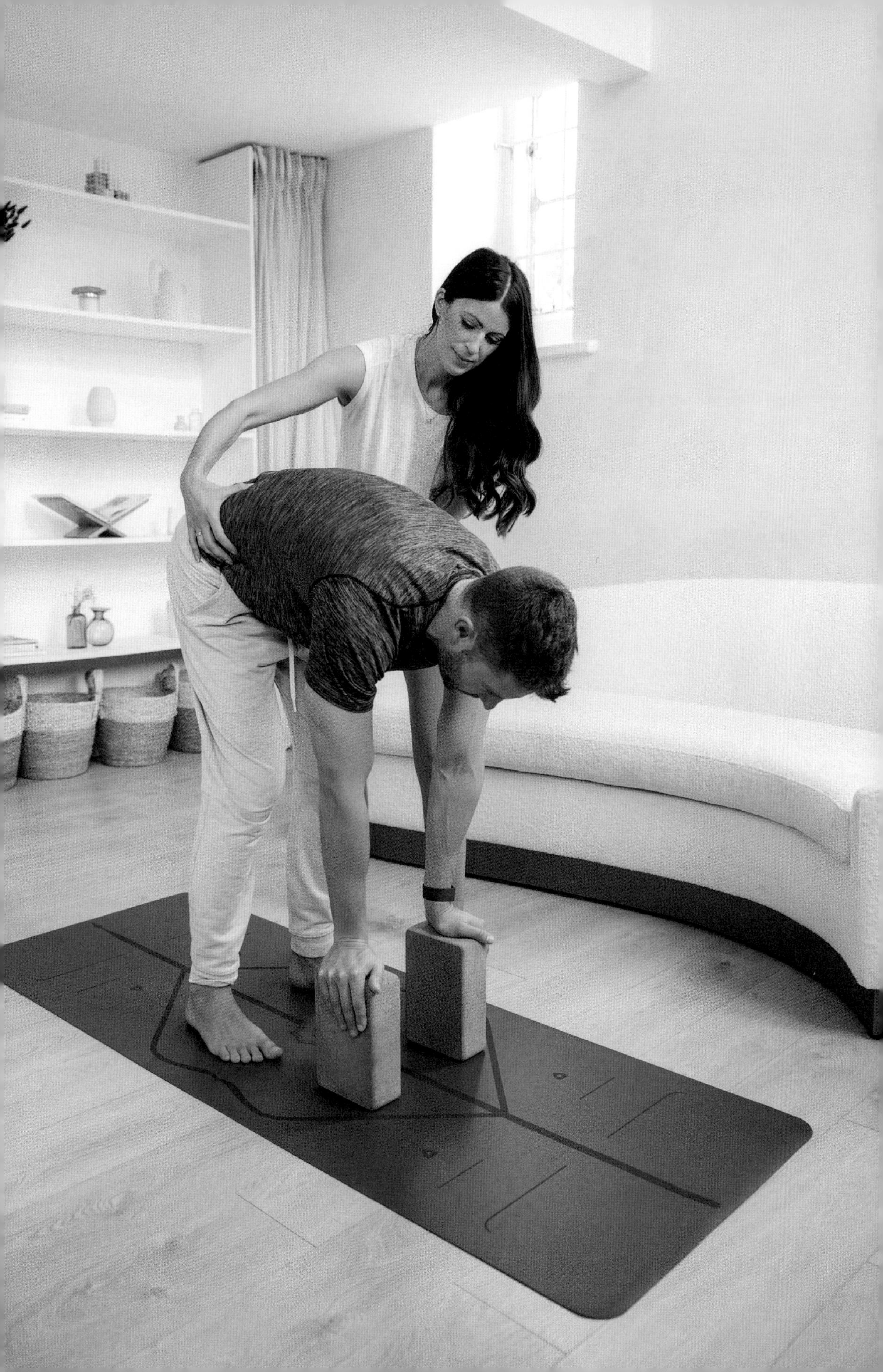

THE BREATH

THE UJJAYI BREATH

When I think about a warrior, I think about someone who stays calm and focused under immense pressure; someone who can act consciously and quickly even in the most difficult of situations. This links so beautifully with the breath as when we learn how to breathe properly, it brings with it many benefits, including increased clarity, focus and calm.

The breathing technique I am sharing this month is the *ujjayi* breath. It's an energising technique that helps to quieten the mind, lengthen and smooth the breath and anchor us to the present moment. It is also known as the victorious or ocean breath and it's an audible breath that's often compared to the sound of the ocean (or some say Darth Vader from Stars Wars!).

Some teachers believe that all *asana* must be practised using *ujjayi*. There are two reasons why I personally don't teach it this way. First, for beginners, it can be difficult enough to link the postures to the breath and therefore throwing *ujjayi* in on top becomes too much for many. Secondly, it has been suggested that in certain cases it can overly strain the vocal chords.

I like teaching *ujjayi* as a breathing practice in isolation at the start of class. This allows students to focus on the technique and how it feels within their bodies. If this breath isn't right for you then I recommend you go back to the three-part breath from month one (see page 31).

Directions:

1. Come into a comfortable seated position, growing tall through the crown of the head and allowing the spine to be neutral and long.
2. As you inhale, feel the belly, the rib cage and all the way to the upper chest gently expand. As you breathe out, aim to make the exhale a similar length to the inhale.
3. Take another deep inhale through the nose then exhale through the mouth making a quiet, whispered 'hahhhh' sound as if you are steaming up a window or mirror. This sound requires a partial closure at the back of the throat.
4. Take another inhale and as you exhale allowing the same faint, whispering sound of constriction to continue, but this time close the mouth and breathe out through the nose. The sound is soft – please don't overly force it.
5. Once you have mastered the exhale, use the same method for the inhale, gently constricting the back of the throat.
6. Repeat for 10–12 rounds.

THE WARRIOR FLOW

This month's signature flow will help you harness both inner and outer strength underpinned by *satya* (truthfulness). Notice how being truthful with your practice brings inner strength and connection. Where can you make small, mindful changes in the postures that make sense for you and your body and nourish you even more?

Aim to practise this flow three or four times per week and if you have more time you can include the seated warm-up flow on page 10 at the start, combine it with month one's mountain flow (see page 33) or repeat the flow multiple times.

PLEASE NOTE
The appendix on page 190 includes a detailed breakdown of each pose, plus variations and modifications. Remember to listen to your body; yoga should never be painful and you can chose to skip any pose that doesn't feel right for you.

As you move around your yoga mat, bring some warrior qualities with you:

- **Perseverance:** The discipline and determination to keep moving forward, even in the midst of obstacles. Don't let challenges in the flow set you back; modify the poses as much as you need and remember child's pose is always there for you to pause and reconnect.
- **Strength:** Just like a warrior, yoga requires both physical and mental strength and the resilience to endure and overcome any difficulties. Be patient with progress and know that over time you will see results.
- **Mindfulness:** Be fully present in the moment and adjust your practice accordingly by being attentive and recognising and listening to your limitations.

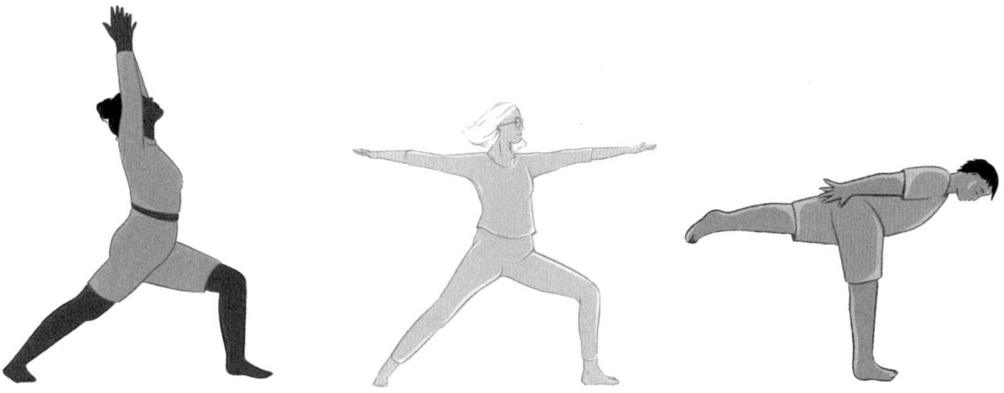

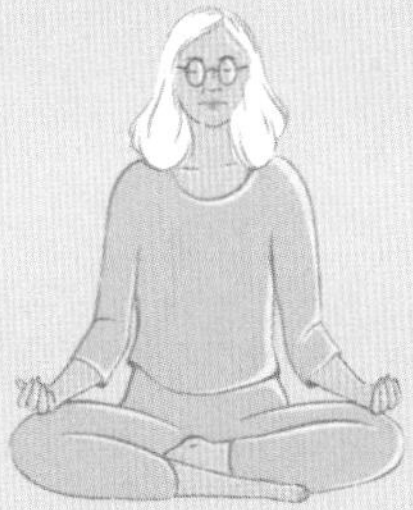

1. SEATED UJJAYI BREATH

In a seated position, take 10 rounds of the ujjayi breath (see page 46).

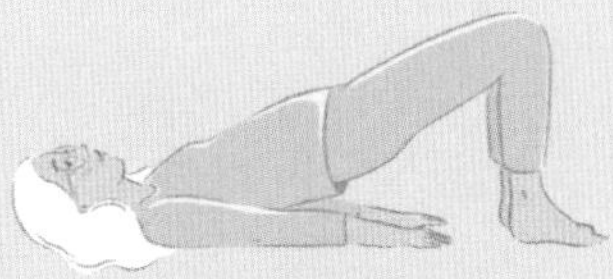

2. BRIDGE

Gently roll onto your back and as you exhale lift into bridge pose for 5 breaths.

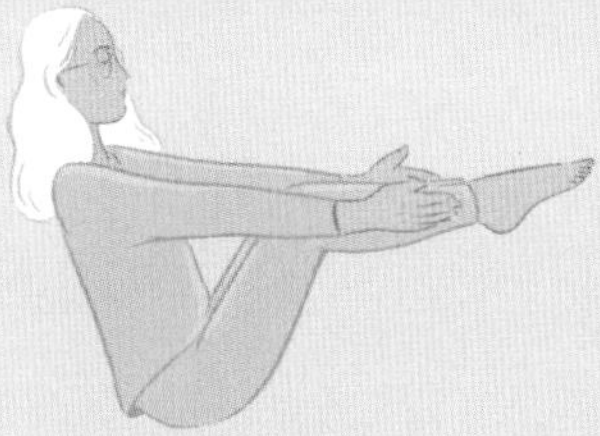

3. BOAT

Come up to sit on the mat. Exhale as you lift into boat pose. Hold for 3 breaths.

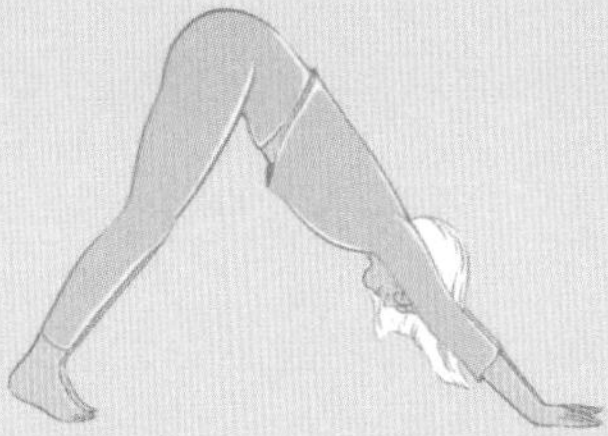

4. DOWNWARD-FACING DOG

Rolling over the knees, exhale as you step back into downward-facing dog for 3 breaths.

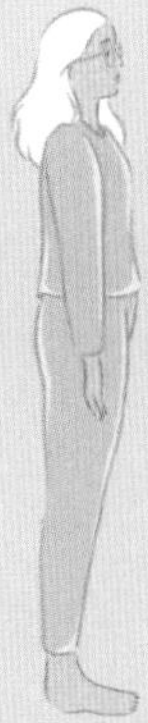

5. MOUNTAIN

Step the feet forward and inhale, lifting into mountain pose for 3 breaths.

SUN SALUTATION B

Complete 1–5 rounds of sun salutation B (see page 16 for details).

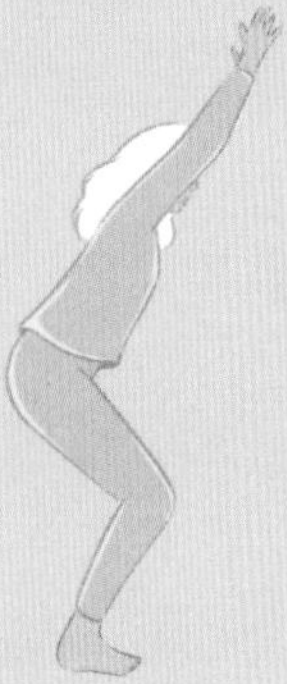

6. CHAIR

Inhale, sweeping into chair pose and hold for 5 breaths.

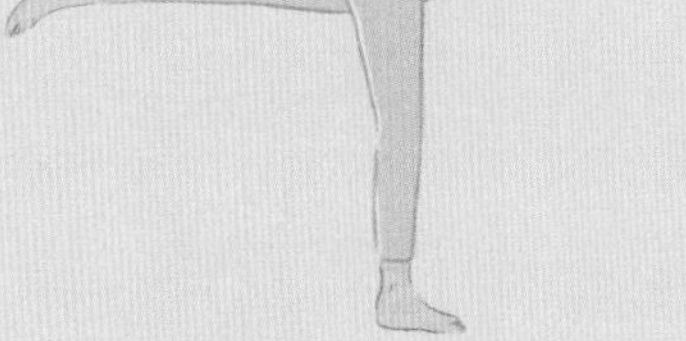

7. WARRIOR III

Exhale, floating the left foot back and finding warrior III. Hold for 3 breaths.

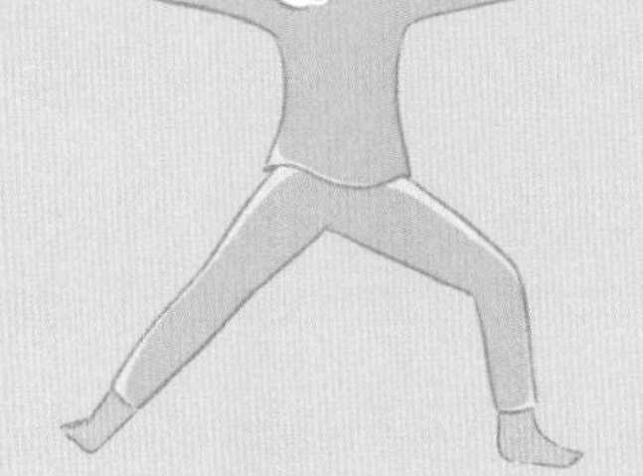

8. WARRIOR II

Gently release the left foot and exhale as you open the body to the left finding warrior II. Hold for 3 breaths.

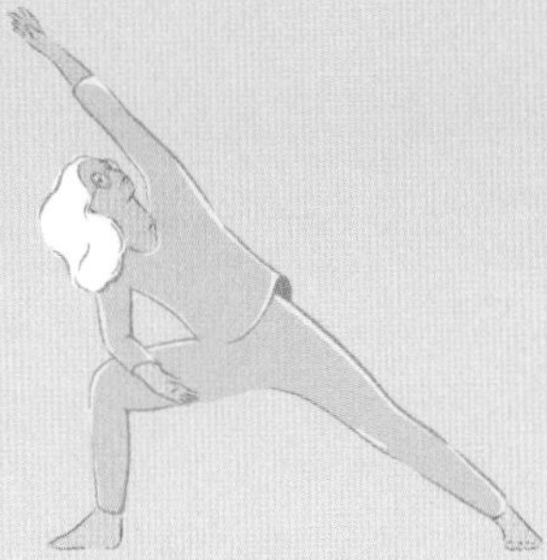

9. EXTENDED SIDE ANGLE

Exhale, releasing to extended side angle and holding for 3 breaths.

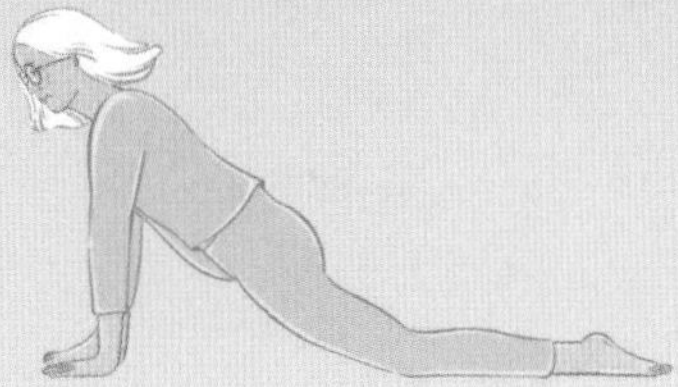

10. LIZARD

Exhale, pivoting onto the back toes and bringing the hands to the inside of the right foot. Hold for 3 breaths.

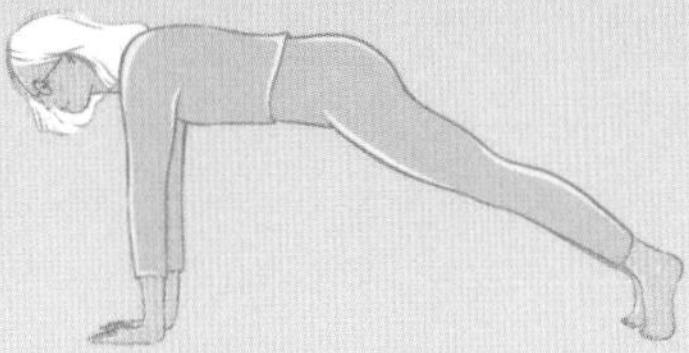

11. PLANK

Exhale as you step back to plank and hold for 3 breaths.

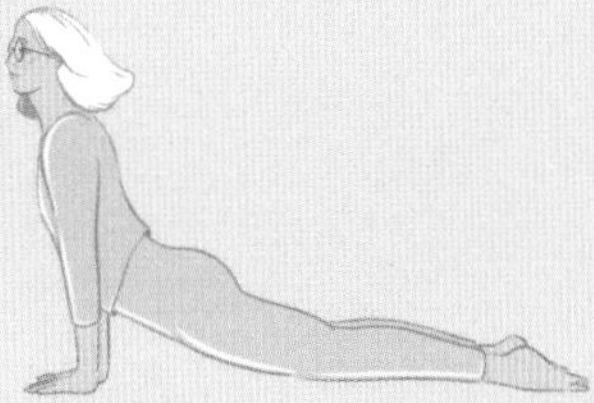

12. UPWARD-FACING DOG

Lowering through yoga push-up, inhale lifting into upward-facing dog or cobra.

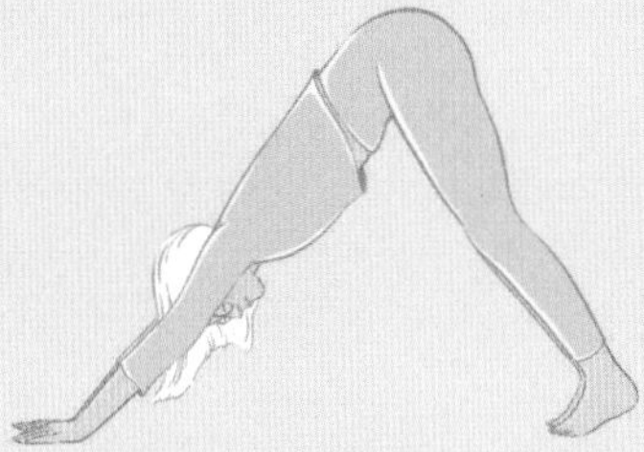

13. DOWNWARD-FACING DOG

Exhale as you move into downward-facing dog and hold for 1 breath.

REPEAT ON THE LEFT SIDE

STEPS 6–13

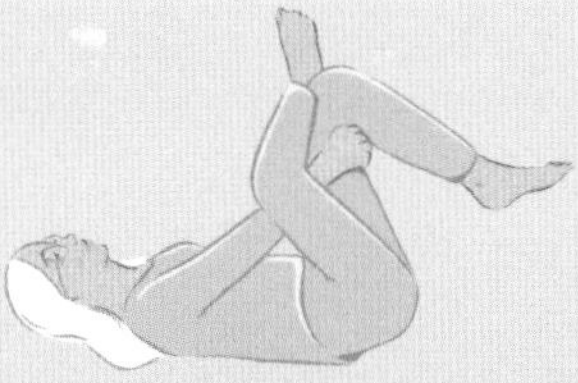

14. RECLINED PIGEON

Coming onto your back, cross the right foot over the left knee and find reclined pigeon. Hold for 5 breaths, then repeat on the opposite side.

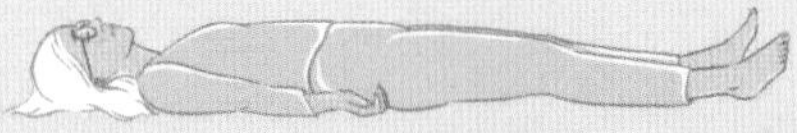

15. SAVASANA

Finally, melt into savasana for 2 minutes or more.

MEDITATION

MANTRA MEDITATION

Meditation helps us cultivate resilience and focus. Just as a warrior trains their body and mind for battles, meditation allows us to train our mind to be more centred, calm and prepared to face the challenges of life.

The meditation I am sharing with you this month is a mantra meditation and it is one of my favourites. A mantra is a phrase you repeat to yourself, typically composed of only a few words or syllables. The mantra is the anchor that keeps the mind steady. I have suggested four different mantras that you can use for this meditation but feel free to use your own if you prefer.

Possible mantras:

▸ **'Aum' or 'Om'**: A sacred sound known as the sound of the universe.

▸ **'So Hum'**: This is a Sanskrit phrase, translated as, 'I am'. It promotes oneness and emphasises our connection to the universe.

▸ **'In me, I trust'**: A mantra that I love because it's a gentle reminder to go within and trust that we have the answers and don't need to turn outwards for them.

▸ **'Let go'**: On each inhale think 'let', and on each exhale think 'go'. The mantra is a reminder to let go of anything you are holding on to that you don't need – tension, your to-do list, let go of them all.

Directions:

1. Come into a comfortable seated position on a chair with an upright spine, somewhere you can be free of distractions.
2. Set a timer for 5 minutes or for as long as you have.
3. Gently close your eyes. If you don't like to close your eyes, you can have your eyes slightly open with the gaze lowered to the floor in front of you to keep your forehead soft.
4. Softly close your lips and let your breath come in through the nose and out through the nose or mouth in its natural rhythm.
5. Before each meditation begins, feel your sitting bones on the chair and your feet on the floor. Imagine roots winding down from these areas, helping you feel secure and grounded.
6. Start to silently repeat your chosen mantra, slowly, softly like you're whispering it within your body.
7. Each time your mind starts to wander, gently bring your awareness back to your mantra.
8. When the timer finishes, take a moment with the eyes still closed to sit and notice how you feel and any thoughts or feelings that arose.

MEDITATION TIPS

FIVE THINGS I WISH I'D KNOWN EARLIER

YOU CAN SIT IN A COMFY CHAIR

Often we have a vision of needing to be sitting in the lotus pose on a hardwood floor. In reality we can meditate anywhere and on anything. All I would recommend is sitting on something where you can have an upright spine to keep a feeling of alertness.

THERE IS SO MUCH VARIETY

Just like styles of yoga, there are a huge number of different meditation types. If you struggle to sit in stillness, try a walking meditation (see page 66). If a breath-based meditation isn't for you, try a body scan (see page 94) or a loving-kindness meditation (see page 149).

IT'S HARD

There's a preconception that meditation is easy because you're not 'doing' anything. Just like everything, it takes practice and commitment. And, spoiler alert, your mind will wander and that's okay; in fact, that is half the point. You realise the mind has wandered and gently bring it back to the present. Remember, you're not doing anything wrong – you're human and our minds do wander!

QUICK MEDITATION BREAKS ARE AMAZING

If you don't have a lot of time, a three-minute meditation break can help you hit pause, find connection and get a needed recharge of your mental batteries.

IT WILL HELP YOU IN WAYS YOU NEVER IMAGINED

I started meditating to reduce stress but a regular meditation practice also helped me become more mindful in everyday life. It also improved my sleep and helped with my creativity and focus.

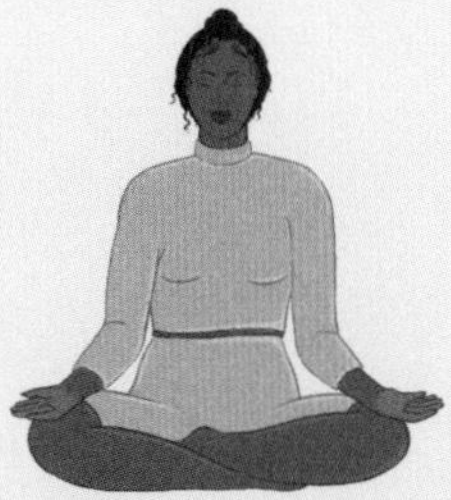

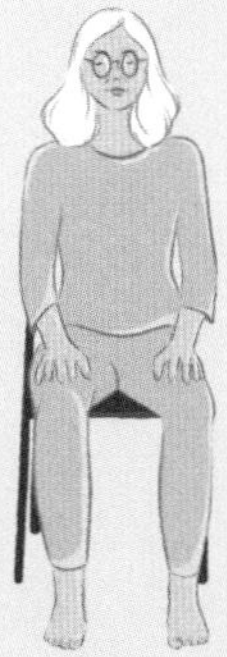

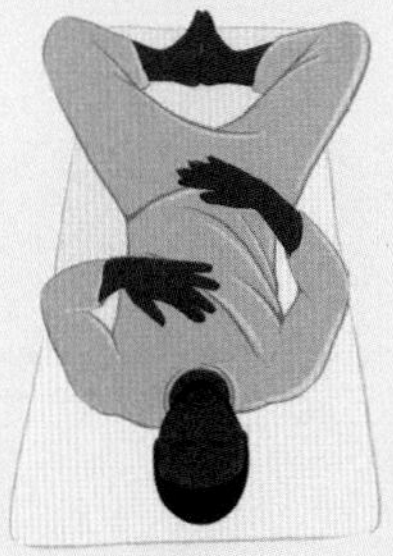

JOURNAL PROMPTS

Below I have given you eight self-reflection questions linked to this month's warrior theme and the yogic concept of *satya*. Try answering two questions weekly alongside the daily journal prompts set out on pages 8–9.

- Think of a challenging situation you are currently facing. How can approaching it with the honesty and integrity of a warrior help you?

- Write about a situation in which you felt tempted to hide or bend the truth. What were the reasons you felt this way and what lessons can you learn for next time?

- Write about someone who embodies the warrior spirit for you. What qualities do you admire in them and how can you integrate those qualities into your own life?

- Consider a time when you received feedback that was difficult to hear. How did you respond and what did you learn about yourself through this experience?

- Consider the connection between authenticity and truthfulness. How does being true to yourself align with your ability to be honest with others?

- Warriors have moments of vulnerability despite their strength and bravery. When have you had a situation where you were vulnerable or asked for help? How did this contribute to your growth and resilience?

- Think about the concept of self-care as an act of self-preservation. How do you prioritise your well-being in a way that aligns with the warrior's commitment to self-nurturing?

- Reflect on the role of empathy in truthful communication. How can you be truthful while still considering the feelings and perspectives of others?

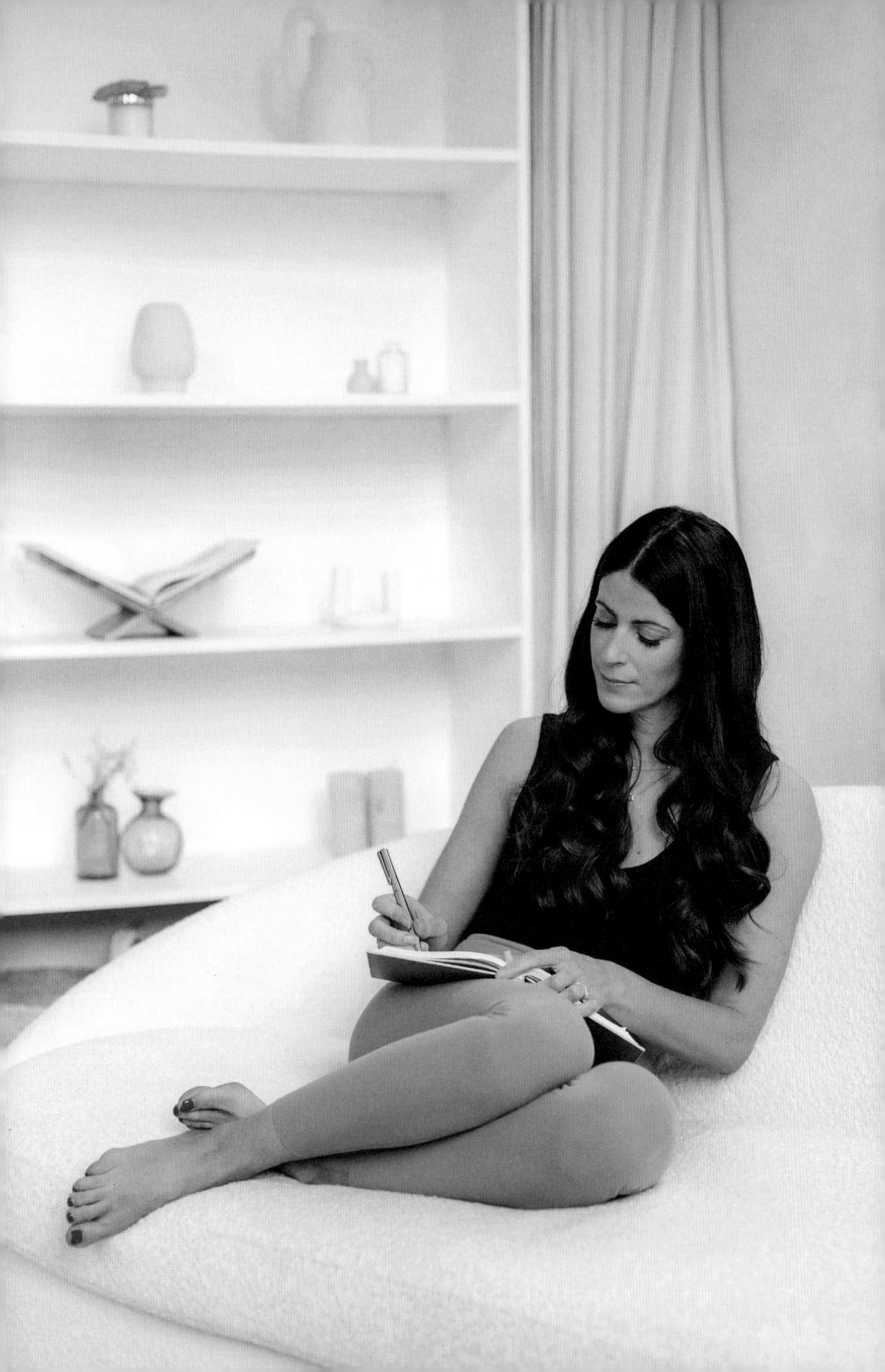

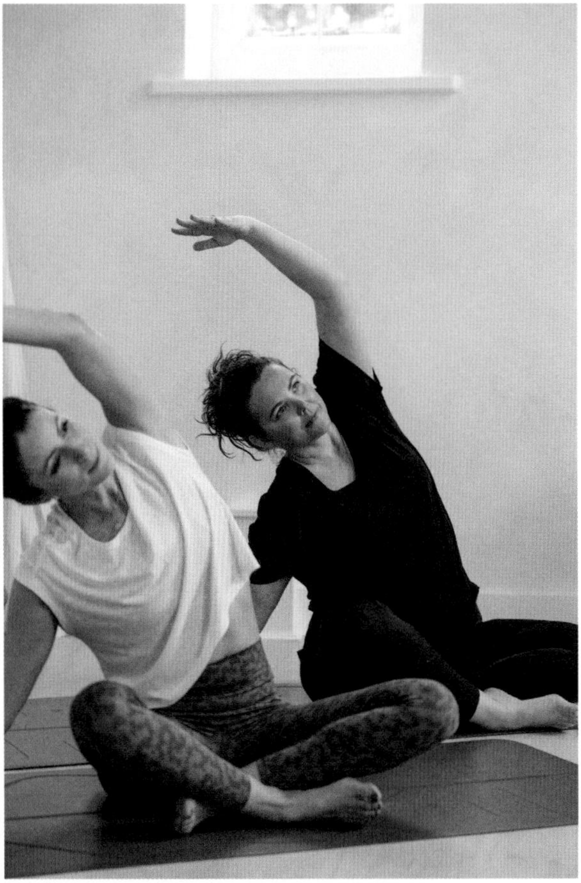
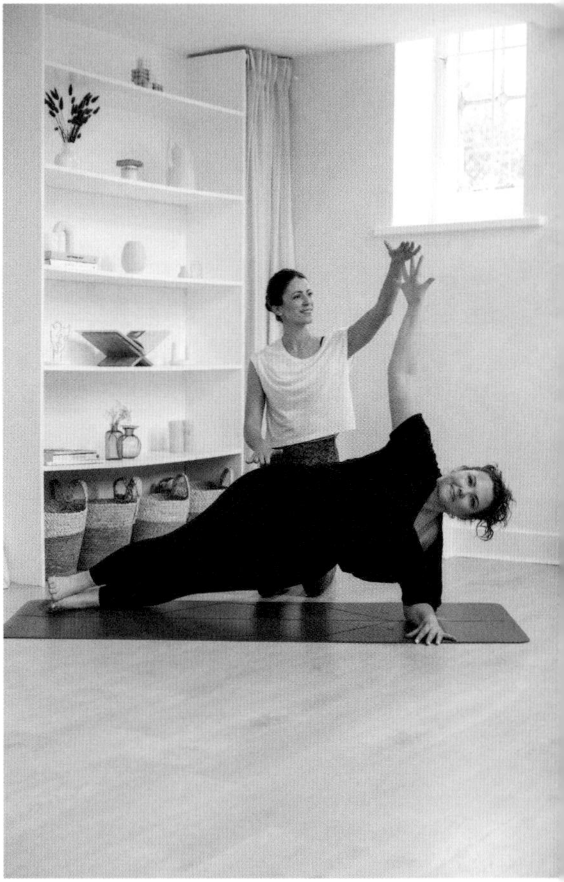
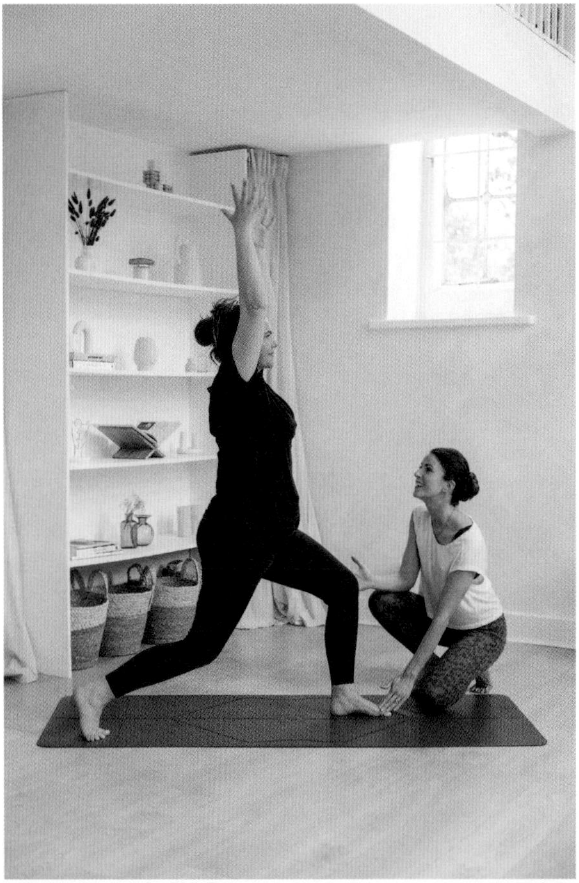
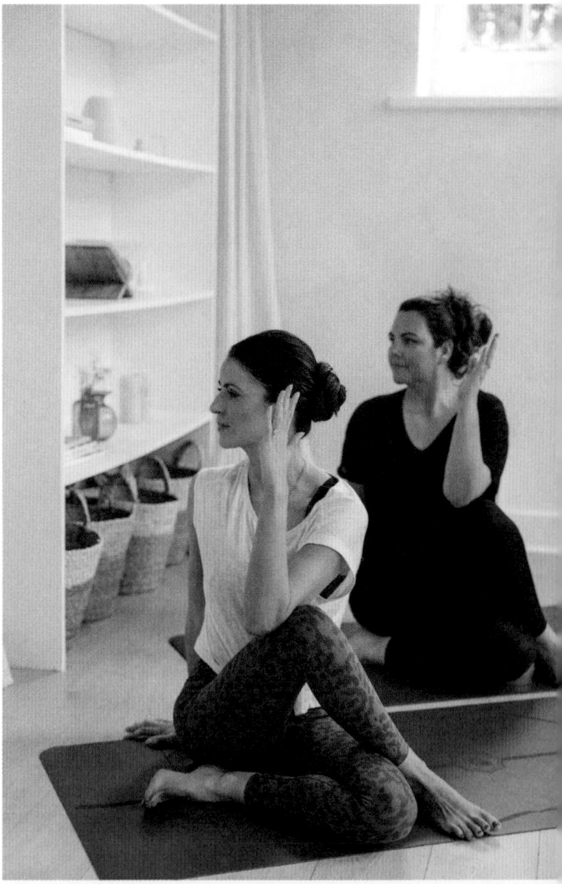

MONTH 3
TORNADO

'IN THE MIDST OF MOVEMENT
AND CHAOS, KEEP STILLNESS
INSIDE OF YOU.'

DEEPAK CHOPRA

TORNADO

This month's theme is the mighty tornado which brings a flow full of twists and strength. I also share more tools to call on for resilience and growth. Part of the reason that yoga changes so many people's lives is because of its ability to instil calm in the midst of chaos. The world we live in is noisy, fast-paced and unpredictable. We spend our lives doing, doing, doing and for many it can be a real struggle to be still and truly rest. Yoga gives us tools to find calm and strength even when life feels like it's moving like a tornado.

In a tornado, there's a centre of intense focus called the 'eye'. In yoga, we aim to cultivate a similar focus and concentration during meditation, breathwork and *asana*. This can at times feel fairly easy, but at others it can feel impossible, with the mind wandering here, there and everywhere. Let this be your reminder that you are human and human beings tend to have busy minds and aren't perfect (which is a *good* thing – we're perfectly imperfect).

If you feel like the silent practices (i.e. the breathing techniques and meditation) are tricky and the mind keeps running away, this month's walking meditation may feel like a welcome break. The meditation is a way to find presence and connection in nature. It can also act as a wonderful reminder of the beauty in the world and give us an opportunity to be grateful for the life surrounding us.

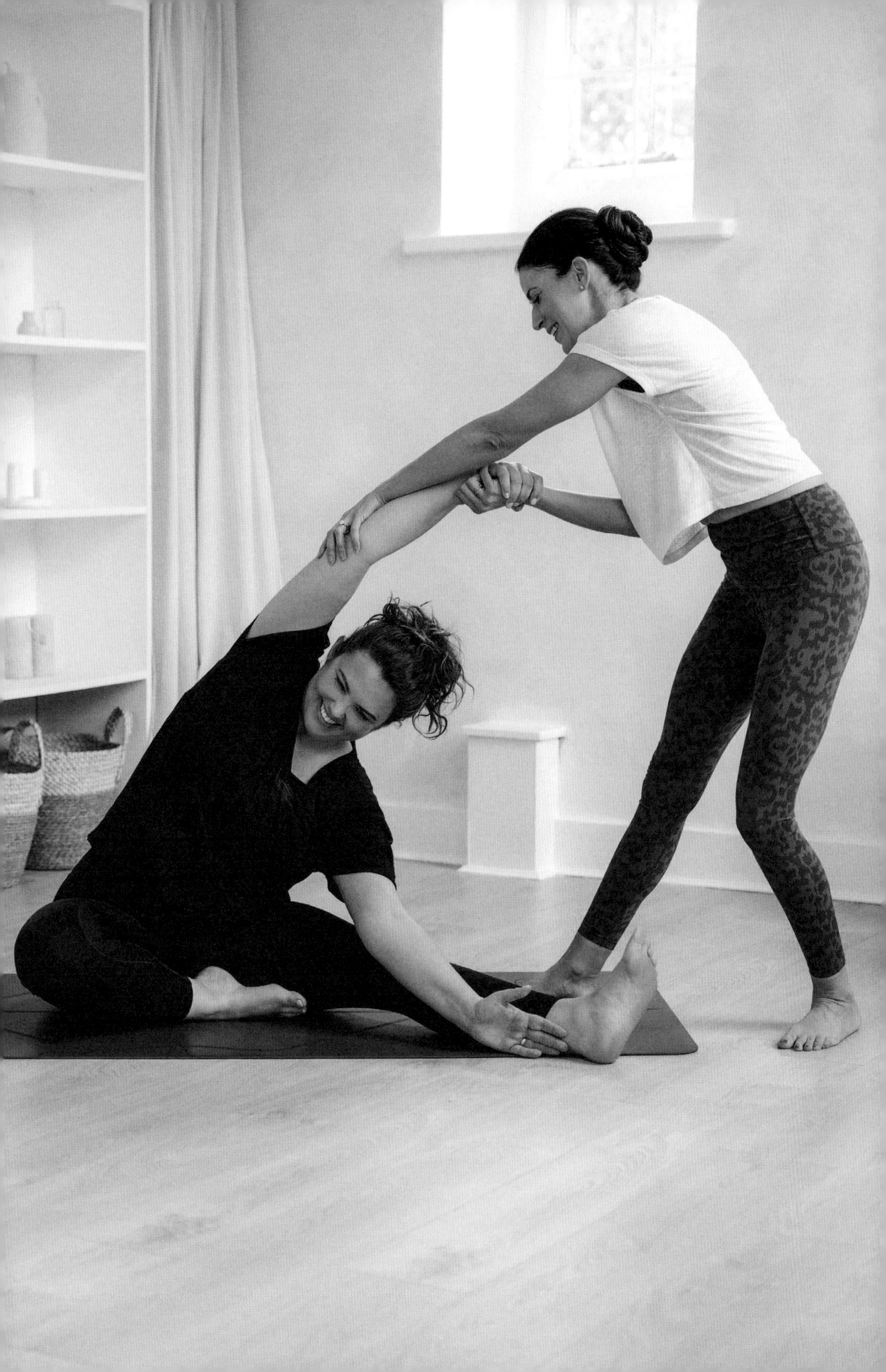

THE PURPOSE OF YOGA

In Patañjali's *Yoga Sutras*, sutra 1.2 states, *'Yogas citta-vritti-nirodhah'*, which can be translated as: 'yoga is the cessation of the fluctuations of the mind'.

This sutra is fundamental to understanding the purpose of yoga: to still the fluctuations of the mind and achieve a state of inner peace, clarity and realisation of the true self. Therefore, the practice of yoga is a means to quieten the mind and attain higher states of consciousness, connection and self-realisation.

On the journey to achieving this stillness, yoga helps us with tools like meditation, mindfulness, *asana*, breathwork and ethical living (through the *yamas* and *niyamas*). In the noise of modern life, stillness and calm can help us to navigate challenges with greater resilience and mindfulness.

Furthermore, by incorporating these practices into our everyday lives, it allows us to develop a more balanced and centred approach to our thoughts and actions. In turn, this allows us to respond to life's situations from a place of inner stability and wisdom.

As students go deeper into their practice, they often experience profound personal growth and transformation. Cultivating the holistic harmony between body, mind and spirit enhances physical and mental well-being and we are better equipped to extend compassion and understanding to others, contributing to a ripple effect and a more peaceful and harmonious world.

ASTEYA (NON-STEALING)

I LIVE IN GRATITUDE FOR ALL THAT I HAVE.

Asteya is the third of the *yamas* and it can be translated as 'non-stealing'. At first glance, this seems like an obvious thing to avoid. However, the meaning of *asteya* goes far deeper than simply not stealing something physical from someone else. It can relate to how much we are taking from the planet, stealing from our yoga practice by moving in a way we aren't ready to do, and stealing people's time or their opportunity to speak, share or be heard.

We can also steal from ourselves, through limiting beliefs, not exercising self-care, a lack of self-trust, supressing our authentic selves and stifling our own growth, for example, by not pursuing our passions and denying ourselves opportunity for personal development.

Asteya involves being honest and maintaining integrity in our actions and interactions with ourselves and with others. If we think about the destructive power of a tornado, it can serve as a metaphor for the harm and suffering caused by dishonesty and theft.

So how can we incorporate *asteya* into our daily lives?

▸ **On the yoga mat:** Cultivate mindfulness, humility and respect for your own body and abilities. Always come from a place of self-compassion. Listen to what your body is telling you and avoid pushing past your limits or into pain. Ask yourself if you are trying to mimic what you think a perfect pose looks like. There isn't one perfect pose; a perfect pose is the one that is right for you in that moment. Practise contentment with where you are in your yoga journey, which is constantly evolving and changing.

▸ **Honesty:** This is a fundamental aspect of *asteya*. We need to be truthful with our words and actions and avoid lying, cheating and deceiving. Living with integrity means we are less likely to engage in behaviours that steal from our own values and principles.

▸ **Mindful consumption:** Be conscious of your consumption habits. Consider the impact of your choices on society and the environment and avoid overindulgence or acquiring more than you truly need.

▸ **Time (others):** Other people's time is as valuable as yours. Be mindful of this by being punctual and considerate and avoid wasting someone else's time unnecessarily.

▸ **Time (our own):** How much are you saying yes to? Do you need to set better boundaries in life? When you constantly say 'yes' to too many commitments or obligations, you can end up stealing time, energy and resources from yourself and stealing from your own self-care.

▸ **Cultivate contentment:** Instead of constantly desiring more or comparing what you have to others, foster a sense of inner abundance.

▸ **Self-care:** Looking after ourselves can sometimes bring immense guilt. Prioritise self-care without this guilt or hesitation. Set aside time for activities that nourish your well-being, just like we would encourage our children, friends or loved ones to do the same.

THE BREATH

THE GOLDEN THREAD BREATH

When I picture a tornado, I picture a swirling energy force, which is why this month I am sharing a breath called the golden thread breath. I learned this from a teacher of mine, Uma Dinsmore-Tuli, many, many years ago and it's a breath I come back to regularly (particularly when life feels chaotic). It's an empowering breath and the lengthened exhalation soothes the nervous system leaving a sense of calm in body and mind. This breathing technique can also be used as a way of controlling pain.

Directions:

1. Come into a comfortable seated position, growing tall through the crown of the head and allowing the spine to be neutral and long.
2. Close the eyes and take a couple of full breaths followed by a big yawn, releasing any tension in the jaw or face.
3. Inhale through the nose and feel the belly, the rib cage and upper chest gently expand.
4. Exhale through thinly parted lips imagining you are blowing out a very fine golden thread of spiralling energy from your lips.
5. If you are using this technique to help control pain, you can imagine the breath coming into the part of the body that's experiencing the pain. Exhaling the golden thread bringing softness and relief, removing that pain bit by bit.
6. Repeat for 10 rounds or more.

THE TORNADO FLOW

This month's signature flow is filled with twists and strength underpinned by the concept of *asteya* (non-stealing). With twists we have a tendency to force the movement from our neck (which is the part of the spine with the biggest range of rotation). Instead, can you bring honesty into the rotational poses through lengthening the spine and leading from the heart, moving with your breath and feeling the twist from the whole spine.

Aim to practise this flow three or four times per week and if you have more time you can include the seated warm-up flow on page 10 at the start, combine it with previous months' flows or repeat the flow multiple times.

As you move around your yoga mat, bring some tornado qualities with you:

▸ **Grounding:** Despite their nature, tornados have a central core. Think about this as you flow. Focus on finding your centre and grounding yourself in each posture. For example, when you're twisting, think about stabilising the hips and lower body and bringing the twist into the spine rather than twisting from the hips.

▸ **Presence:** Tornados' destructive nature means that they require our attention and awareness. Be mindful in each practice, staying present using the breath, the body and the sensations within it.

▸ **Fluidity:** Tornados are powerful but move with a sense of fluidity and grace. Work towards fluid movements and transitions, slowing down and following the breath as much as you need to.

PLEASE NOTE

The appendix on page 190 includes a detailed breakdown of each pose, plus variations and modifications. Remember to listen to your body; yoga should never be painful and you can chose to skip any pose that doesn't feel right for you.

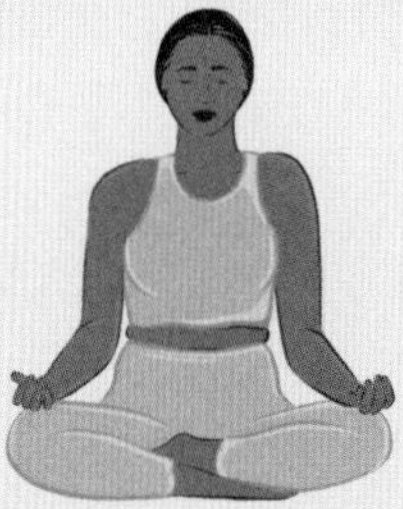

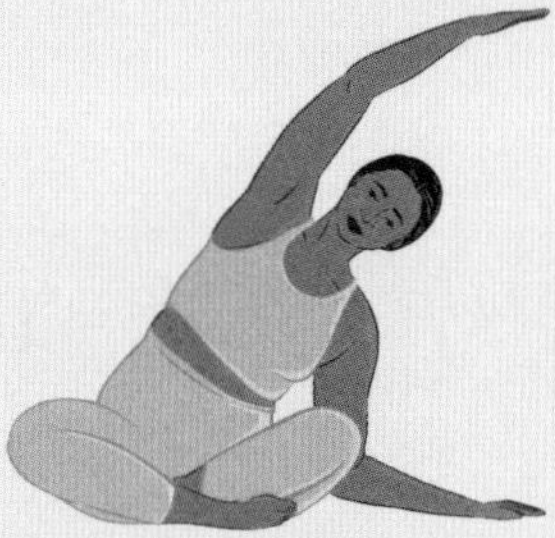

1. GOLDEN THREAD BREATH

In a seated position, take 10 rounds of the golden thread breath (see page 60).

2. SEATED SIDE STRETCH

Gently take 5 side stretches on both sides.

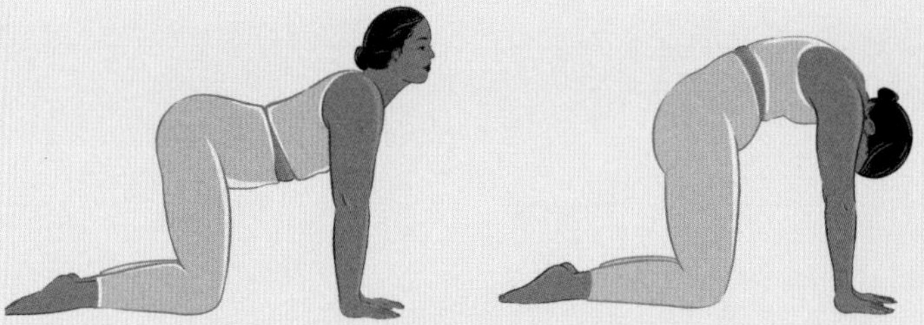

3. CAT AND COW

Coming onto all fours, inhale into cow pose and exhale into cat pose. Repeat 3 times.

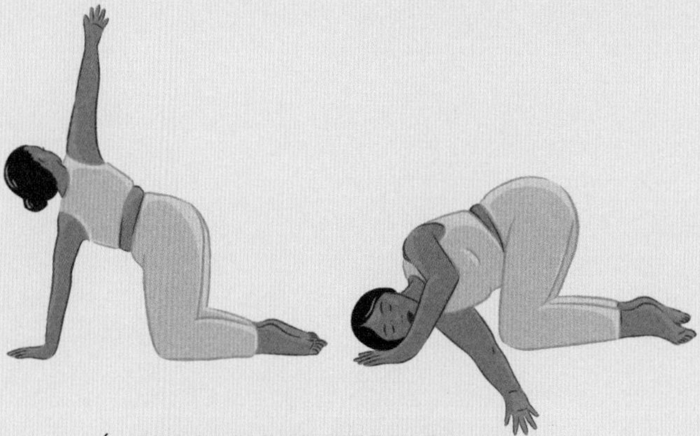

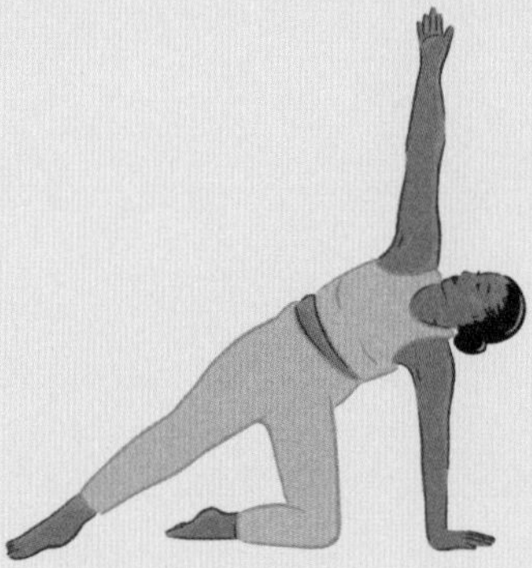

4. THREAD THE NEEDLE

Inhale, reaching the right arm high. Exhale, threading the right arm underneath the body. Repeat 3 times.

5. SIDE PLANK KNEE DOWN

Inhale reaching, the right fingers high finding side plank and hold for 5 breaths.

REPEAT ON THE LEFT SIDE

STEPS 4 AND 5

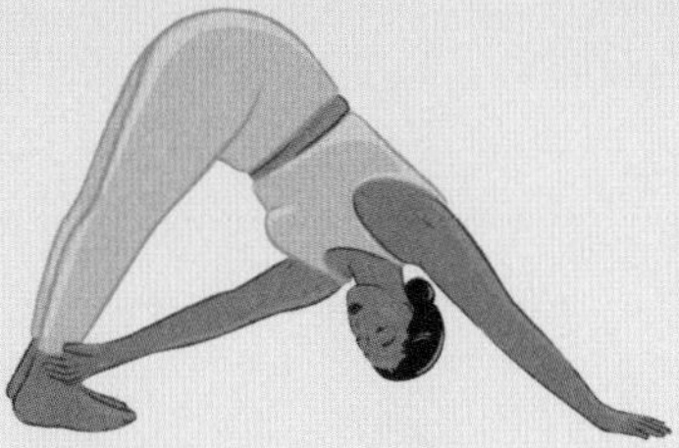

6. DOWNWARD-FACING DOG TWIST

Finding downward-facing dog, lift the left hand and twist, holding for 3 breaths. Repeat on the other side.

SUN SALUTATIONS A & B

Option to include sun salutations A and B (see pages 16–20).

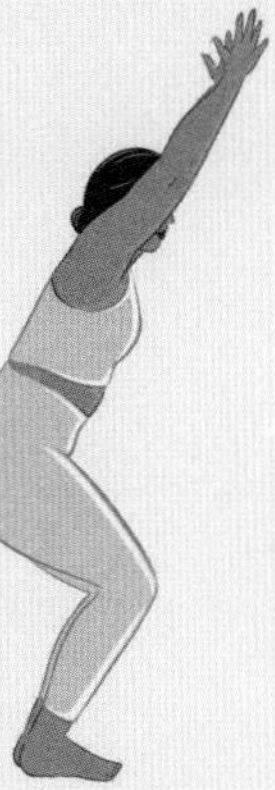

7. CHAIR

Inhale, sweeping into chair pose and hold for 3 breaths.

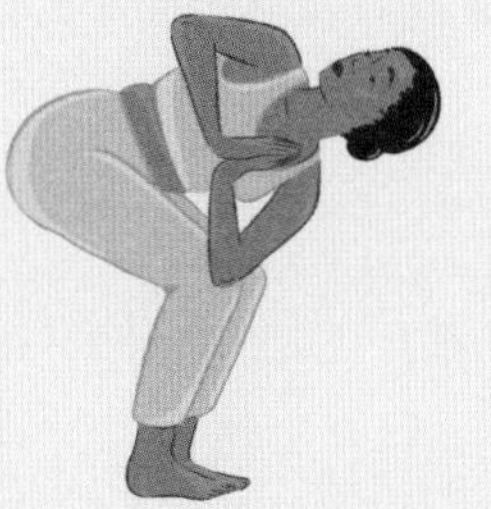

8. TWISTED CHAIR

Exhale, twisting to the right and hold for 5 breaths.

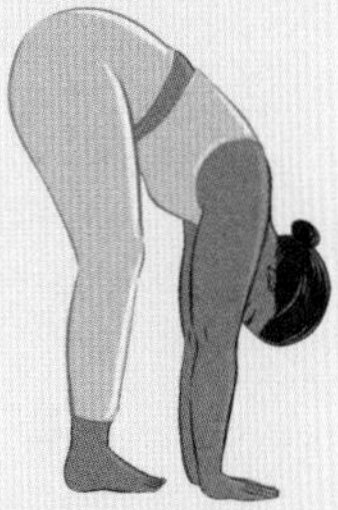

9. STANDING FORWARD BEND

Exhale as you hinge from the hips and fold to the floor.

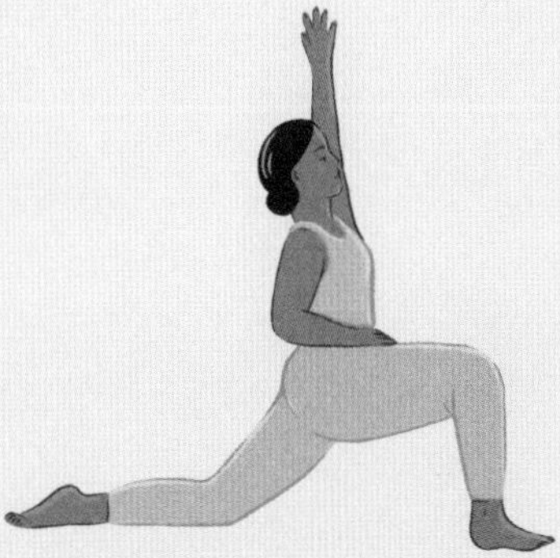

10. LOW LUNGE

Step the left foot back and inhale into low lunge. Hold for 3 breaths.

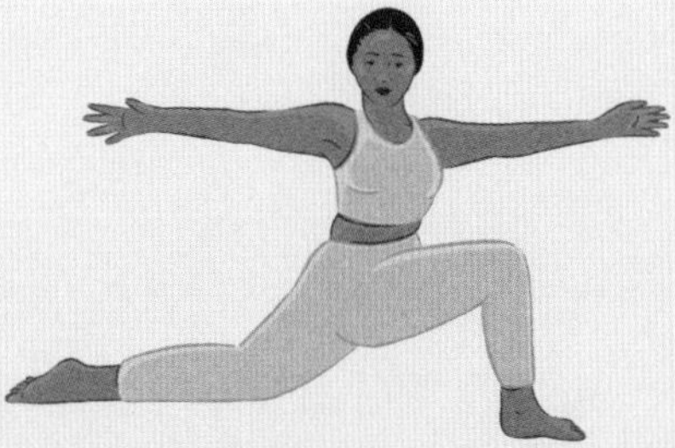

11. LOW LUNGE TWIST

Exhale and reach the right hand back and left arm forwards parallel to the ground. Hold for 5 breaths.

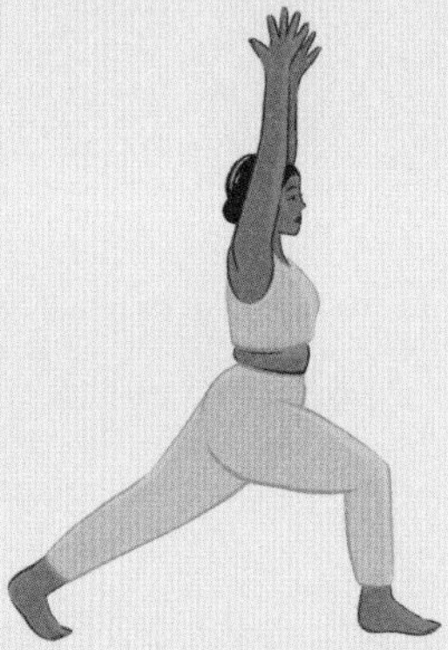

12. HIGH LUNGE

Inhale sweeping the arms up and lifting to high lunge.

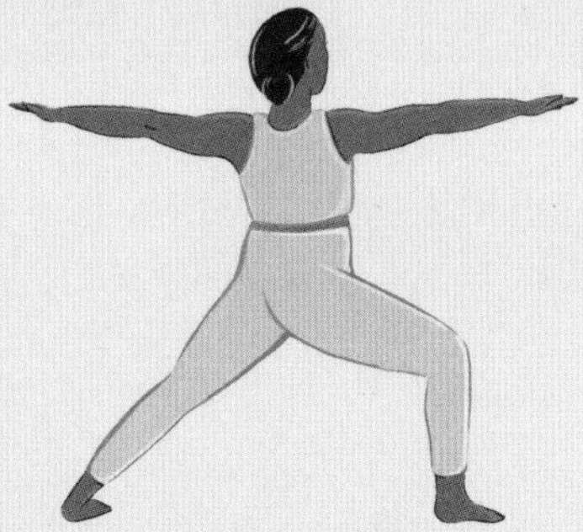

13. WARRIOR II

Exhale, opening the body to the left and finding warrior II. Hold for 5 breaths.

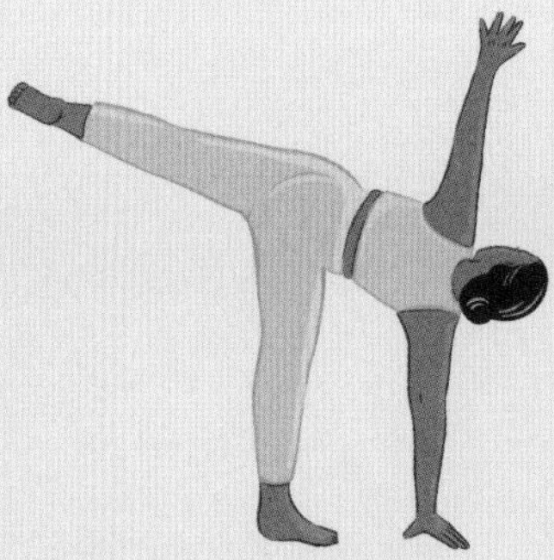

14. HALF MOON

Exhale, shifting the weight forward and lifting the left leg up into half moon. Hold for 3 breaths.

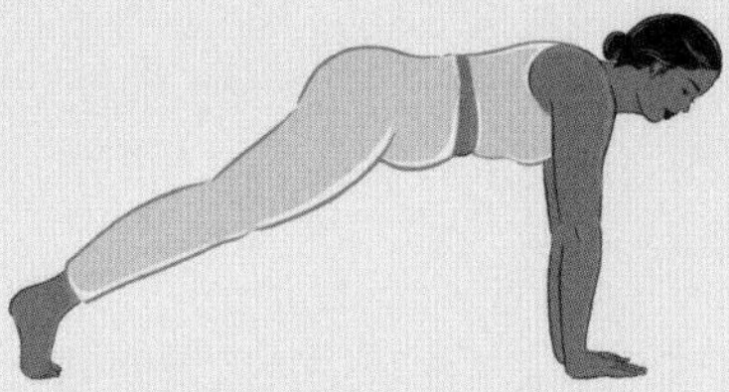

15. PLANK

Slowly release, windmill the hands to the floor and step back to plank for 1 breath.

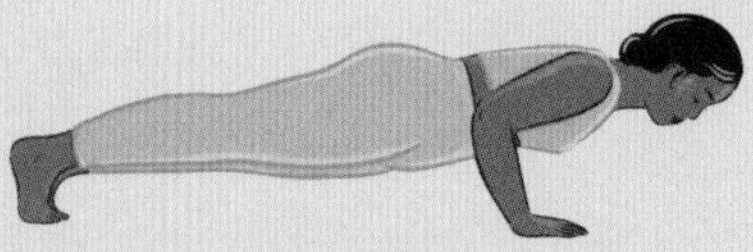

16. YOGA PUSH-UP

Exhale as you lower through yoga push-up.

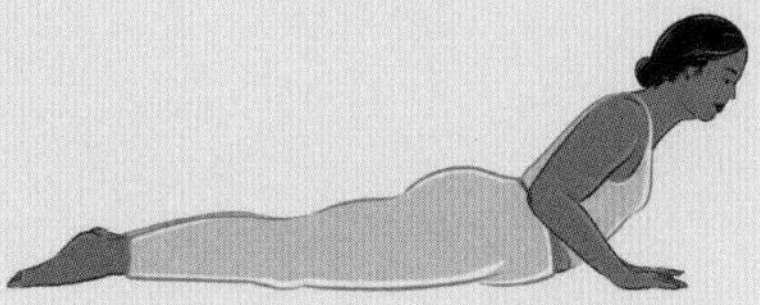

17. COBRA

Inhale, opening the chest into cobra or upward-facing dog.

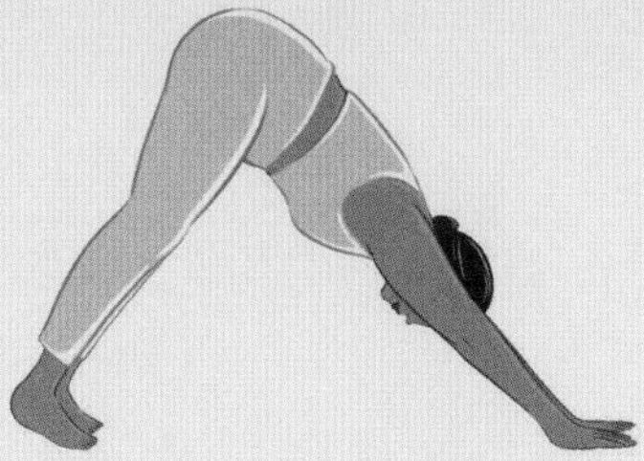

18. DOWNWARD-FACING DOG

Exhale, lifting the hips to the sky to find downward-facing dog. Hold for 5 breaths.

REPEAT ON THE OTHER SIDE

STEPS 7–18

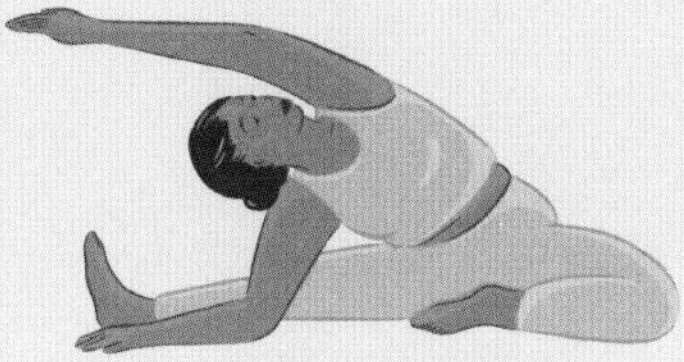

19. REVOLVED HEAD-TO-KNEE

Hop to a seated position with the right leg straight finding revolved head to knee and hold for 5 breaths.

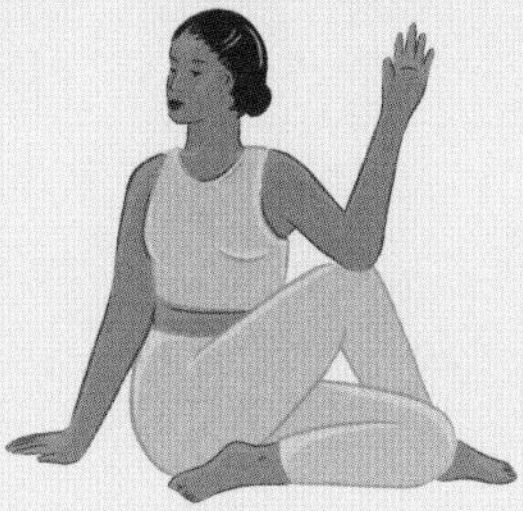

20. HALF LORD OF THE FISHES

Step the right foot over the left thigh and twist. Hold for 5 breaths.

REPEAT ON THE LEFT SIDE

STEPS 19 AND 20

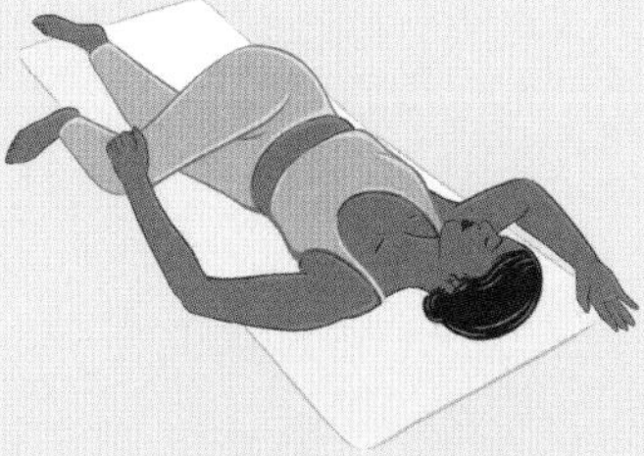

21. SUPINE TWIST

On your back, exhale as you find your supine twist and hold for 5 breaths. Repeat on the other side.

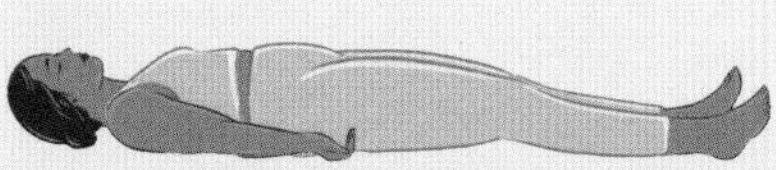

22. SAVASANA

Come back to centre and melt into savasana for 2 minutes or more.

MEDITATION

WALKING MEDITATION

This month's meditation is a moving meditation. It connects body and breath by bringing awareness to your physical sensations to anchor you in the present. We can so often walk (and breathe) on autopilot. In a walking meditation you focus the attention fully on the sensations in the soles of your feet or in the muscles and joints of your legs. Some people favour this form of meditation as it enables them to engage their bodies while meditating. It's helpful, for example, if you sit a lot for work.

This month I have talked about how life can be chaotic, just like a tornado. When thinking about this walking meditation imagine the tornado as your life and you are heading to its central eye for a sense of calm and stillness.

Directions:

1. Set a timer for 10 minutes or more.
2. The best location to practise is outdoors – a back garden, park or even a quiet pavement. Choose a place where you are safe, won't be interrupted and where you don't need to make decisions as to where you walk.
3. As you walk, bring your full focus into the present moment. Walk at a slightly slower-than-regular pace, observing the change in sensations in your feet as you walk.
4. Be mindful of all sensations: the feeling of your breath, any tension or discomfort, the effect of the movements on your mind and body; be open to them all.
5. Feel free to intentionally move your attention to any sounds, objects and smells, but the key is intention. Intentionally allow the mind to explore and observe them.

JOURNAL PROMPTS

Below I have given you eight self-reflection questions linked to this month's tornado theme and the yogic concept of *asteya*. Try answering two questions weekly alongside the daily journal prompts set out on pages 8–9.

▸ Reflect on a recent time when you felt content with what you had. What contributed to that feeling?

▸ Like a tornado, what inner strengths and qualities do you possess that allow you to navigate life's challenges with resilience and power? What could you work on?

▸ Have there been moments when you crossed someone's boundaries, knowingly or unknowingly? How can you work towards greater respect for others' space, time and possessions?

▸ Tornados can reshape landscapes. Think about someone who's changed your life for the better and why? Can you send them a random note of kindness reminding them how much they mean to you.

▸ Think about your consumption habits. How can you better strike a balance between wanting and needing?

▸ Like the eye of a tornado, consider the idea of finding your 'centre' or inner calm amid life's storms. Think of three ways you can try to cultivate inner peace and balance, even when external circumstances are chaotic?

▸ Are there instances when you've been less than honest or where your integrity was compromised? What can you learn from these experiences?

▸ A tornado can be thought of as both destructive and cleansing. Are there aspects of your life that need to be 'cleared away' to make room for renewal and growth?

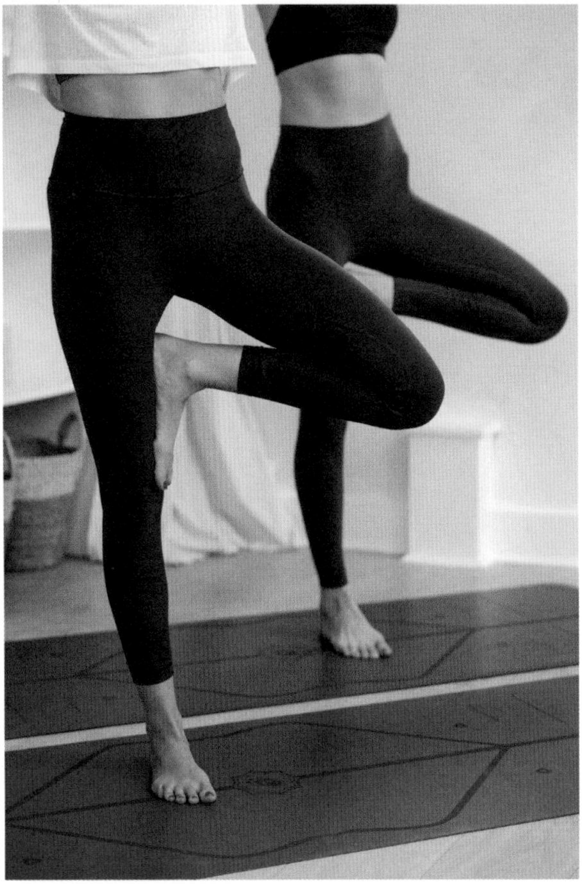
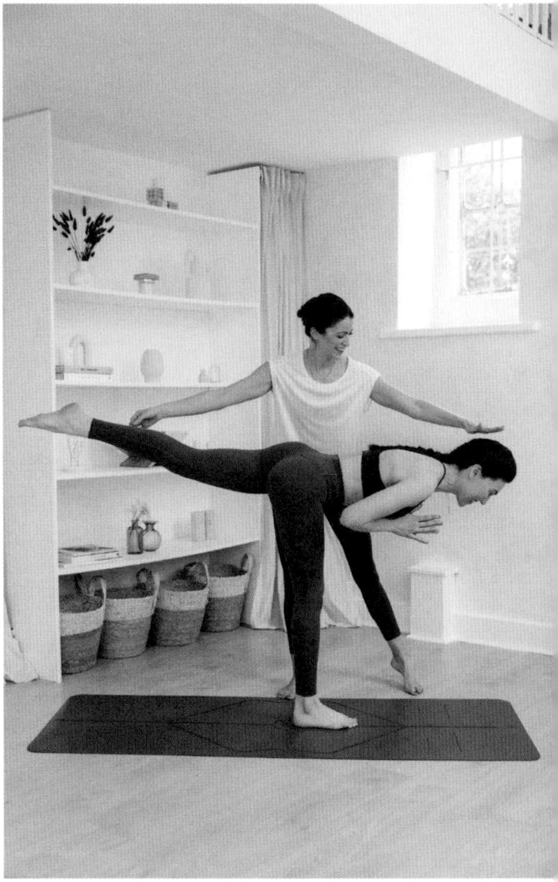
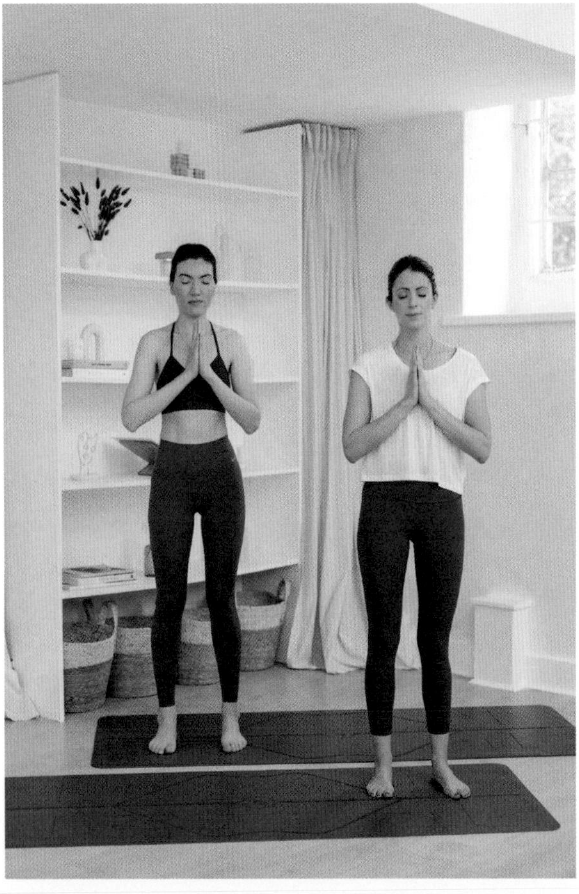
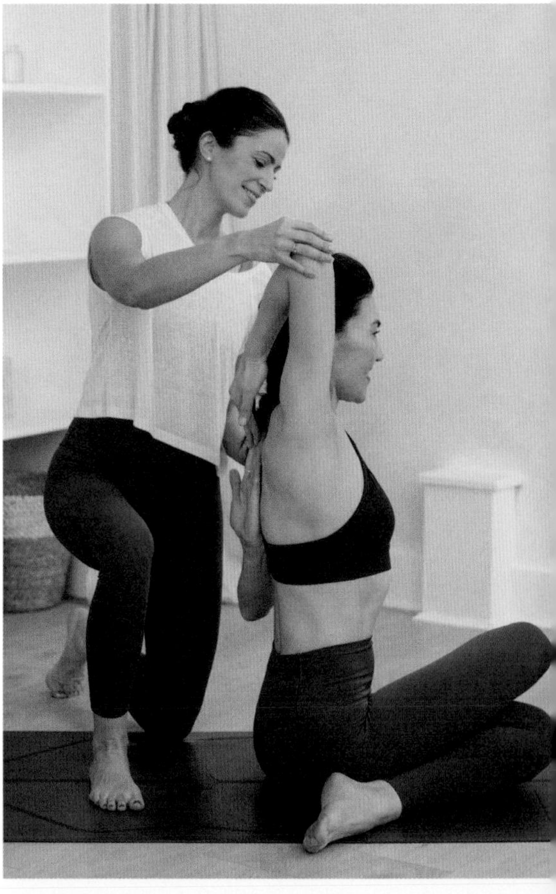

MONTH 4
TREE

'WE DO NOT INHERIT THE EARTH
FROM OUR ANCESTORS; WE
BORROW IT FROM OUR CHILDREN.'

CHIEF SEATTLE

TREE

This month we embrace the serenity and strength of the tree as we play with balance, inner stability and connection to the earth. Trees are rooted and graceful, strong and adaptable. We can be inspired by these qualities on the yoga mat, continuing our focus of strong foundations, finding grace in our transitions and being open to change or modifications.

We also delve into the yogic concept of *brahmacharya,* meaning 'moderation'. Trees remind me of this concept in the way that they conserve their energy during seasons when resources are limited, by reducing their growth or casting off leaves. This mirrors the focus on *brahmacharya* and on channelling our energy more efficiently, recognising where we may be expending energy where it isn't needed and identifying where it may be better directed.

The signature flow this month does of course include the iconic tree pose, as well as a number of other balancing poses and trickier transitions. As always, if these feel challenging it's because they are. Please be kind to yourself, modify and know that in time your practice will become easier.

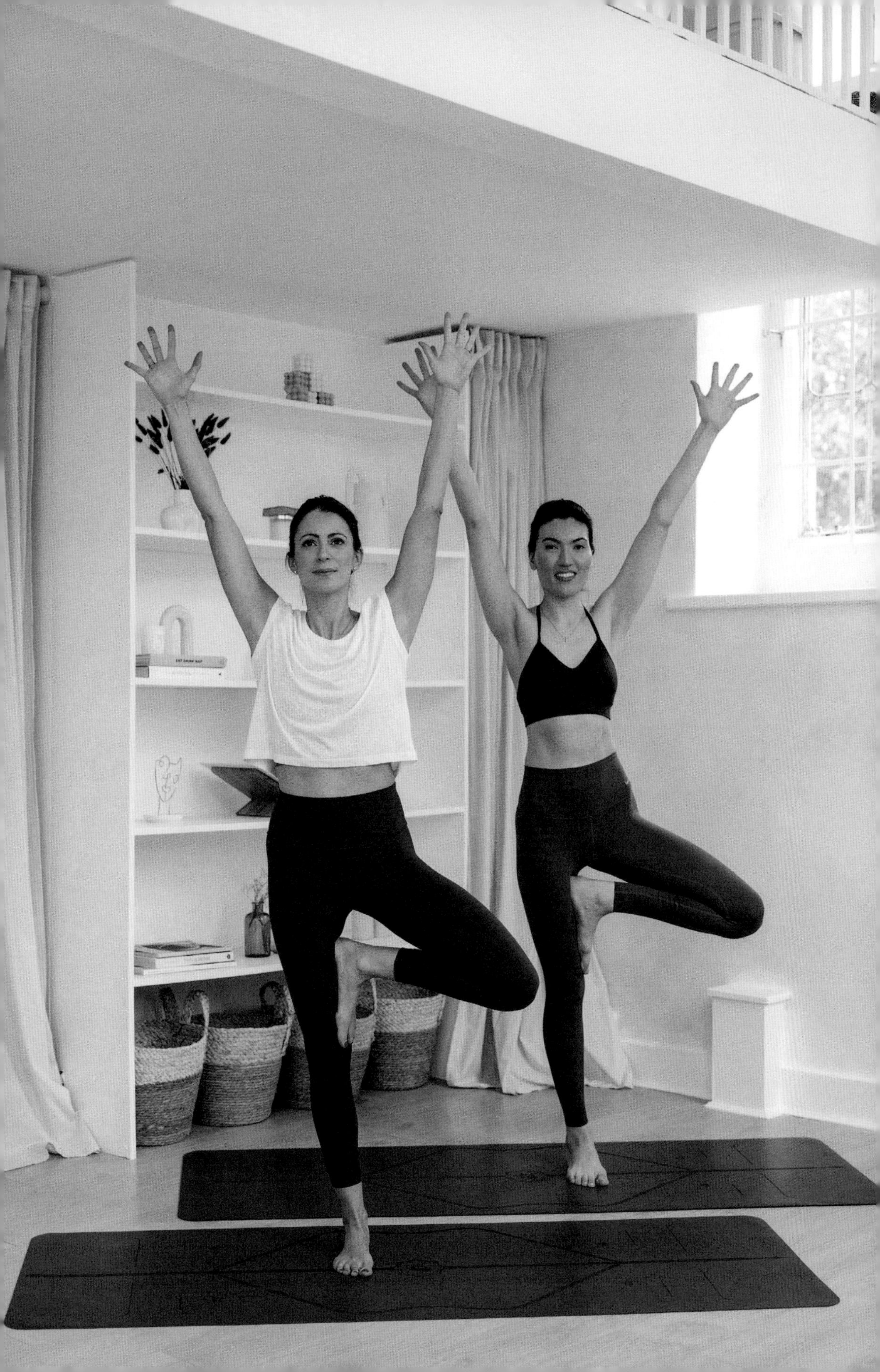

EFFORT AND EASE

Sutra 3.46 of Patañjali's *Yoga Sutras* states: *'sthira-sukham asanam'*, which roughly translates as: 'postures should be stable and comfortable' and another translation is 'finding the balance between effort and ease'.

Sthira, steadiness, encourages us to establish a stable foundation in our practice, just as a tree firmly roots itself into the earth. A tree stands tall and unwavering, whatever the external conditions, and in the same way *sthira* asks us to maintain unwavering presence both on the yoga mat and in our daily lives when we are faced with challenges or distractions.

Sukha, ease or comfort, can be thought of as graceful adaptation or a happy/pleasant state of mind. Despite their strength, trees also need the flexibility and ease to sway with the wind and adapt to the changing seasons. Similarly, yoga invites us to bring a sense of fluidity and graceful adaption into the practice as opposed to simply force and tension.

Draw inspiration from the concept of *sthira-sukha* on and off the mat. It will help you to work towards a balanced and sustainable yoga practice and life, which will ultimately foster a deeper sense of well-being and mindfulness.

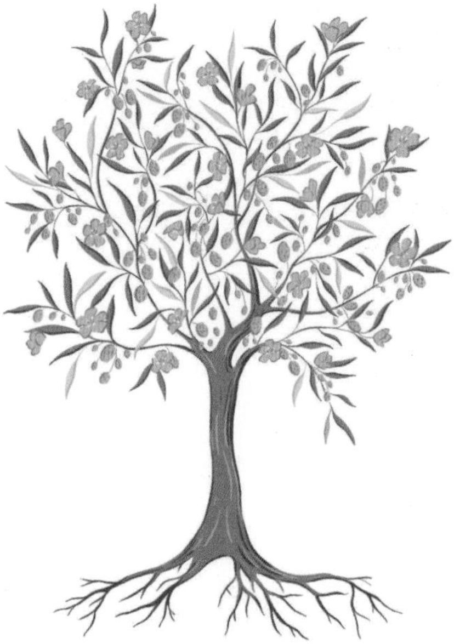

BRAHMACHARYA (MODERATION)

I AIM TO CHANNEL MY VITAL ENERGY MINDFULLY AND APPROPRIATELY.

Brahmacharya is the fourth of the *yamas* and the traditional translation is celibacy – striving for non-excess in our sexual desires and passions. *Brahmacharya* can also be thought of as the 'right use of energy' and finding moderation and balance in life.

Although energy can be renewed, it isn't infinite. *Brahmacharya* reminds us to make sure we are not pushing ourselves too much (or perhaps too little). We have become a society prone to excess, whether that is through exercise or food, bingeing TV box sets or overworking; the list goes on. *Brahmacharya* is linked to the yogic concept of *santosha*, or contentment (see page 114), as when you are content there is no need for excess.

Mindfulness is a key practice in maintaining *brahmacharya* as it can help us go into each action with consciousness and an intention of balance (not indulgence). The mindfulness exercise for this month (see page 79) will help you tune in to how an action you are taking (eating that second chocolate bar, for example) really makes you feel and whether it's actually what you need in that moment.

So how can we incorporate *brahmacharya* into our daily lives:

▸ **On the yoga mat:** Every time you step onto your mat, use your breath to guide your movement. It will help you realise when you are overexerting yourself and when you can channel more energy into the movements. Practise *asana* with a sense of moderation and self-awareness by listening to your body and finding the balance between effort and ease in each pose.

▸ **Know what's enough:** Be mindful of what you're eating, how much you're working and how much time you spend connected to technology. Can you find balance and pinpoint what level is enough before you reach excess?

▸ **Balance in relationships:** Can you promote healthy boundaries, mutual respect and practise mindful and compassionate communication. Think about how you spend quality time in your relationships – could you be more present?

▸ **Energy conservation:** Are you practising self-care and do you need to slow down? Life is sacred and so often we move quickly from one thing to the next not taking enough time to pause and appreciate life. Rest and self-care are necessary, not selfish.

▸ **Find your creativity:** Directing energy away from excessive distractions means you'll have more to plug into creative pursuits at work and in your hobbies.

▸ **Eyes of a child:** Have you ever been with a child who sees something that is seemingly normal for us for the first time and they find it absolutely magical? Notice the beauty in everyday life that we often overlook.

THE BREATH

THE SAMA VRITTI BREATH

Sama vritti, or equal ratio breathing, is a simple yet highly effective breathing technique you can practise anywhere. *Sama* means 'equal' and *vritti* means 'fluctuations', so, with *sama vritti* we create a breathing pattern whereby the inhalation and exhalation are equal in duration as well as intensity. It's an excellent technique to calm the mind and bring our nervous system back into balance. The rhythmic breathing pattern can also improve focus and concentration and enhance respiratory function.

Sama vritti reminds me of the grounded nature of trees as it helps to provide a stable foundation for the body and mind and foster a sense of inner stability and grounding.

Directions:

1. Come into a comfortable seated position, growing tall through the crown of the head and allowing the spine to be neutral and long.
2. Take a few breaths, tuning in and observing the body and mind.
3. Inhale softly and slowly through the nose for a count of 4 and exhale softly and slowly through the nose for a count of 4.
4. You can increase or decrease the length of the inhale and exhale to suit you as long as they are equal.
5. Repeat for 10–12 rounds or more.

THE TREE FLOW

This month's signature flow will help you to cultivate balance, strength and mindfulness. Think about the concept of *brahmacharya* throughout the flow:

▸ Use the rests in child's pose to reflect on the importance of these moments in helping us to find balance in our practice.

▸ Work on the transition between warrior II and half moon, making it as fluid and graceful as you can. Can you strive to lift into half moon with minimal momentum and land a warrior II so softly you can't hear the step?

▸ As you flow, can you make mindful tweaks to postures using your breath as a guide to help you balance effort and ease?

Aim to practise this flow three or four times per week and if you have more time you can include the seated warm-up flow on page 10 at the start, combine it with the previous months' flows or repeat the flow multiple times.

As you move around your mat, bring some tree-like qualities with you:

▸ **Stability:** Trees are deeply rooted and stable. In the standing and balance postures, press your feet / foot firmly into the mat as you grow tall through the crown of your head. This will help you to automatically connect with your core and stability muscles.

▸ **Patience:** Trees grow slowly. Patience in our practice is important. Balancing postures can be challenging, so modify as needed, avoid rushing and allow your body to adapt over time.

▸ **Connection to nature:** Can you practise outside at least once this month? Practising yoga outdoors, near trees, can deepen your connection to nature and enhance your sense of well-being.

PLEASE NOTE

The appendix on page 190 includes a detailed breakdown of each pose, plus variations and modifications. Remember to listen to your body; yoga should never be painful and you can chose to skip any pose that doesn't feel right for you.

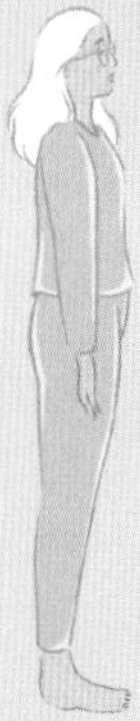

1. STANDING SAMA VRITTI

Standing in mountain pose, take 10 rounds of *sama vritti* (see page 74).

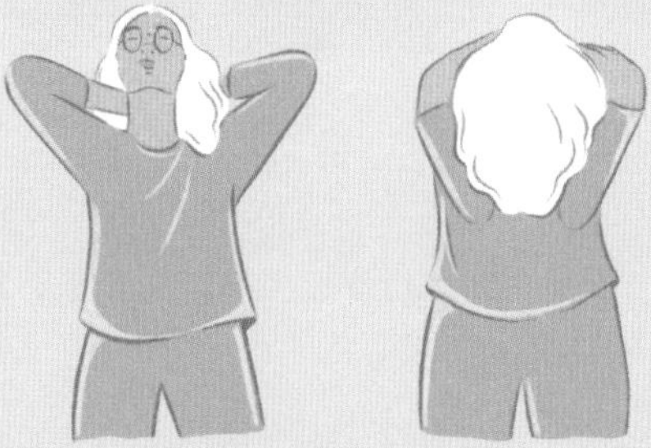

2. STANDING HEART OPENER

Inhale opening the heart and exhale rounding the back. Repeat 5 times.

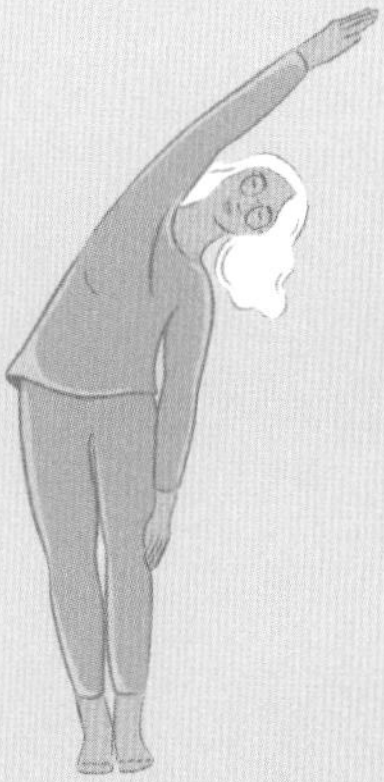

3. STANDING SIDE STRETCH

Inhale lifting the right fingers to the sky and exhale take a side bend to the left. Repeat on the opposite side, then repeat 3 times each side.

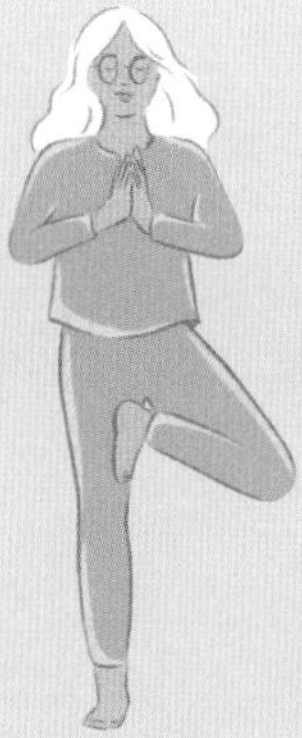

4. TREE

Inhale lifting the left leg and bringing the foot to the inside of the right ankle, shin or thigh. Hold for 5 breaths.

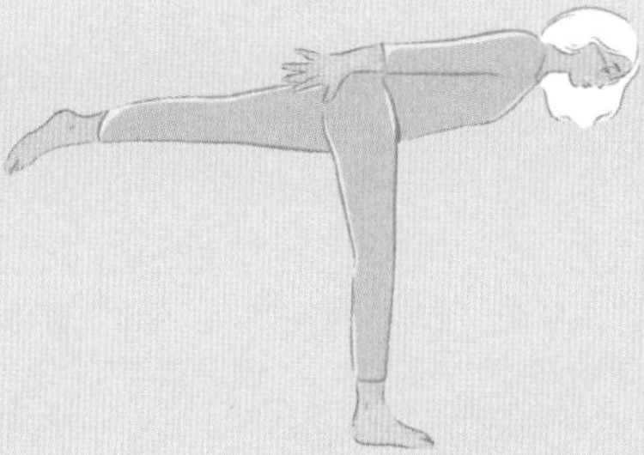

5. WARRIOR III

Exhale as you send the left leg back behind you to warrior III. Hold for 5 breaths.

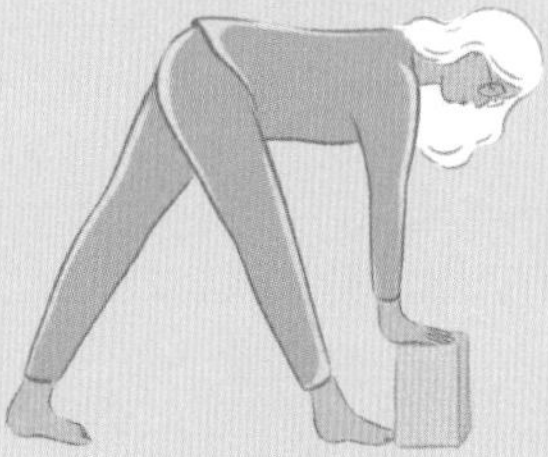

6. PYRAMID

Exhale releasing the left foot to the floor and folding into pyramid pose. Hold for 5 breaths.

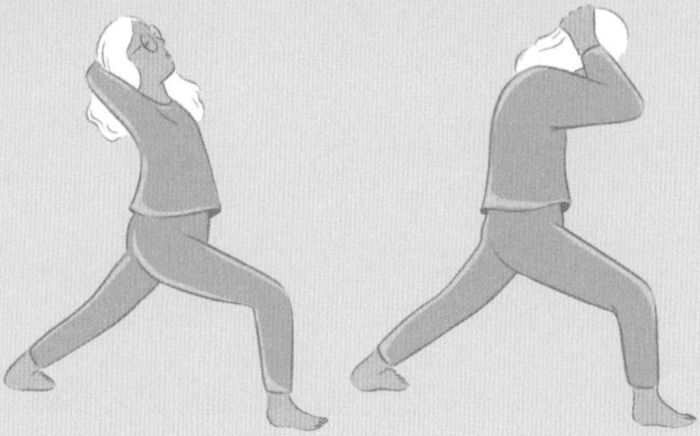

7. HIGH LUNGE HEART OPENER

From high lunge, inhale opening the heart and exhale rounding in. Repeat 3 times.

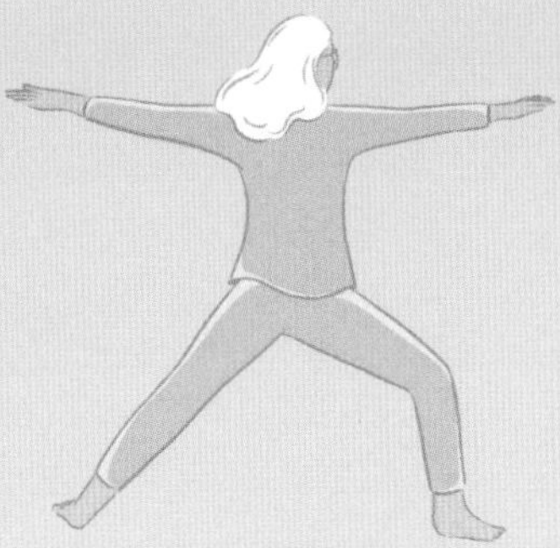

8. WARRIOR II

Exhale opening into warrior II. Hold for a full breath.

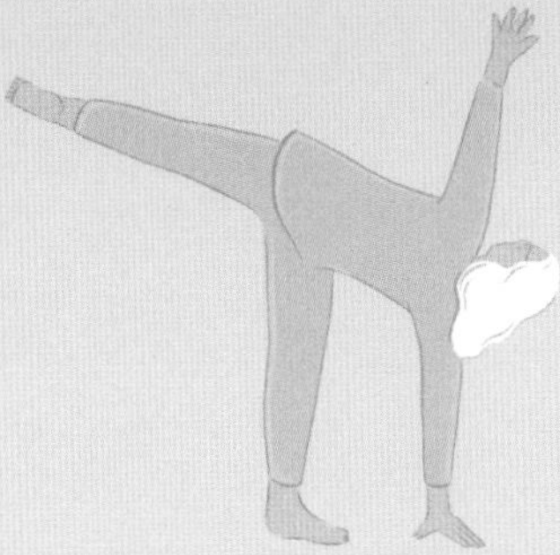

9. HALF MOON

Inhale reaching the torso forward, exhale and lift into half moon pose. Hold for a full breath.

REPEAT 3 TIMES

STEPS 8 AND 9

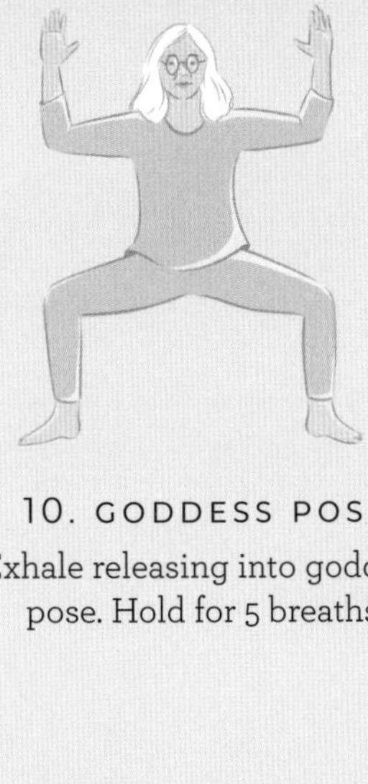

10. GODDESS POSE

Exhale releasing into goddess pose. Hold for 5 breaths.

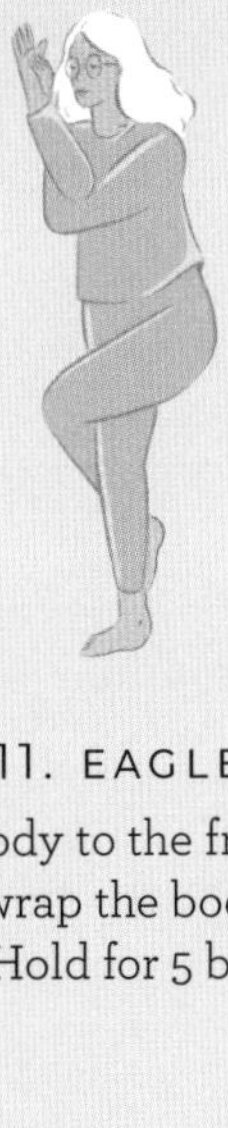

11. EAGLE

Turning the body to the front of the mat, exhale and wrap the body into eagle pose. Hold for 5 breaths.

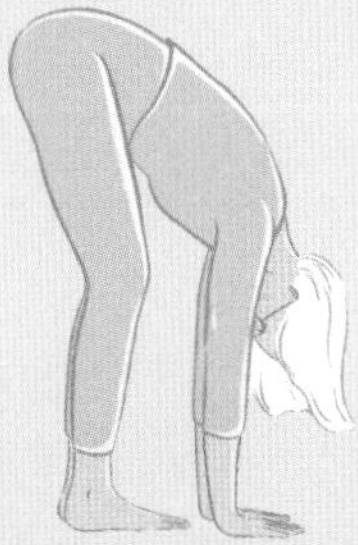

12. STANDING FORWARD BEND

Inhale to unravel, exhale and fold the body down into a standing forward bend. Hold for 5 breaths.

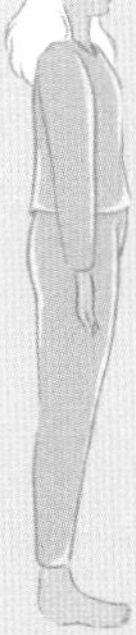

13. MOUNTAIN

Grounding down through the feet, inhale into mountain pose.

REPEAT ON THE OTHER SIDE

STEPS 4–13

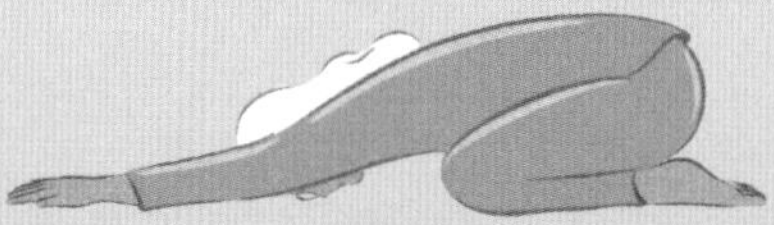

14. CHILD'S POSE

Release the hands to the floor and step back, melting down into child's pose for 5 breaths.

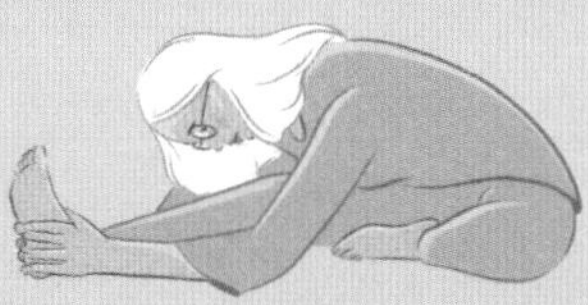

15. HEAD-TO-KNEE FORWARD FOLD

Inhale into a seated position, releasing the right leg long and exhale fold forward. Hold for 5 breaths.

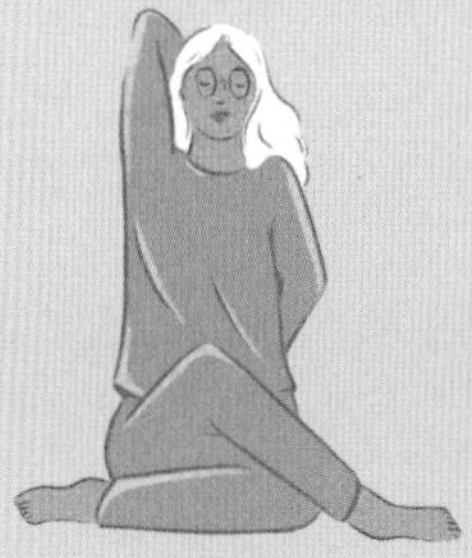

16. COW FACE

Stack and cross the right leg over the left finding cow face pose. Hold for 5 breaths.

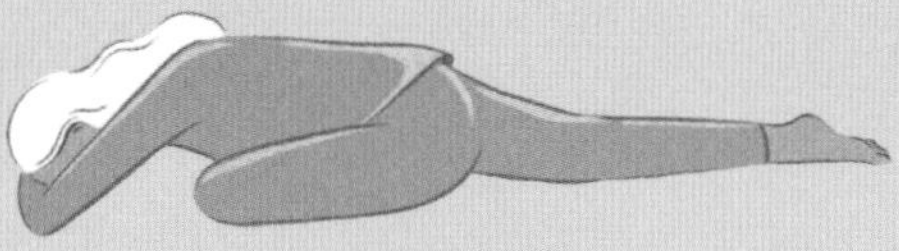

17. PIGEON

Release the right leg and send it back behind you into pigeon pose. Hold for 5 breaths.

REPEAT ON THE LEFT SIDE

STEPS 15–17

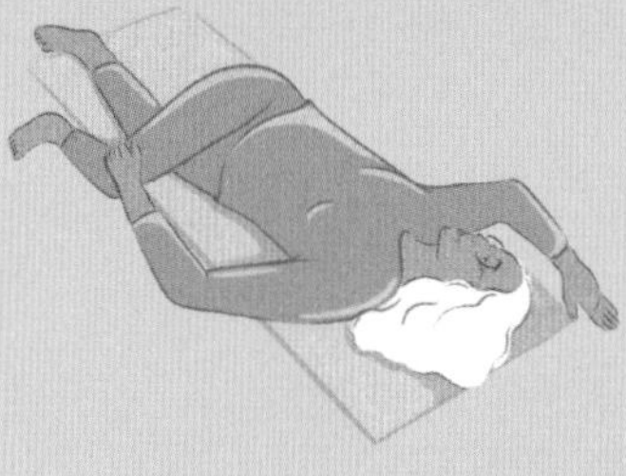

18. SUPINE TWIST

Coming onto your back, hug the right knee in and come into a supine twist. Hold for 5 breaths before repeating on the opposite side.

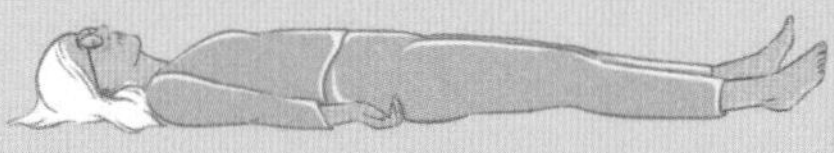

19. SAVASANA

Release and melt into savasana for 2 minutes or more.

MINDFULNESS

QUIT THE AUTOPILOT

How often do you find yourself switching onto autopilot for parts of your day. Doing a task without even noticing what you're doing, whether it's during your journey to work, when eating your dinner or even washing your hair? Bringing mindfulness into everyday tasks can enhance your quality of life and benefit your mental, emotional and physical well-being (see page 7).

We might think a mindfulness practice should be easy, but paying attention can be surprisingly tough. Our minds want to run off to future worries or thoughts of the past. I find it helpful to remember that part of mindfulness is recognising when the mind has wandered and then gently bringing it back without judgement, just compassion. Over time, mindfulness can help us become calmer, more productive and creative.

This month's task is in fact more of a challenge. I want you to grab a pen and paper and write down as many daily tasks you can think of in which you switch to autopilot. Each day can you be mindful during one of these tasks? Carry out each element of the task slowly, paying full attention to what you're doing. Notice how this makes you feel.

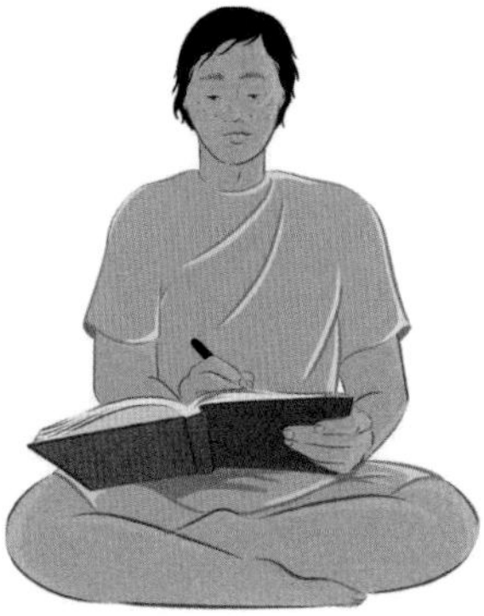

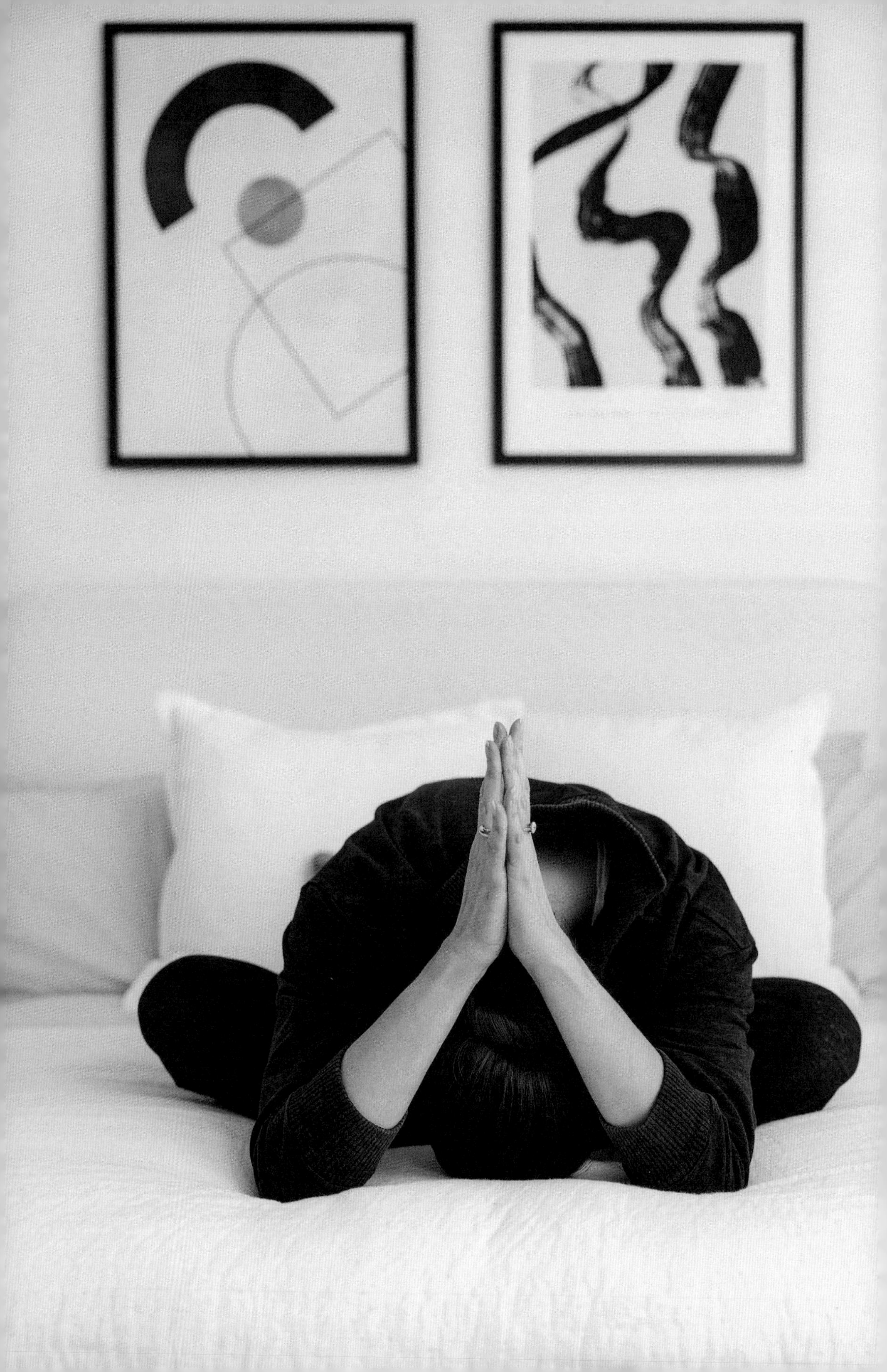

JOURNAL PROMPTS

Below I have given you eight self-reflection questions linked to this month's tree theme and the yogic concept of *brahmacharya*. Try answering two questions weekly alongside the daily journal prompts set out on pages 8–9.

▸ Trees adapt to the changing seasons. Think about how you adapt to changes in your life and what lessons you can draw from the resilience of trees.

▸ Think about ways you overindulge. Where could you benefit from increased moderation and self-control?

▸ Trees provide shelter and support for many creatures. Reflect on the people in your life who offer you support and a sense of belonging. How can you nurture these relationships?

▸ Consider your use of technology and social media. How can you practise moderation and be more mindful in your usage to avoid excessive distractions and wasted time?

▸ Trees often symbolise strength and resilience. Reflect on a challenging experience in your life (big or small) and how you were able to draw on your inner strength to navigate it.

▸ Are there any patterns of excessive attachment or dependency in your relationships? How can you maintain healthier boundaries?

▸ Just like how nature is interconnected, think about how you are you connected to the world around you. How can you deepen your sense of connection to others and the environment?

▸ Reflect on the balance in your life. Are you neglecting other important aspects of your life by spending too much focus on work or something similar? How can you find a healthier balance?

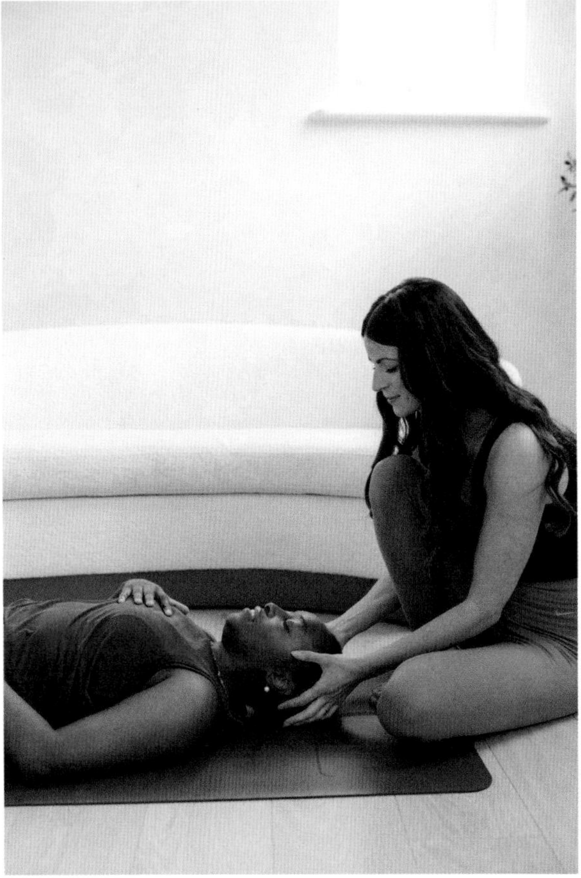
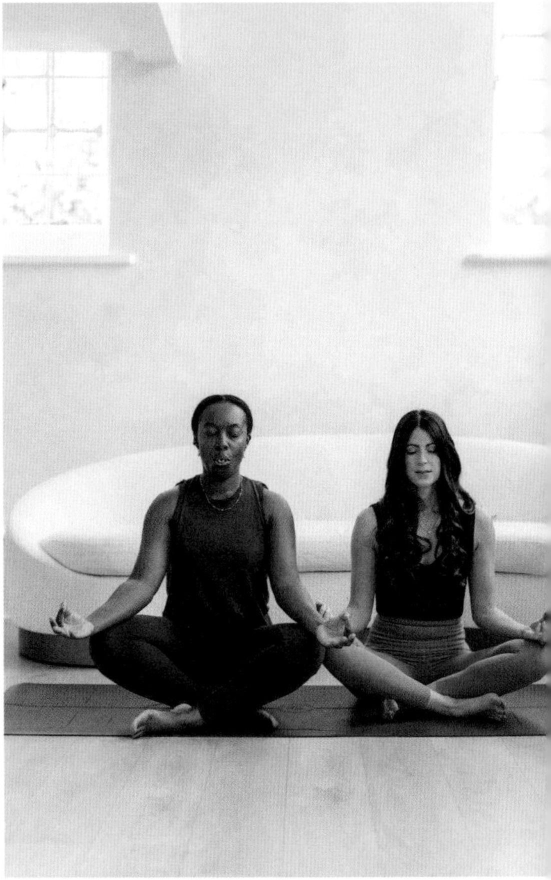
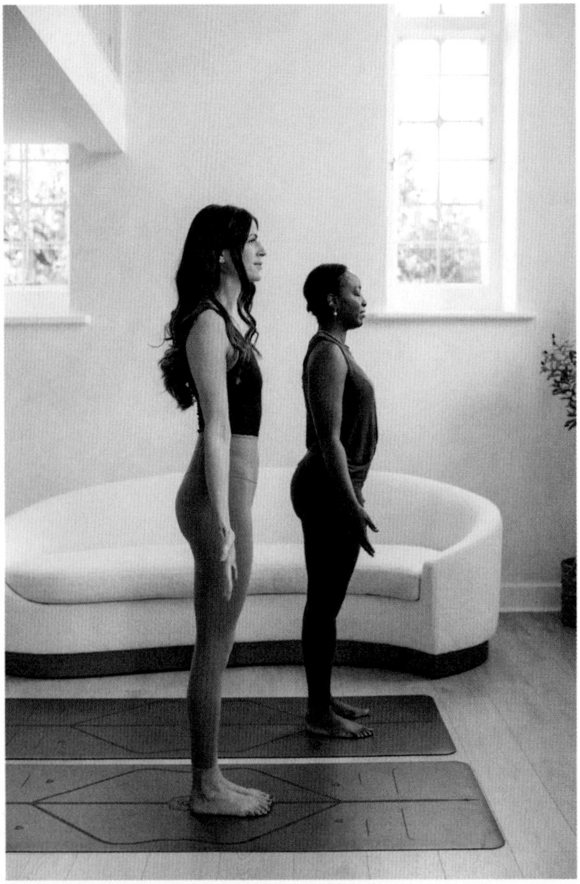
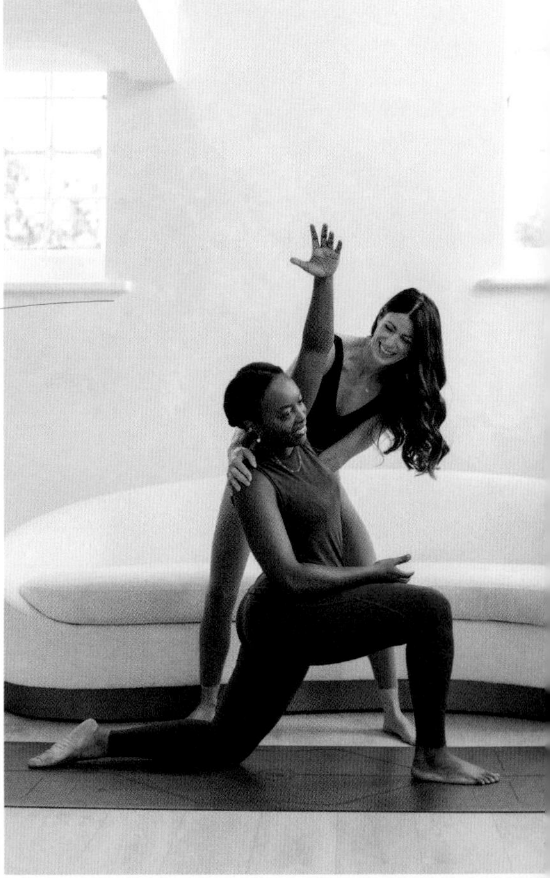

MONTH 5
SQUIRREL

'THERE'S ENOUGH ON THIS PLANET
FOR EVERYONE'S NEEDS BUT NOT
FOR EVERYONE'S GREED.'

MAHATMA GANDHI

SQUIRREL

It may sound a little strange having a month themed around small, furry acrobats, but let me explain. This month we explore the last of the *yamas*, *aparigraha*, which is often interpreted as the practice of non-attachment and non-greed. Greed weighs us down, makes us heavy and doesn't necessarily equate to happiness. Although squirrels may appear greedy to humans, their behaviour of collecting and storing nuts is driven by survival instinct and their place in the ecosystem rather than greed. They don't hoard excessive amounts and they have also been known to share, so in my eyes they embody the idea of *aparigraha*.

In this month's signature flow, we are working towards camel pose (*ustrasana*). This is a more advanced heart-opening posture which has lots of modifications to make it work for all bodies. We can explore the theme of non-attachment by paying attention to the sensations within this pose rather than what we think it should look like. Camel pose also takes a degree of surrender and trust as you lean back and open your heart.

We are now a third of the way through the year and you are still going, which is *amazing*. Be proud of your hard work and dedication. Even if you've fallen off the wagon at times, that's okay. Keep up your practice, keep exploring your body, try not to compare yourself to others and remember that you can substitute this month's flow with any from the previous months when you would like to.

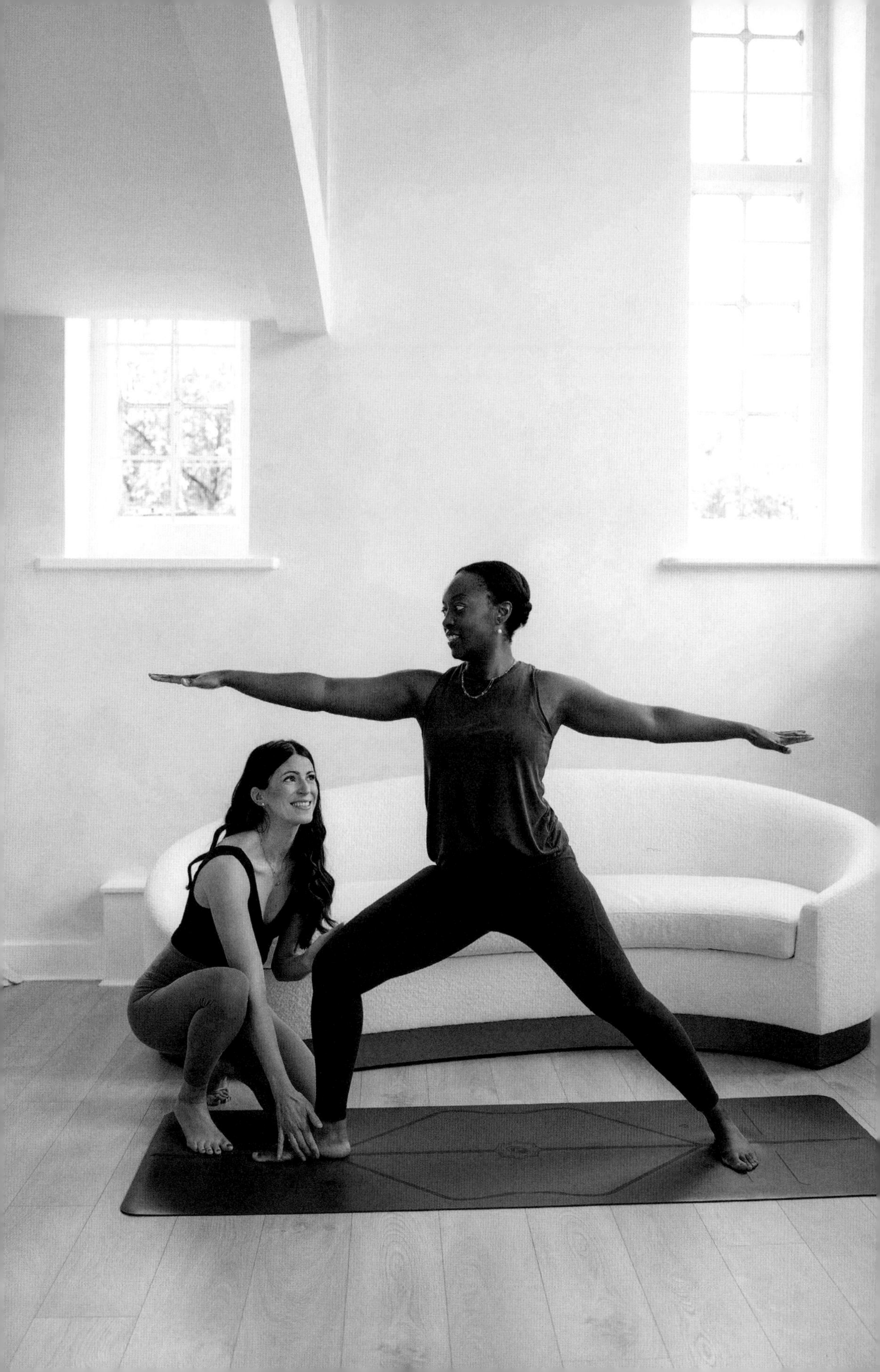

APARIGRAHA (NON-ATTACHMENT)

EMBRACE THE FREEDOM IN LETTING GO.

We need to remember that nothing stays the same. Life is constantly moving and changing and therefore attaching oneself to how things are at present is going to end in suffering. But change isn't the reason for the suffering, it's the attachment. By letting go of attachment, we can find freedom. This concept of non-attachment or letting go is our fifth *yama: aparigraha.*

When thinking of *aparigraha* and letting go I often use the example of clutter in the home, such as a wardrobe full to bursting with clothes (some may even still have their price tags). You find yourself shopping for more, even though you have plenty. This habit of constantly wanting more can of course lead to clutter but also financial issues and dissatisfaction. We need to let go of the want for more and find contentment in what we have (leading us back to the concept of *santosha;* see page 114).

If we relate this to this month's squirrel theme, a squirrel's instinctive behaviour of non-greed reflects the wisdom of letting go of excess. Squirrels remind us that although life's offerings are abundant, it is possible to maintain balance and contentment without succumbing to greed or materialistic desires.

So how can we incorporate *aparigraha* into our daily lives:

▸ **On the yoga mat:** Let go of ego. *Aparigraha* encourages us to leave our ego at the door and accept where we are in our practice today, without thinking about what yesterday or last week looked like. Find contentment in your current capabilities and you will find freedom in your practice. For more about letting go of the ego, see opposite.

▸ **Declutter regularly:** Room by room, set aside time to declutter your living spaces. What are you holding on to that you haven't used in the past year. Can you give that object a home where it'll be loved and used? Ask yourself, how much stuff do I need? Keeping your home uncluttered creates a sense of spaciousness that can reduce attachment to material possessions.

▸ **Do you really need this?:** Can you be mindful in the way you consume and ask yourself if you genuinely need that new purchase. Think long-term when you buy something and also consider where it's come from and what's it made from to assess how its journey may have affected others or the natural world.

▸ **Create memories:** Shift your focus from accumulating possessions to creating memorable experiences. What hobbies, activities or places bring you joy and nurture your personal growth?

▸ **Forgive:** There's a quote from Buddha that states: *'Holding on to anger is like grasping a hot coal with the intent of throwing it at someone else; you are the one who gets burned.'* Embrace non-attachment in your relationships by letting go of resentments, freeing the mind and practising forgiveness.

▸ **Digital detox:** *Aparigraha* sits alongside *brahmacharya,* or moderation (see page 73) and encourages non-greed and moderation in consumption. Practise non-attachment by regularly taking breaks from your digital devices, which may have become a source of attachment and clutter in your life. This may also help you realise how attached you are to them and how much time you can waste using them.

LETTING GO OF EGO

The concept of ego is often referred to in yoga because it plays such a vital role in how students approach their practice and interact with the world around them.

The ego believes that our identity is our body, mind, thoughts and feelings. It's driven by many things, including fear, insecurity, competition and the need for recognition, success and achievement. The ego craves validation and approval and often relies on external sources to affirm its self-worth. It feeds on 'more, more, more'.

One way ego can manifest itself in students is as competitiveness: they strive to perform poses 'perfectly', pushing the body into positions it isn't ready for or comparing its ability to that of other yogis. This competitive mindset can lead to frustration, even injury, and misses the purpose of yoga.

To progress in our yoga practice, we need to overcome the grip of the ego. Identifying the nature of the 'I, me, my, mine' type of thought and discerning what is necessary (protection and boundaries) and what is driven by desire, want and aversion.

The ego can often be viewed as an obstacle to fulfilling our potential because it can hinder our personal growth and instil a fear of failure and/or comparison, stopping us trying new things and stepping out of our comfort zone. It is also resistant to change, preferring familiarity.

Here are four things you can work on to help tame the ego from your yoga practice (and life):

1. Practise mindfulness and self-awareness on the yoga mat. You can do this through observing your thoughts, emotions and physical sensations without judgement as you practise. Embody the concept of *satya* (truthfulness) and be honest with yourself about how things really feel and what you are or aren't ready for.
2. Set intentions and keep the long-term goal clear in your mind. Why are you practising yoga and what do you really want to get out of your practice?
3. Let go of attachments to outcomes. Enjoy the process and everything it teaches you.
4. Embrace imperfection because no one is perfect, perfection doesn't exist. Allow yourself to make mistakes and to learn from them. Fail without judgement.

As well as the above, all the practices in this book, such as meditation and self-study, are aimed at transcending the ego. They aim to help you dissolve a false sense of self.

THE BREATH

THE SITALI AND SITKARI BREATH

While squirrels may pant or seek out cool surfaces to dissipate heat from their bodies, we can call on the breathing technique for this month to achieve the same thing. *Sitali* and *sitkari* are breathing techniques that can cool the body, have a calming effect on the mind and reduce frustration. They are especially beneficial in hot weather.

Refrain from practising *sitali* and *sitkari* when you are ill as these techniques lose all the benefits of nasal breathing (like filtering of air, warming and humidifying, which all help to prevent further irritation and infection). And if you are unable to roll your tongue then *sitkari* is used in place of *sitali*.

Directions:

1. Come into a comfortable seated position, growing tall through the crown of the head and allowing the spine to be neutral and long.
2. Take a few breaths, to find stillness and observe the body and mind.
3. For *sitali*, roll the tongue and stick it out of the mouth like a straw. Inhale through the tongue, briefly hold the breath as you put the tongue back into the month and close the lips. For *sitkari*, press the teeth together and the tongue against the back of teeth. Inhale and slowly draw the inhale through the teeth and over the tongue.
4. Exhale through the nose.
5. Repeat for 10 rounds.

THE SQUIRREL FLOW

This month's signature flow will help you open your heart and build up to a new more advanced posture, camel pose (*ustrasana*). Embrace *aparigraha* by letting go of what poses should look like and focusing on how they feel. Have all your props to hand and remember the appendix sets out a number of modifications to help the pose feel right for you (see page 190).

Use child's pose to encourage the theme of letting go between the more dynamic poses. Release the core and breathe into the belly and ribs to help surrender, and reflect on how the flow is feeling for you and your body. Practise mindfulness using the breath and body to help you stay present and avoid clinging to expectations or judgment.

Aim to practise this flow three or four times per week and if you have more time, you can include the seated warm-up flow on page 10 at the start, combine it with the previous months' flows or repeat the flow multiple times.

As you move around your yoga mat, bring some squirrel-like qualities with you:

▸ **Adaptability:** Squirrels adapt to various environments and the changing seasons, much like yoga invites us to adapt to the ever-changing circumstances of life. Tune in to how you are feeling each time you step onto your mat, and this will help you determine what you need in your practice to find balance.

▸ **Fearlessness:** Have you ever seen a squirrel jump from one branch to another? They are bold, graceful and seem to have little fear. When we are faced with a new challenging pose it can feel intimidating. Can you approach the new poses this month with some squirrel grace and fearlessness, bringing curiosity and a knowledge that you can adjust each posture to make it right for you.

▸ **Playfulness:** Squirrels are often seen engaging in playful activities. Infuse the quality of playfulness in your practice, approaching each pose and transition with a sense of curiosity and play.

PLEASE NOTE
The appendix on page 190 includes a detailed breakdown of each pose, plus variations and modifications. Remember to listen to your body; yoga should never be painful and you can chose to skip any pose that doesn't feel right for you.

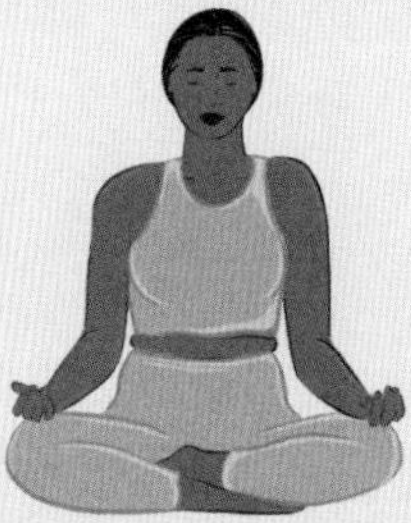

1. SEATED THREE-PART BREATH OR SITALI/SITKARI

In a seated position, take 10 rounds of the three-part breath (see page 31) or *sitali/sitkari* (see page 88).

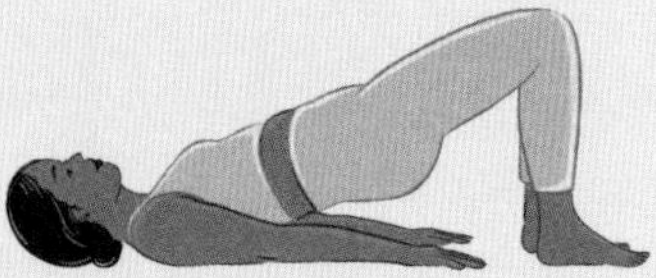

2. BRIDGE

Releasing onto the floor, exhale lifting up into bridge and hold for 5 breaths.

BEGIN WRIST SEQUENCE

See page 221.

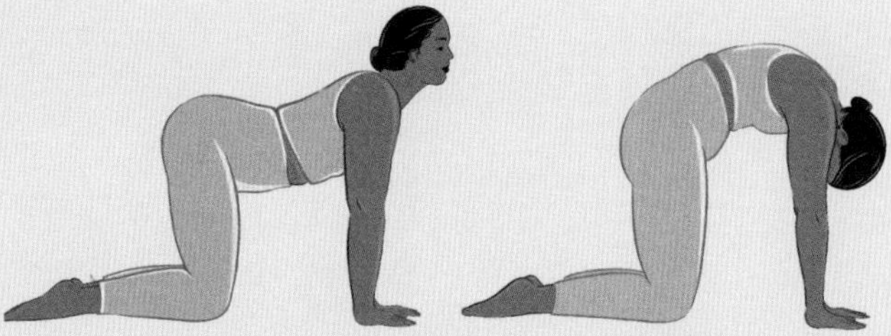

3. CAT AND COW

Inhale into cow pose and exhale into cat pose. Repeat 5 times.

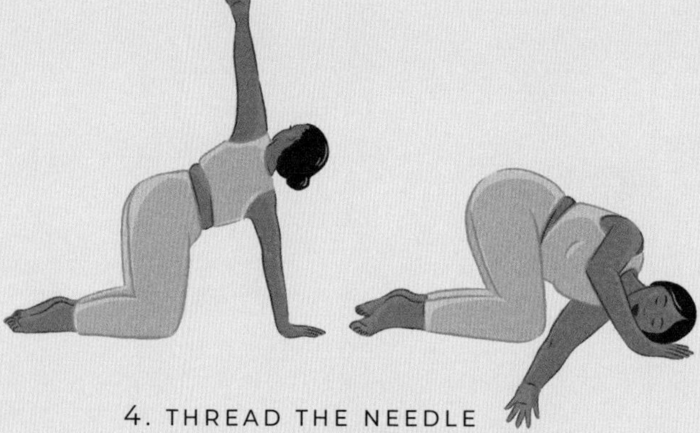

4. THREAD THE NEEDLE

Inhale reaching the left fingertips to the sky and exhale threading the arms underneath the body. Repeat 5 times on each side.

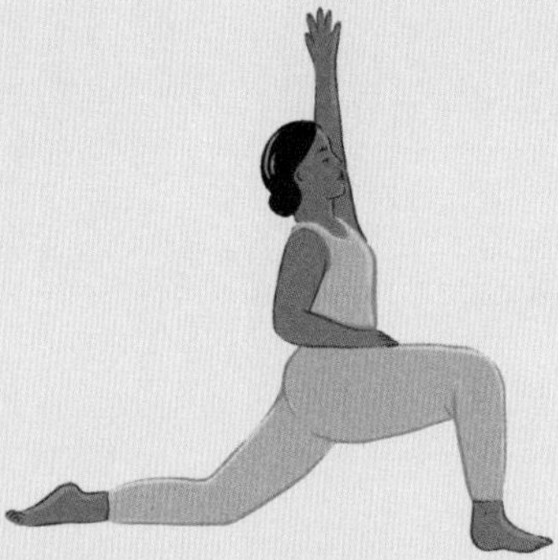

5. LOW LUNGE SIDE STRETCH

Step the right foot forward, inhale taking the left fingers to the sky and exhale taking a side stretch to the right. Hold for 5 breaths.

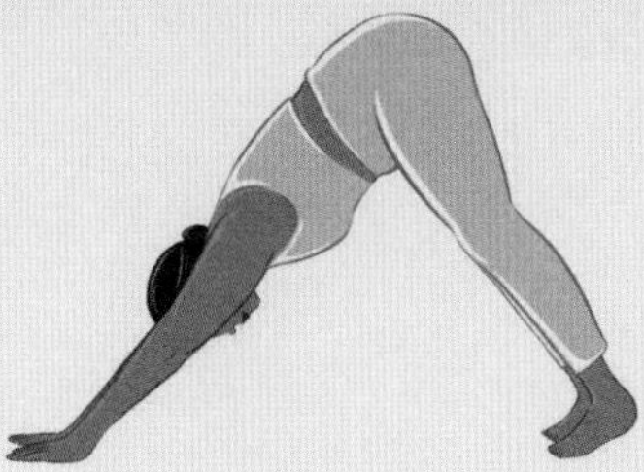

6. DOWNWARD-FACING DOG

Frame the front foot and step back to downward-facing dog. Hold for 5 breaths.

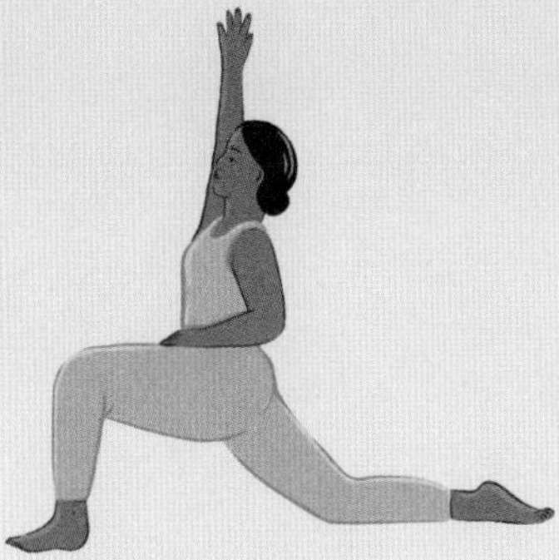

7. LOW LUNGE SIDE STRETCH

Step the left foot forward, inhale the right fingers to the sky and exhale taking a side stretch to the left. Hold for 5 breaths.

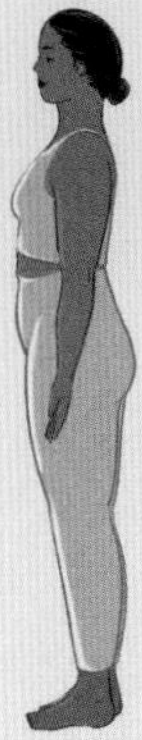

8. MOUNTAIN

Step the right foot forward and inhale to rise to mountain pose. Hold for 2 breaths.

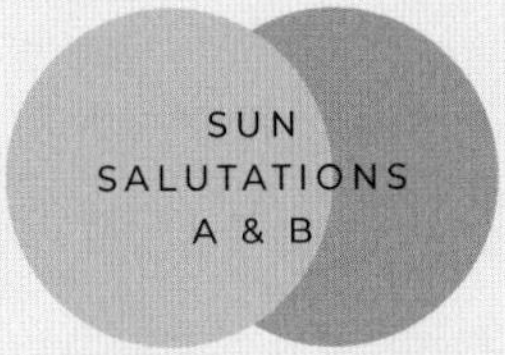

Option to include sun salutations A and B (see pages 16–20).

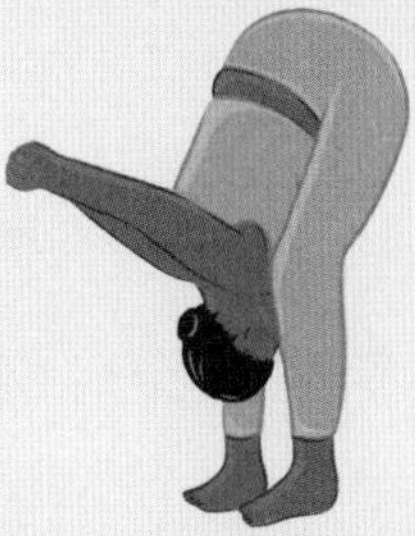

9. STANDING FORWARD BEND WITH LOCK

Exhale and fold the body down into a standing forward bend interlacing the hands behind the back. Hold for 5 breaths.

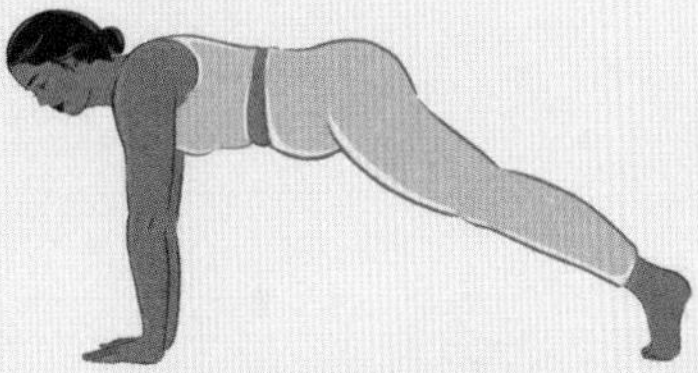

10. PLANK

Plant the hands and step back to plank. Hold for 3 breaths.

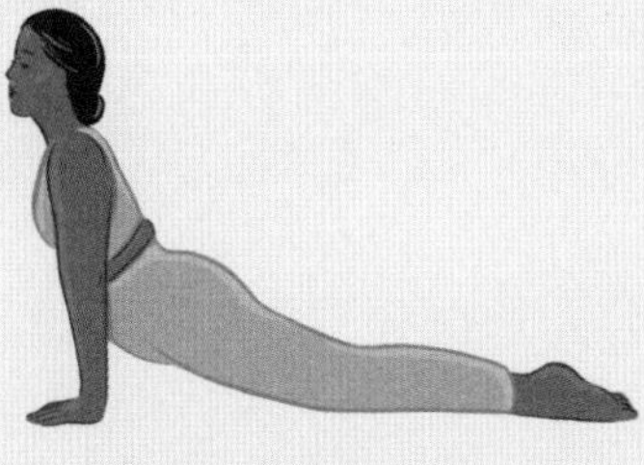

11. UPWARD-FACING DOG

Exhale through yoga push-up, inhaling into upward-facing dog or cobra. Hold for 3 breaths.

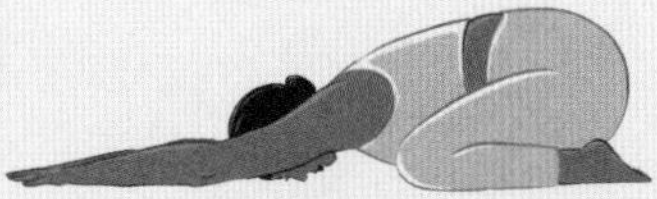

12. CHILD'S POSE

Exhale dropping the knees and sitting the hips to the heels. Hold for 5 breaths.

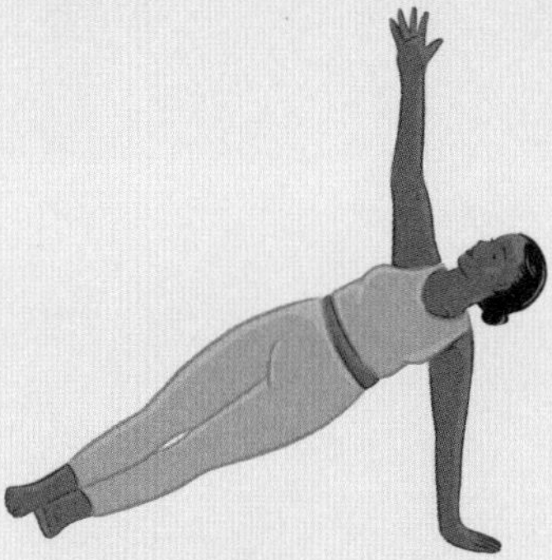

13. SIDE PLANK

Inhale to plank and exhale lifting the right fingertips to the sky finding side plank. Hold for 3–5 breaths.

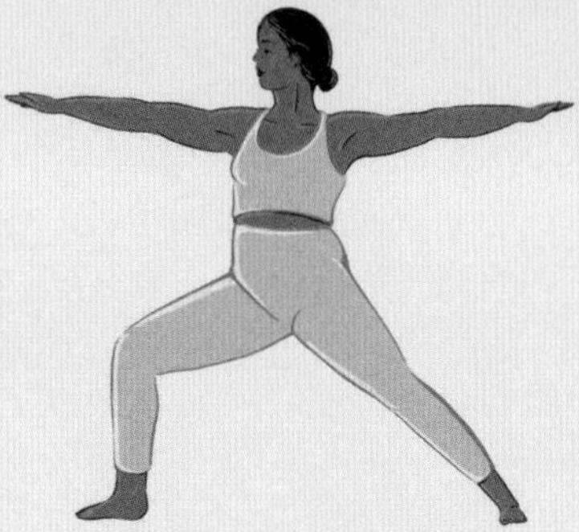

14. WARRIOR II

Step the right foot forward and windmill up into warrior II. Hold for 5 breaths.

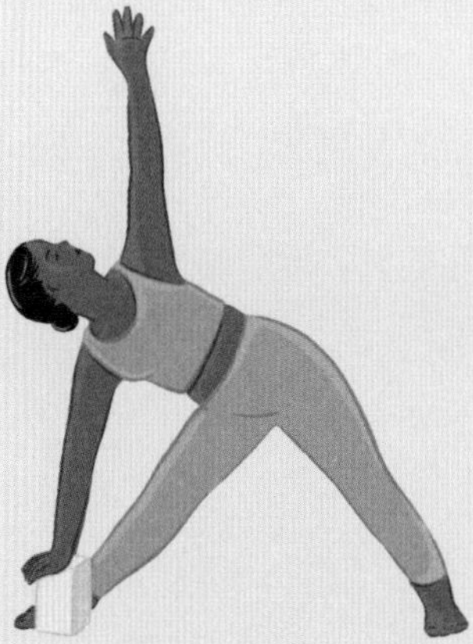

15. TRIANGLE

Straighten the front leg, inhale reaching forward and exhale opening up into triangle pose. Hold for 5 breaths.

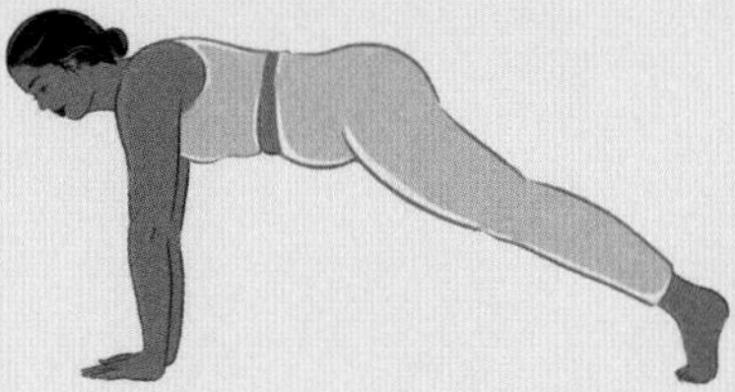

16. PLANK

Windmill the hands to the floor and step back to plank. Hold for a full breath.

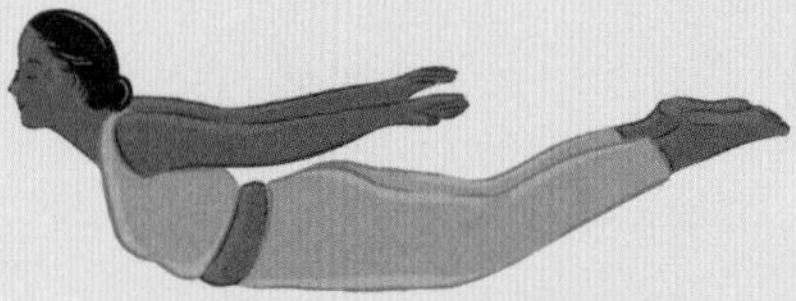

17. LOCUST

Exhale onto the belly and inhale lifting into locust pose. Hold for 3 breaths.

REPEAT ON THE LEFT SIDE

STEPS 13–17

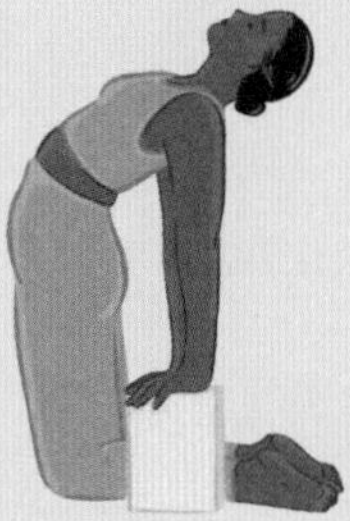

18. CAMEL

Coming onto the knees, inhale and lift the chest into camel pose. Hold for 3–5 breaths.

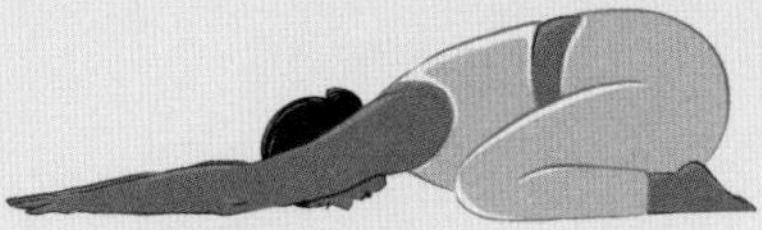

19. CHILD'S POSE

Exhale, melting down into child's pose. Hold for 5 breaths.

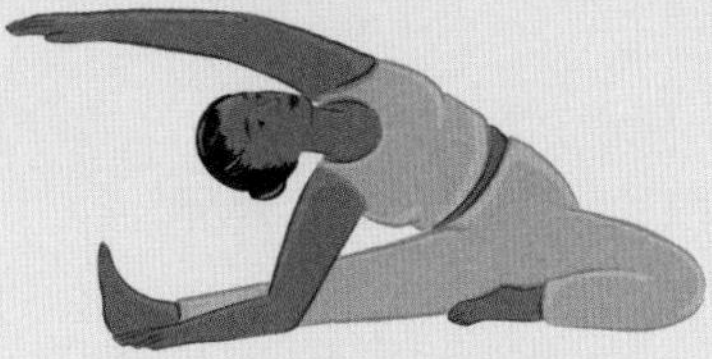

20. REVOLVED HEAD-TO-KNEE

Inhale into a seated position, releasing the right leg long and exhale, taking a side bend to the right. Hold for 5 breaths.

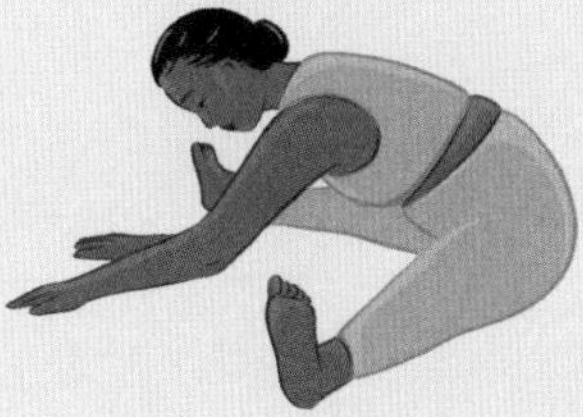

21. WIDE-ANGLE SEATED FORWARD BEND

Release the left leg long, inhale and open the chest, exhale and fold forward between the legs. Hold for 5 breaths.

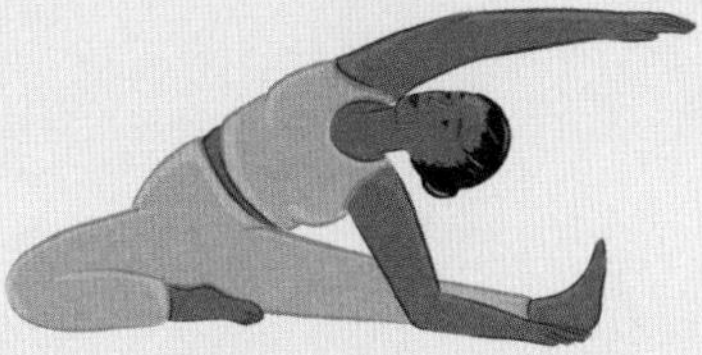

22. REVOLVED HEAD-TO-KNEE

Inhale into a seated position, bringing the right foot in, and exhale taking a side bend to the left. Hold for 5 breaths.

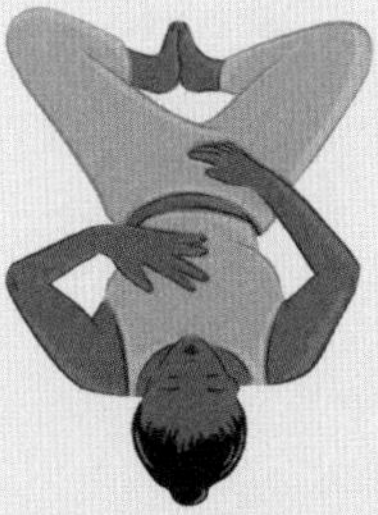

23. RECLINED COBBLER'S

Release into reclined cobbler's pose for 10 breaths.

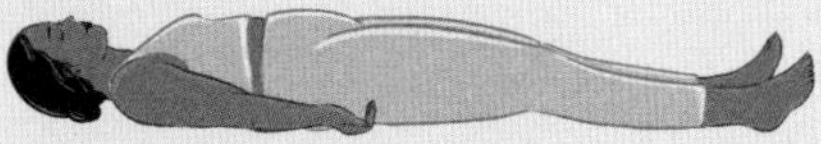

24. SAVASANA

Finally, melt into savasana for 2 minutes or more.

MEDITATION

BODY SCAN MEDITATION

The meditation this month is a body scan meditation. It is linked to the concept of non-attachment as we systematically move our attention through different parts of the body, observing physical sensations without judgment. This practice cultivates non-attachment by teaching us to witness sensations, both pleasant and unpleasant, without clinging to or resisting them.

Directions:

1. Come into a comfortable seated position on a chair with an upright spine, somewhere you can be free of distractions.
2. Set a timer for 5 minutes or for as long as you have.
3. Gently close your eyes. If you don't like to close your eyes, you can have your eyes slightly open with the gaze lowered to the floor in front of you to keep your forehead soft.
4. Softly close your lips and let your breath come in through the nose and out through the nose or mouth in its natural rhythm.
5. Before each meditation begins, feel your sitting bones on the chair and your feet on the floor. Imagine roots winding down from these areas, helping you feel secure and grounded.
6. Tune into all sensations of the feet, feeling the weight of them resting on the ground, noticing any pressure or heat from the toes up through the ankles. Notice any sensation on the skin and from within. Now let the feet be soft and release.
7. Start to trace your awareness up through the body in exactly the same way: through the legs, pelvis, torso, shoulders, arms and right up to the crown of the head.
8. At each point notice all sensations, whether there is any tension, maybe even noticing vibrations or tingling energy from within, then let the body area be soft and release it fully.
9. To end this meditation, become aware of your whole body, soft and supported.
10. When the timer finishes, take a moment with your eyes still closed to sit and notice how you feel and any thoughts or feelings that arose.

JOURNAL PROMPTS

Below I have given you eight self-reflection questions linked to this month's squirrel theme and the yogic concept of *aparigraha*. Try answering two questions weekly alongside the daily journal prompts set out on pages 8–9.

▸ Consider the material possessions you hold on to with a strong sense of attachment that are not necessities. How do those attachments affect your daily life and well-being?

▸ Squirrels require intense focus when foraging for food. How do you cultivate focus and concentration in daily activities and goals and what distractions do you need to minimise?

▸ Reflect on your digital consumption habits. Do you need to be more mindful and set boundaries?

▸ Squirrels are naturally curious creatures. Consider whether you are open to new experiences and opportunities for learning and how you might nurture this going forwards.

▸ Think about the people in your life. Are there any relationships where attachment or expectations have caused discomfort or suffering, either to you or to them? Where might you be able to release some of those ties?

▸ Squirrels often share their resources with other squirrels. Ask yourself how you engage with your community, and whether you are open to collaboration and sharing without expecting anything in return?

▸ What are three things you're grateful for in your life right now that are not related to material possessions? Can you consider this question every day this week and bring more gratitude into your life?

▸ Squirrels diligently prepare for the future by storing food. What one or two steps are you taking to prepare for your future (financial, personal growth or career-related)?

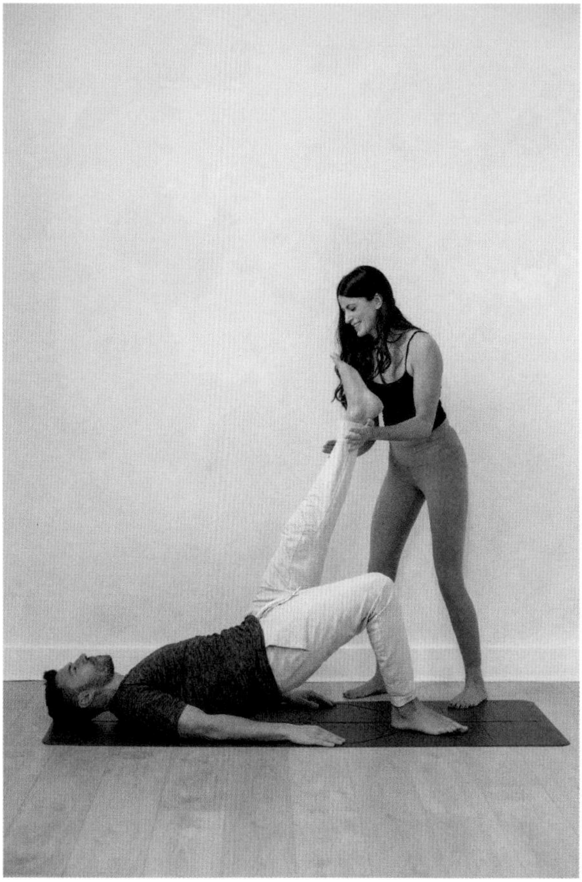
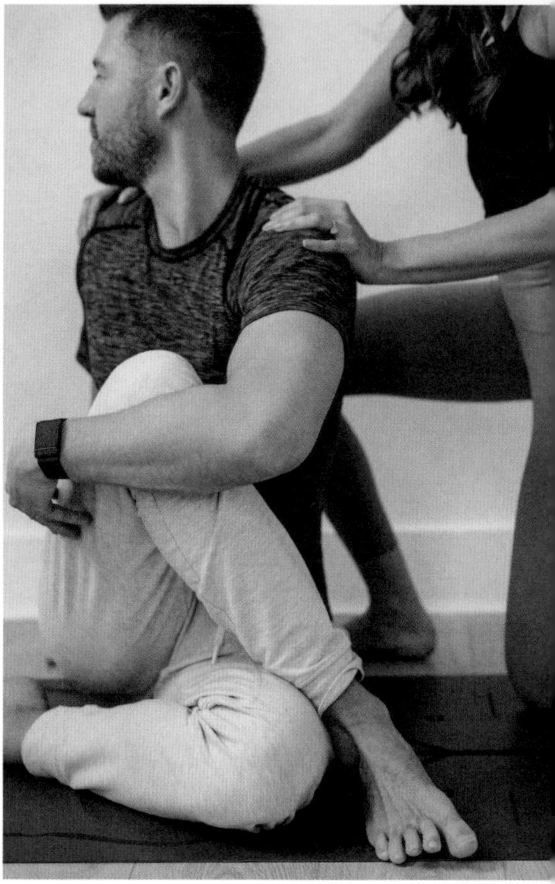
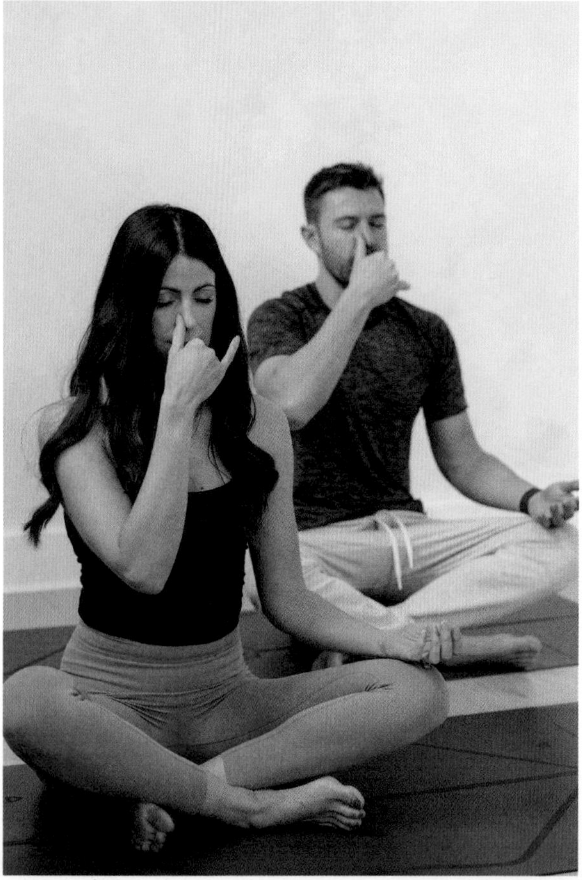
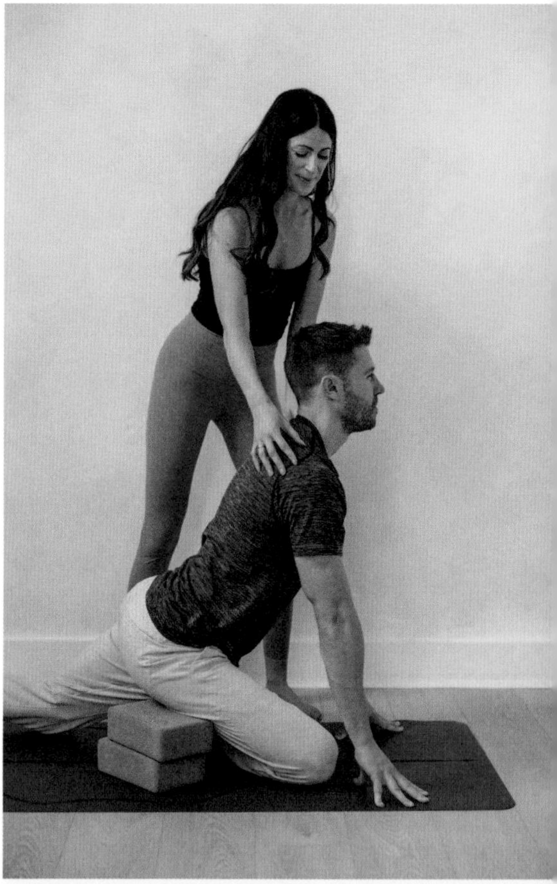

MONTH 6
OCEAN

'DANCE WITH THE WAVES, MOVE WITH THE SEA, LET THE RHYTHM OF THE WATER SET YOUR SOUL FREE.'

CHRISTY ANN MARTINE

OCEAN

Close your eyes for a moment and imagine you are on the beach looking out at the ocean. Feel the sand in your toes, the soft breeze on your skin, smell the salty air and hear the waves gently coming into shore. Take three soft, slow breaths as you continue to imagine yourself by the sea and notice how it makes you feel.

This month's theme is the ocean. The ocean is vast, powerful and free. It reminds us of the need for fluidity in life and riding the currents (life's ups and downs) with grace and balance. In the ebb and flow of both the ocean and our practice, we can be guided towards a deeper understanding of ourselves and the world around us. This month is your reminder that there will be an ebb and flow in your practice. You'll take five steps forward and then it may feel like you take six steps back. Keep moving and keep practising, because even those steps back are teaching you something.

In yoga, water is one of the five fundamental elements that are believed to make up the physical and energetic world. These elements are earth, water, fire, air and ether (space). Each is associated with certain qualities, characteristics and energies; water is associated with adaptability and flexibility. This month's signature flow is fluid and energising, full of twists and lightness, like the waves of the ocean.

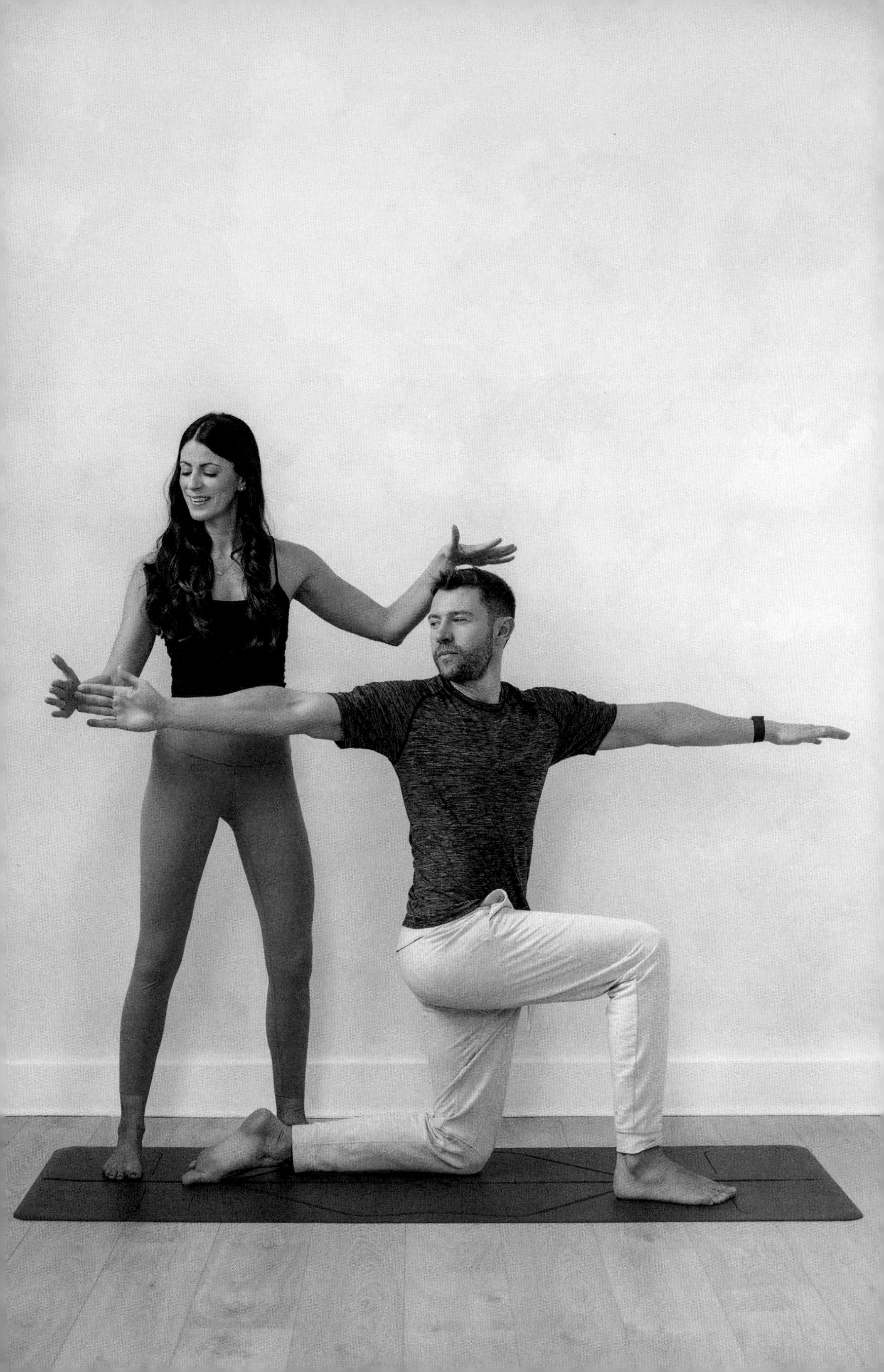

SAUCHA (PURITY)

CREATE SPACE IN YOUR MIND AND CREATIVITY WILL FLOW NATURALLY.

The second of Patañjali limbs (see page 26) are the five *niyamas*, set out below. The *niyamas* can be thought of as internal *yamas* as they are ethical principles that bring our focus to our body and surroundings and guide how we behave in a compassionate manner towards ourselves. Just like with the *yamas*, the more we practise the *niyamas*, the more these positive ripples of change spread to others to emulate.

1. ***Saucha*** – cleanliness of the body, heart, mind and surroundings
2. ***Santosha*** – contentment
3. ***Tapas*** – discipline or to practise causing positive change
4. ***Svadhyaya*** – study of the self and/or sacred texts
5. ***Ishvara pranidhana*** – humility, faith, surrender to a higher being

The first of the *niyamas* is *saucha*; it translates to 'cleanliness' or 'purity' and invites us to purify everything – our body, thoughts, words, actions and everything in our life. Have you ever noticed how a messy room creates a hectic mind and vice versa? When our body and minds are clear, we become lighter.

Children are wonderful teachers of purity as they approach life with innocent curiosity and playfulness. Their actions and expressions are often genuine and untainted by external influences. Their ability to be amazed by the world around them should be a lesson to us all to see the beauty and purity in everyday experiences.

Here are some ways can we incorporate *saucha* into our daily lives:

▸ **On the yoga mat:** Come to the mat with a clear intention helping to create a mental environment that aligns with *saucha*. As you move, think about mindful movement. Practise with awareness, paying attention to the alignment of your body and what tweaks you need to make to ensure the practice is right for you.

▸ **Environment:** To reduce mental and physical distractions, maintain a clean and organised living space, ensuring you declutter regularly.

▸ **Nourish your body:** Prioritise a balanced diet, choosing fresh, whole food wherever possible and avoiding excessive processed and/or unhealthy options.

▸ **Mindful consumption:** Be aware of how much and what you are consuming, not just in terms of food but social media, news, entertainment and information. Choose content that uplifts and sustains you rather than drains you.

▸ **Bird's-eye view:** Take an overview of your life and note down what truly matters to you. Recognise any habits and thought patterns that don't serve you well. Can you simplify your life to focus on your priorities and let go of those things that don't contribute to your well-being?

▸ **Giving:** When we give to others through acts of kindness and service, without expecting anything in return, it creates a purity in our actions and contributes to the well-being of our community.

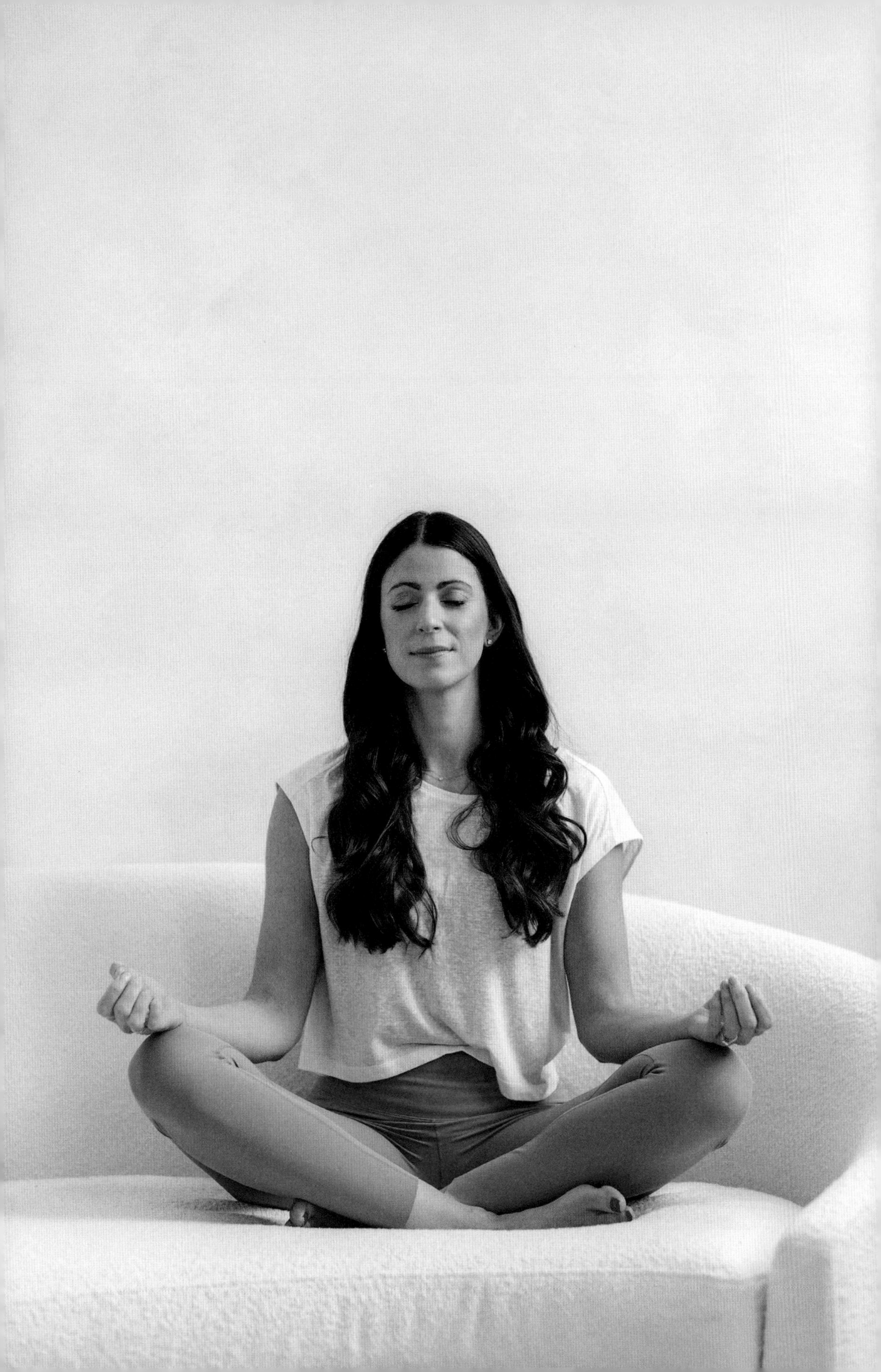

THE BREATH

NADI SHODHANA

This month I've chosen a yogic breathing technique called *nadi shodhana*, or alternate nostril breathing.

The word *nadi* in Sanskrit refers to the channels through which *prana* (life force energy) flows, and *shodhana* translates to 'purification'. This breathing technique is thought to create a sense of purification and balance. It's a technique that calms the nervous system, balances the hemispheres of the brain and is a perfect tool to use when you're feeling stressed and seeking stability. Imagine each breath mirroring the soothing cadence of ocean waves, the dance between the rise and fall of the sea.

Directions:

1. Come into a comfortable seated position, growing tall through the crown of the head and allowing the spine to be neutral and long.
2. Take a few breaths, tuning in and observing the body and mind.
3. Tuck the index and middle fingers of your right hand into your palm (*vishnu mudra*) and exhale fully to begin. Alternatively, you can place the index finger and middle finger between the eyebrows (to the third eye) if more comfortable.
4. Bring the right thumb to your face and close the right nostril. Take a full, soft and slow inhale through the left nostril. Close the left nostril with the ring finger then release the right nostril and exhale slowly and fully. Take a full and slow inhale through the right nostril. Close the right nostril with the thumb then release the left nostril and exhale slowly and fully. This is one cycle.
5. Repeat for eight to ten cycles, trying to even out the breath, aiming for an equal length of inhale and exhale.
6. After your practice ends, bring the breath back to a natural rhythm and take a moment to tune in and notice how you're feeling and any sensations that arose.

THE OCEAN FLOW

This month's signature flow is cleansing and energising. It plays with the theme of the ocean, and you can add sun salutations (see pages 16–20) for extra heat and purification whenever you have time. This flow will allow you to release tension and open the hips, a place where many of us feel tense or stuck.

When you look out to the ocean there is so much more going on than what you see on the surface. If you have ever been snorkelling or scuba diving you have had a taste of this. Much of the ocean's life and beauty lie beneath the surface. The reason I am sharing this is because the beauty of yoga isn't in what it looks like. Someone might be able to do the whole of this month's flow, looking exactly like the pictures in the book; however, they may hobble off the mat feeling dreadful. They may have pushed themselves into what they believe the pose 'should' look like without regard for their body and what they truly needed.

Please take this piece of advice into every practice as it is fundamental in the practice of yoga: *'Yoga is not about what it looks like. It is about how it feels in your body.'*

Really consider whether you need that extra sun salutation or whether you're pushing yourself to do it because you think you should. This shift in perspective is crucial to ensure that you are fostering a sustainable and nourishing movement practice. It will remind you that every individual's body is unique, and what may work for one person might not be suitable for another. What may feel good for your body one day may not the next! It encourages a compassionate and intuitive approach to movement and the breath, promoting overall well-being on and off the mat.

Aim to practise this flow three or four times per week and if you have more time, feel free to include the seated warm-up flow on page 10 at the start, combine it with the previous months' flows or repeat the flow multiple times.

As you move around your yoga mat, bring some ocean qualities with you:

▸ **Strength:** Channel the power of the ocean's waves, feeling the core support your movements and using your foundations (the part of the body touching the ground) to ground down to keep you stable and strong.

▸ **Adaptability:** Just as the ocean adapts to changing tides and different environments, be open to modifications and variations in your practice. Explore different ways of moving to help adapt your practice to your body's needs.

▸ **Fluidity:** Channel fluidity and grace on the yoga mat by imagining you are moving through water as you move from one pose to another. Be less elephant (clunking the feet or hands down) and more ocean. For example, take the transition from downward-facing dog to low lunge. Can you step the foot forward lightly without a sound (using the hand to help you move the foot forward if needed)? This control and mindfulness in your movement is a huge part of the practice and can help ensure you are using the muscles you need to.

PLEASE NOTE
The appendix on page 190 includes a detailed breakdown of each pose, plus variations and modifications. Remember to listen to your body; yoga should never be painful and you can chose to skip any pose that doesn't feel right for you.

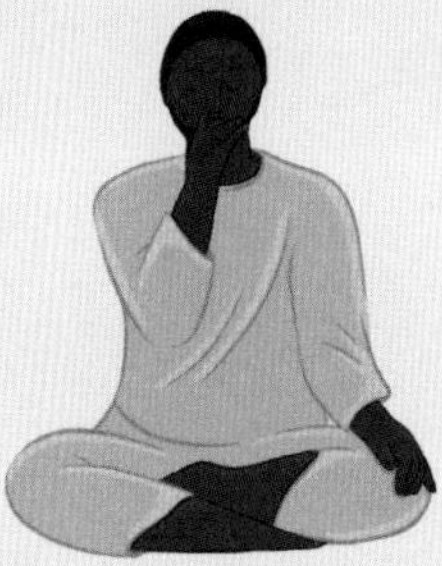

1. SEATED NADI SHODHANA

In a seated position, take 10 rounds of *nadi shodhana* (see page 102).

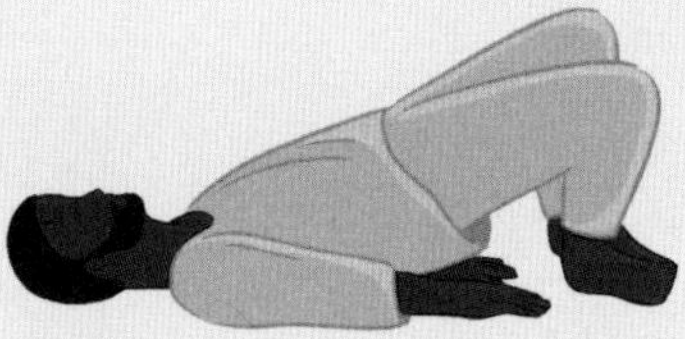

2. COBBLER'S BRIDGE

Releasing onto the floor, bring the soles of the feet together, exhale lifting the hips up and hold for 5 breaths.

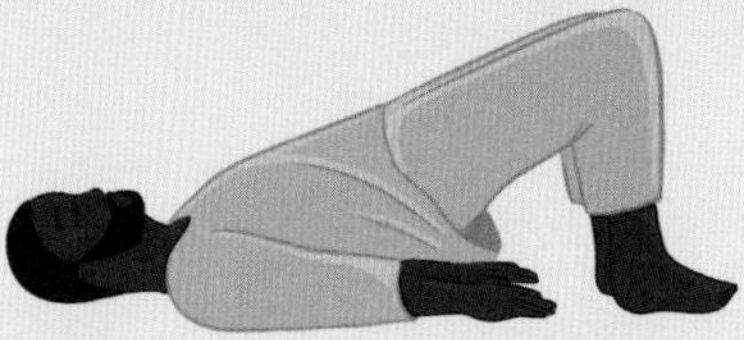

3. BRIDGE LIFTS

Bringing the feet onto the floor, exhale to lift the hips into bridge and inhale to lower.
Repeat 10 times.

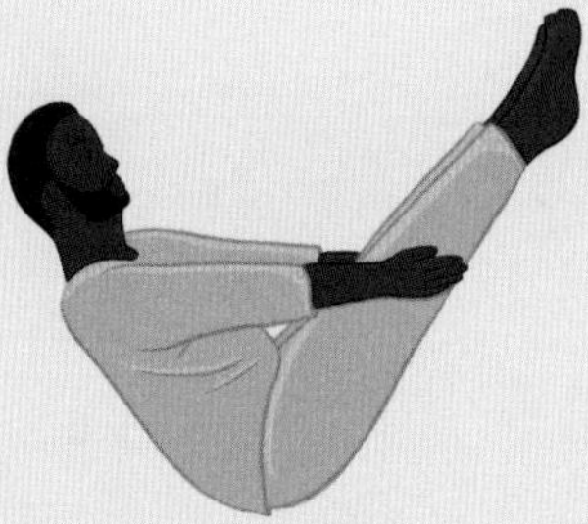

4. BOAT

Come up to sit on the mat. Exhale as you lift into boat pose. Hold for 3 breaths.

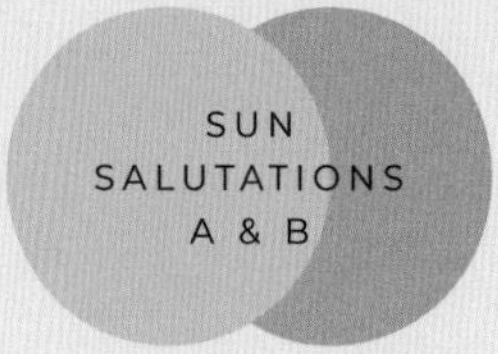

Option to include sun salutations A and B (see pages 16–20).

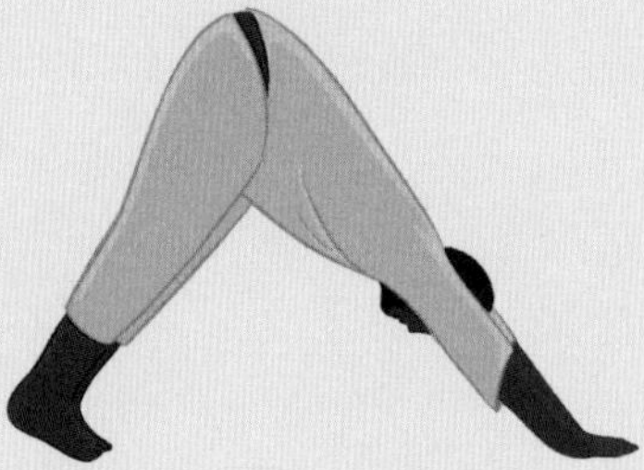

5. DOWNWARD-FACING DOG

Exhale lifting the hips into downward-facing dog and hold for 5 breaths.

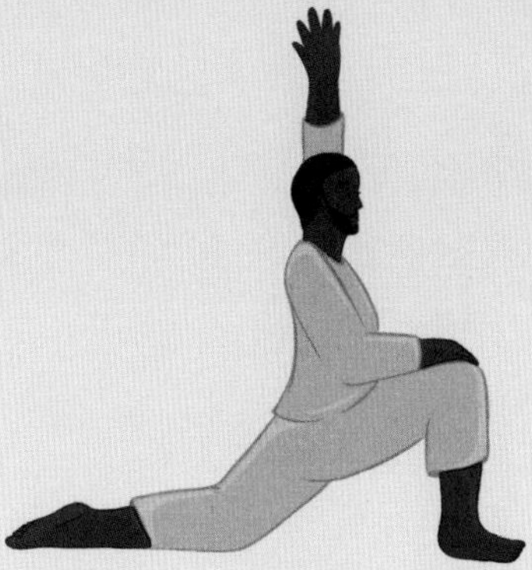

6. LOW LUNGE SIDE STRETCH

Step the right foot forward, inhale the left fingers to the sky and exhale taking a side stretch to the right. Hold for 5 breaths.

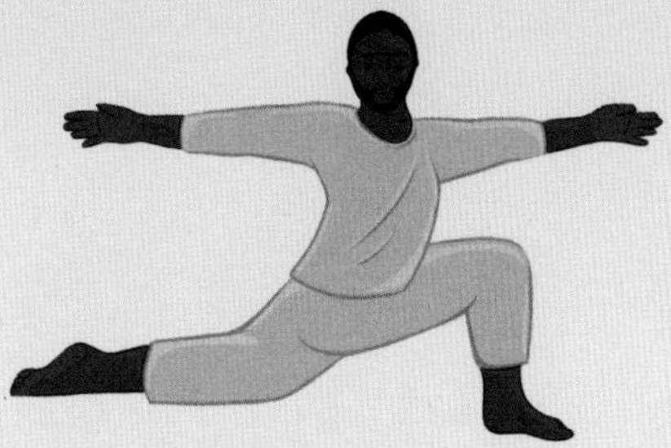

7. LOW LUNGE TWIST

Inhale to centre and exhale to twist. Hold for 5 breaths.

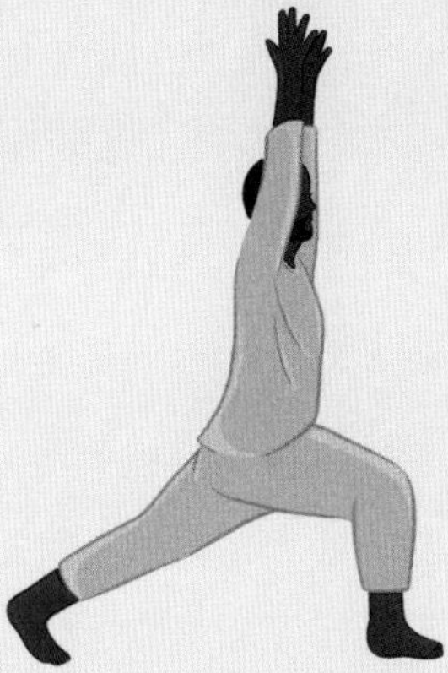

8. HIGH LUNGE

Inhale to centre and lift into high lunge. Hold for a full breath.

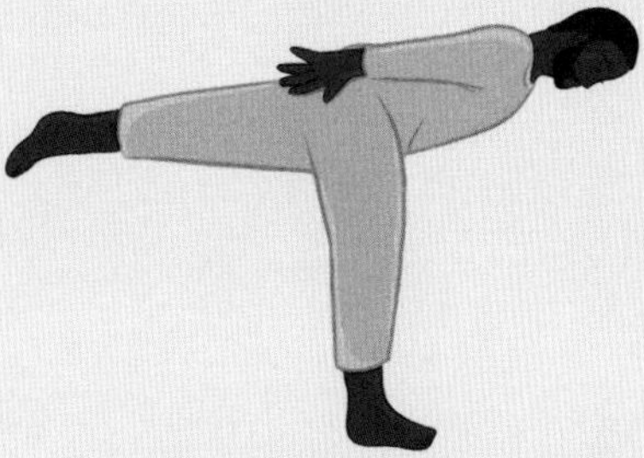

9. WARRIOR III

Exhale shifting the weight forwards and lifting into warrior III. Hold for 3 breaths.

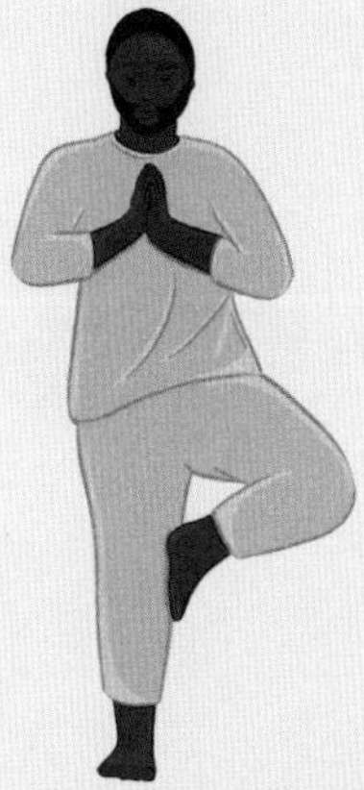

10. TREE POSE

Inhale to stand, bringing the left foot to the inside of the right ankle, shin or thigh. Hold for 5 breaths.

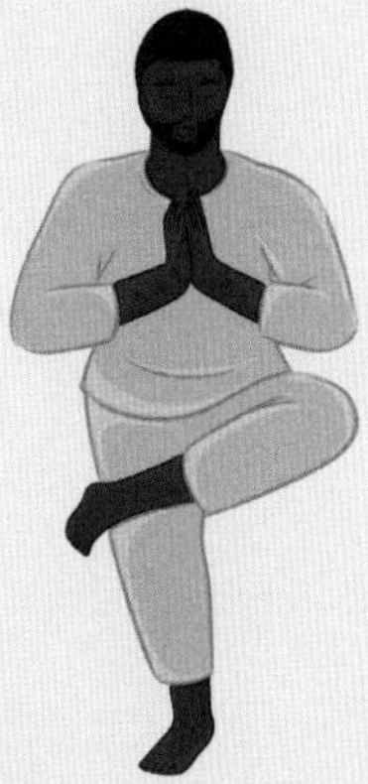

11. FIGURE FOUR CHAIR

Exhale into chair and figure four the left ankle above the right knee. Hold for 3 breaths.

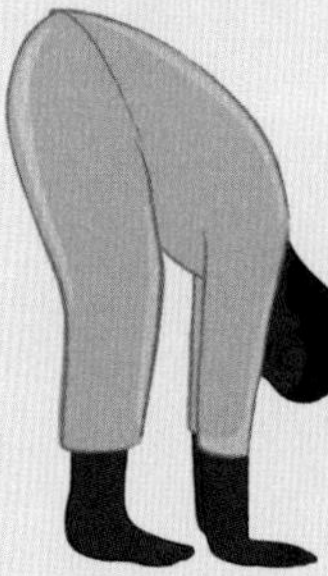

12. FORWARD FOLD

Exhale, releasing the left foot and folding forwards. Hold for 5 breaths.

REPEAT ON THE LEFT SIDE

STEPS 5–12

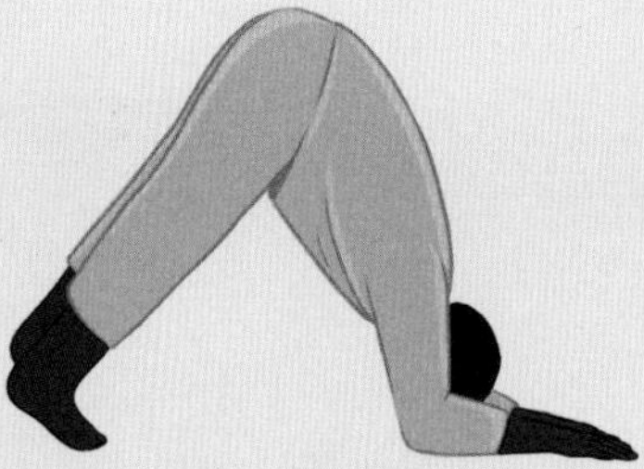

13. DOLPHIN

Step into tabletop and release the forearms down to the ground, lifting the hips to the sky. Hold for 5 breaths.

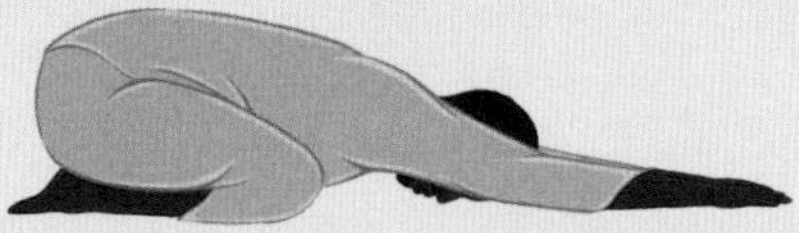

14. CHILD'S POSE

Exhale, melting down into child's pose. Hold for 3 breaths.

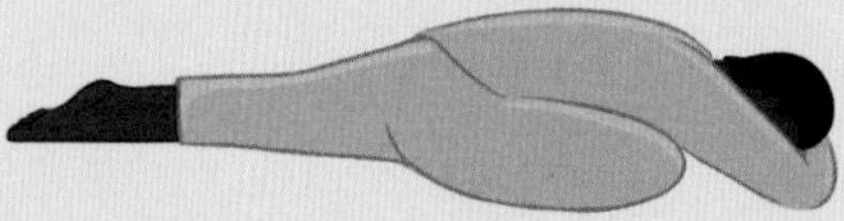

15. PIGEON

Placing the right shin across the front of the mat, find pigeon pose. Hold for 5–10 breaths.

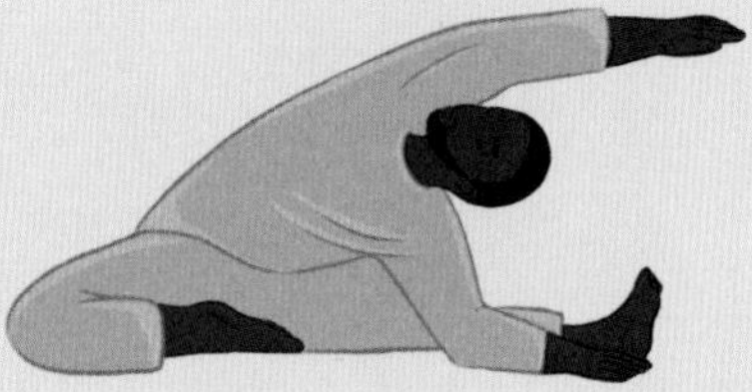

16. REVOLVED HEAD-TO-KNEE

Swing the left leg forwards and side bend into revolved head-to-knee pose. Hold for 5 breaths.

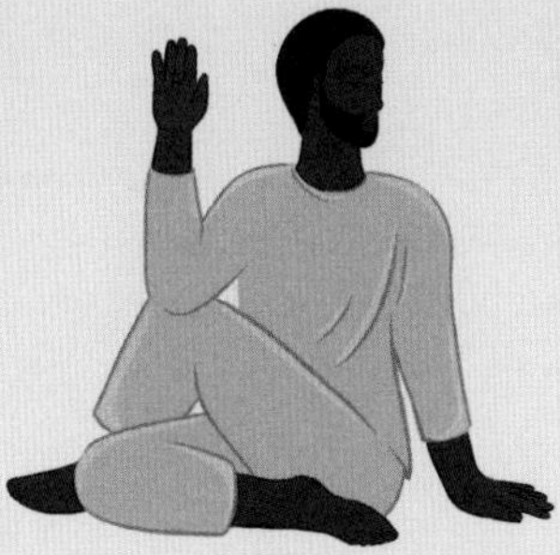

17. HALF LORD OF THE FISHES

Step the left foot over the right thigh, inhale to lengthen and exhale to twist. Hold for 5 breaths.

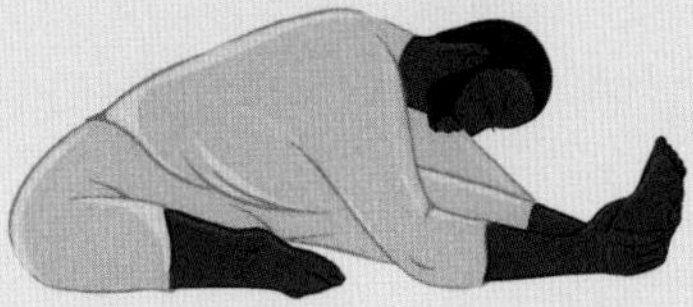

18. HEAD-TO-KNEE FORWARD FOLD

Release the left leg straight forwards, inhale to lengthen, exhale and fold. Hold for 5 breaths.

REPEAT ON THE OTHER SIDE

STEPS 15–18

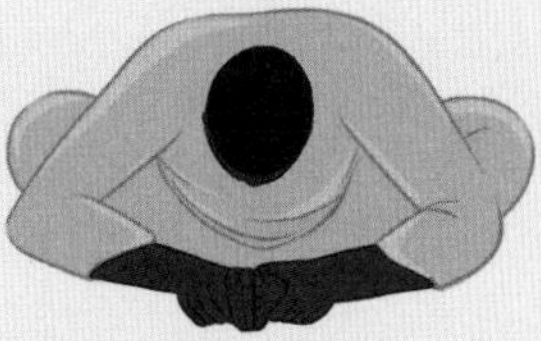

19. COBBLER'S POSE

Bring the soles of the feet to touch finding cobbler's pose. Hold for 10 breaths.

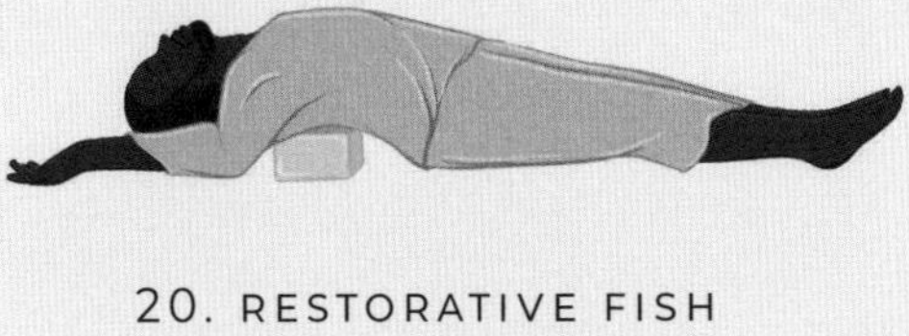

20. RESTORATIVE FISH

Placing a block or cushion under the thoracic spine, melt over the prop and release. Hold for 10 breaths.

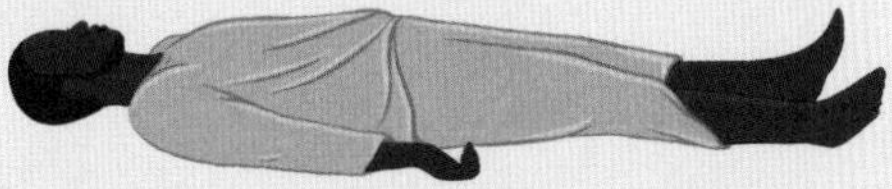

21. SAVASANA

Remove the prop and melt into savasana for 2 minutes or more.

MINDFULNESS

MINDFUL CLEANING

The mindfulness exercise this month is mindful cleaning. It's simple but powerful as it allows us to turn mundane chores into purposeful and calming activities. These opportunities for mindfulness and presence can have a whole host of benefits, such as improved concentration, heightened mind–body connection, enhanced productivity and improved mental clarity.

Directions:

1. Your intention for this task is to create a clean and organised space that promotes a sense of calm and well-being.
2. Eliminate any distractions by turning off the TV, switching off your phone or putting it on silent, and create a quiet environment.
3. Take a few moments to practise mindful breathing and ground yourself in the present. Softly and slowly breathe in through the nose, and softly and slowly breathe out through the nose.
4. As you clean, pay attention to the sensations in your body. Notice the feeling of your muscles working and the texture of the things you touch. Try to slow down, giving your full attention to what you're doing and noticing if you have a tendency to rush.
5. Express gratitude for the items you're cleaning and the space you're organising. It sounds simple but this mindset shift can make the cleaning task more enjoyable and meaningful.
6. Notice if the mind starts wandering away and whenever this happens, gently bring it back to the present.
7. Once the cleaning is complete, take a moment to appreciate the result. Notice how the space looks and feels after your mindful attention and effort and notice how the exercise felt for you.

JOURNAL PROMPTS

Below I have given you eight self-reflection questions linked to this month's ocean theme and the yogic concept of *saucha*. Try answering two questions weekly alongside the daily journal prompts set out on pages 8–9.

▸ Consider your physical cleanliness and health. Are there any changes you can make to your daily routine to improve your overall well-being?

▸ What small steps can you take to incorporate the soothing qualities of the ocean into your daily life?

▸ Do you have any mental clutter or negative thought patterns that are weighing you down? What practices help you deal with these feelings?

▸ Reflect on how marine ecosystems are interconnected, research it if needed. How does understanding this connection deepen your appreciation for sea life and the importance of conservation?

▸ Take a walk around your house and look at how clean and tidy your space is. Does it support your well-being or do you need to make some changes?

▸ Consider how actions and choices impact the global issue of climate change and rising sea levels. Think of three changes you can make to contribute to a sustainable future for our planet.

▸ What daily practices, rituals or routines can you add to your life to help you maintain *saucha*?

▸ Reflect on the soothing sounds of the ocean. What music or sounds bring you joy or calm and can you incorporate them into each day this week and notice how they make you feel?

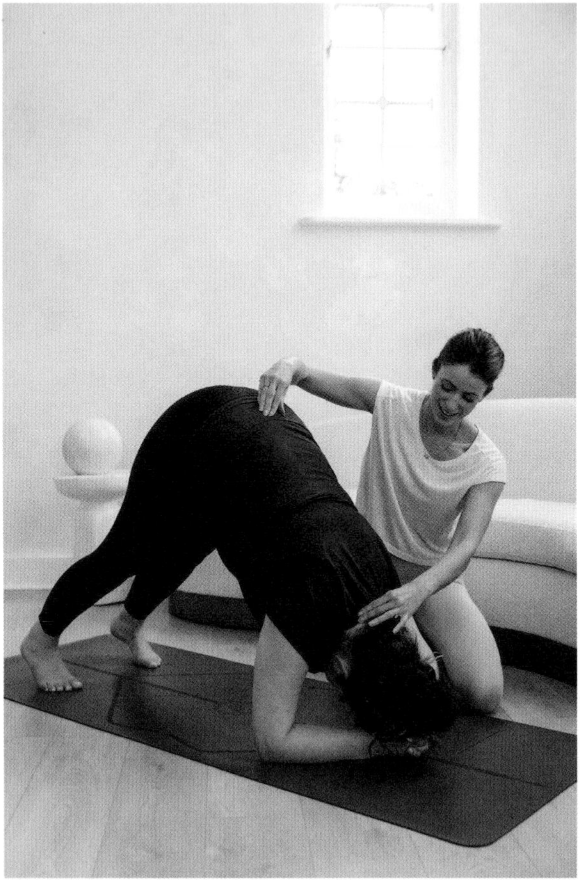
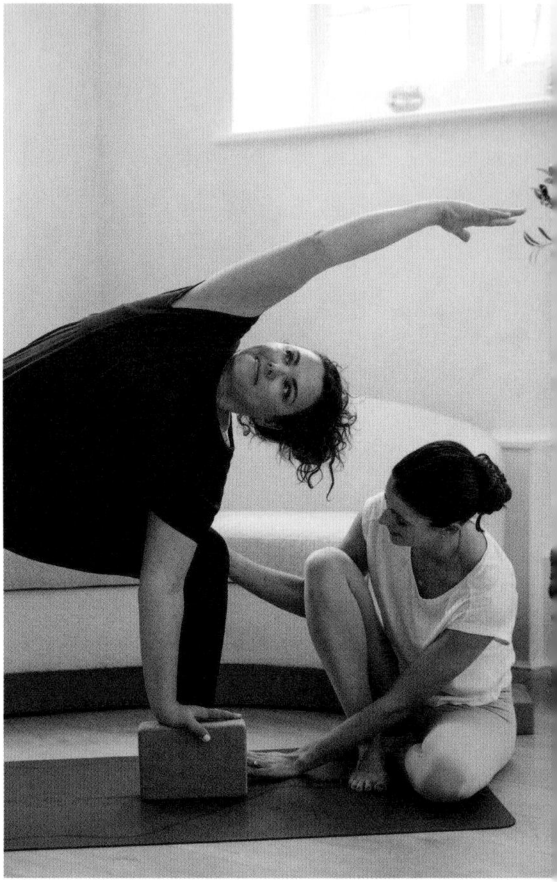
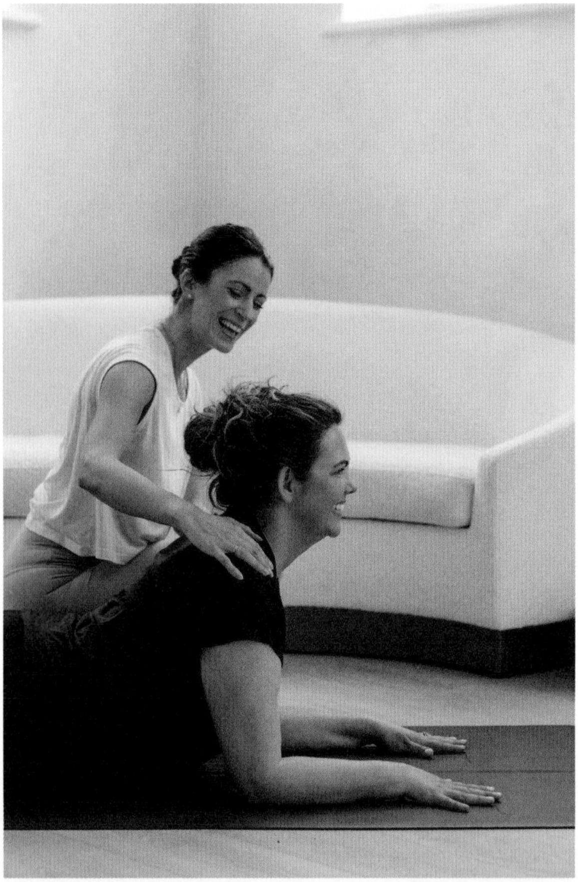
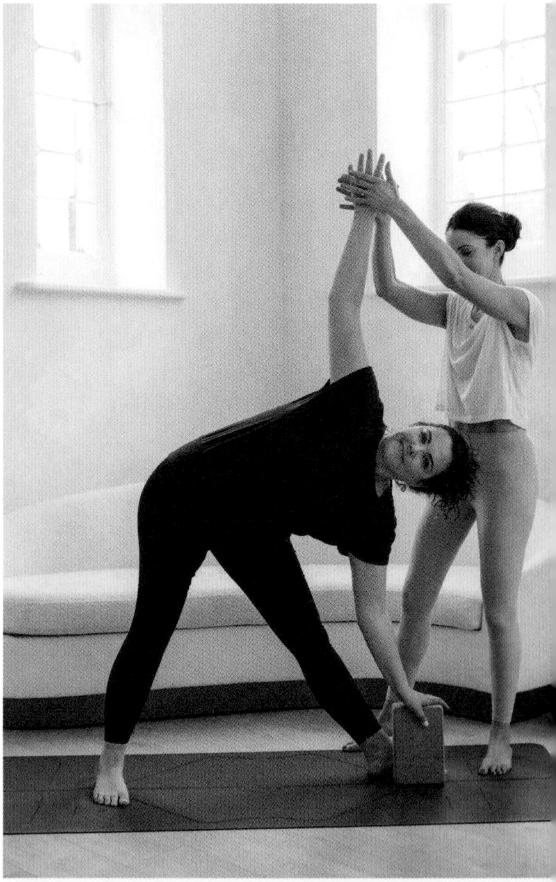

MONTH 7
CLOUD

'DON'T FORGET: BEAUTIFUL SUNSETS NEED CLOUDY SKIES.'

PAULO COELHO

CLOUD

You are halfway through your Yoga Happy year and I would like you to take a moment to close your eyes and ask yourself the following question: *In what way has yoga made the biggest difference to my life so far?*

You've committed six months of dedication and hard work to your practice and yes, perhaps you've fallen off the wagon at times, but you're still here. Maybe certain postures now seem more accessible; perhaps your strength and flexibility are improving, but what about your emotional well-being and stress levels? How is your sleep quality and how is your mental focus? Maybe you can't put your finger on a specific thing, it's simply that yoga makes you *feel better* – that's how it was for me at the start.

Over the past six months you've learnt an array of tools to help you stay strong, calm and resilient in the chaos of life. Call on these tools whenever you need them as well as the new techniques from this and future months.

This month is themed around the clouds and here's why: One morning I was leaving to take my two children to school and as we left the house, the sky was grey and the rain falling. I said to the kids, 'Oh no, what a miserable day outside.' My son turned to me and said, 'but Mummy, think how happy and grateful the trees and flowers are for the rain.' I have never looked at the clouds and rain in the same way since. Perspective is everything.

This month we look at the yogic concept of *santosha*, or contentment, alongside an open-hearted gratitude flow.

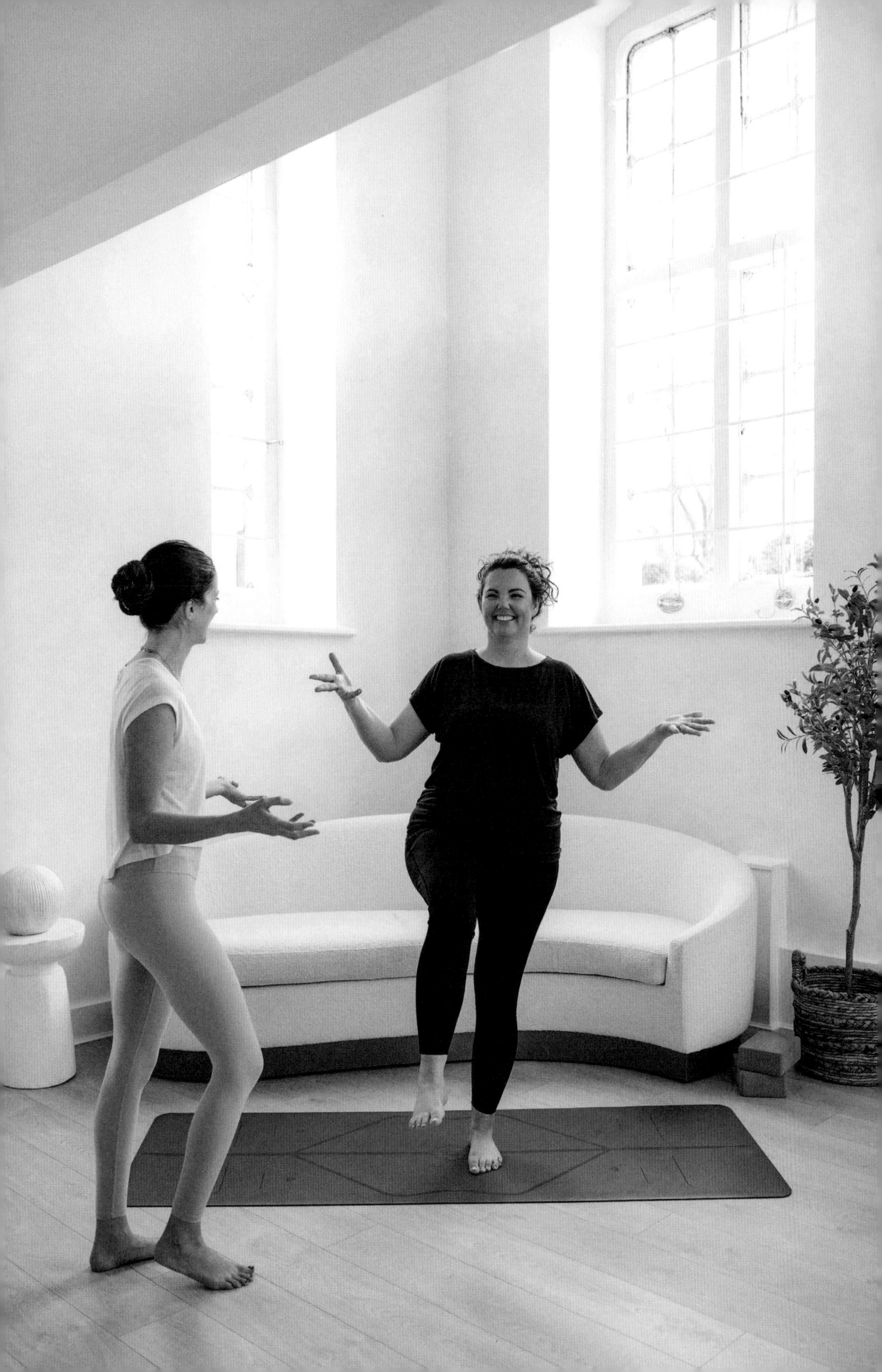

SANTOSHA (CONTENTMENT)

EMBRACING AND FINDING JOY IN THIS MOMENT HERE AND NOW.

Santosha is the second *niyama* and translates to 'contentment'. It invites us to find gratitude and contentment in what we have rather than seeking what we don't. I want to share up front that *santosha* isn't about pretending that everything is okay. Nor is it about denying that life can be extremely challenging at times. *Santosha* is accepting the present and finding a balanced perspective where we can see that there is gratitude even in the midst of heavy times and uncertainty. Even in the darkest times, can you seek those pockets of sunlight through the clouds that are trying to break free?

True happiness comes from allowing life to change from moment to moment; not searching for what we don't have but instead feeling content with what we have at this moment. We live in a society where we link happiness to future achievements or external conditions. Thinking, 'I'll be happy when I get that job,' or, 'I'll be happy when I find a partner.' This mindset places happiness in the futures and creates a cycle of longing for the next achievement or possession. It also means that we are dependent on reaching specific goals or acquiring certain things to find happiness.

Practising *santosha* helps us to break free from that cycle. It helps us realise that true contentment is found within, irrespective of external achievements. It invites us to live life mindfully, appreciating and savouring the moment right now because in reality it is the only moment that we know is certain. This doesn't mean you can't have goals or aspirations, but *santosha* encourages balance – working towards a goal without sacrificing current happiness.

Here are some ways that we can incorporate *santosha* into our daily lives:

▸ **On the yoga mat:** Cultivate gratitude for the opportunity to move on your yoga mat. Each pose can become a moment to express thanks for the capabilities of your body. So often we forget to be grateful for the seemingly simple gift of movement or can even be cruel to our bodies, but when you think about it, our bodies are incredible and movement is such a blessing.

▸ **Gratitude list:** Set aside time each day to write down what you're grateful for. A gratitude practice has incredible benefits backed by research (see page 8). If you haven't started one yet, give it a try each day this month and witness the positive impact it has on your life.

▸ **Limit comparisons:** Repeat after me: 'I will not compare myself to a stranger on the internet.' Why? Because that picture you're seeing is a fraction of someone's life and with the current editing tools available, so little of what we see online is real. Stop comparing yourself to those online and to people in real life too. Focus on you and your unique journey and accomplishments without getting caught in the comparison trap.

▸ **Smell the roses:** Savour the small moments in your day. Take time over that hot cup of tea, smell the flowers on your daily walk or pause to gaze at a beautiful sunset. Cultivate awareness and appreciation for the simple joys in life – I guarantee it will make your life fuller.

▸ **Mindful eating:** Do you often rush your food, not really taking in the experience? It is easily done. Instead, practise mindful eating by finding gratitude for the food on your plate, savouring the flavours and textures and being fully present during each meal (no phones allowed).

▸ **Find peace with the clouds:** Just like my story at the start of this chapter, instead of wishing for a perfectly clear sky, observe the clouds without judgement. Embrace the beauty of the ever-changing patterns and colours they create and how each moment is a one-of-a-kind masterpiece. Thank the rain for the nourishment it gives to the earth, and take this concept into the cloudy parts of life too.

▸ **Perfectly imperfect:** Accept and embrace imperfection in yourself and in others. Once we recognise that perfection is not a realistic or sustainable goal, it is freeing.

THE BREATH

THE BOX BREATH

Box breathing or square breathing is a simple yet highly effective breathing technique that I personally find amazing for stress reduction and focus. It's a variation of the *sama vritti* technique we learned in chapter 4 (see page 74). Just like the calming effect of watching clouds, practising box breathing can help bring a sense of tranquillity and peace to the mind, allowing you to find stillness amid life's storms. You can even use the clouds as a visualisation during this breath: as you hold the breath, picture the clouds and how they seem to pause, momentarily holding their shape, before transitioning.

Please note: This breathing technique is generally a safe and beneficial practice for most people. However, there may be some contraindications or situations in which it should be used with caution or avoided. In pregnancy, individuals should avoid holding the breath for extended periods as it can reduce oxygen flow to the baby. Always consult a healthcare professional or qualified instructor if you have concerns about practising box breathing, especially if you have underlying medical conditions.

Directions:

1. Come into a comfortable seated position, growing tall through the crown of the head and allowing the spine to be neutral and long.
2. Take a few breaths, tuning in and observing the body and mind.
3. Inhale through the nose for a count of four.
4. Hold your breath for a count of four.
5. Exhale through the nose for a count of four.
6. Hold your breath for a count of four.
7. This is one round. You can visualise the breath as a square: you inhale up the side, hold as you go across, exhale down the side and hold as you go back across to the start.
8. Repeat for 10–12 rounds or more.

THE CLOUD FLOW

This month's signature flow is an open-hearted gratitude flow. The flow includes poses that require longer holds, such as chair, during which it can be difficult to find gratitude. I challenge you to summon gratitude in those moments and notice how it makes you feel. Also notice the places in your body where you feel stuck in the flow, perhaps the hips or shoulders or somewhere different. Can you imagine breathing into these areas to help release some of that tension?

With the signature flow, embody the theme of clouds. Imagine your heart space expanding and a feeling of lightness, just as the clouds float weightlessly in the sky. Focus in particular on the breath, making sure it stays open and free, especially in the back-bending postures. If the breath starts to feel stuck or forced, ease gently out of the posture until you find space to breathe.

Aim to practise this flow three or four times per week and if you have more time, feel free to include the seated warm-up flow on page 10 at the start, combine it with the previous months' flows or repeat the flow multiple times.

As you move around your yoga mat, bring some cloud qualities with you:

- **Flowing transitions:** Mirror the way clouds seamlessly shift and change form in the sky. Embrace a sense of flow and ease in your movements. You can even add sun salutations into the flow at the points I've suggested as a form of continuous, fluid movement.
- **Weightlessness:** Cultivate a feeling of lightness in your practice. Whether this is through spinal extension, grounding down through the feet as you lift through the crown of the head, or through backbends to create a sense of space and floating the chest open and upwards.
- **Tranquillity:** Clouds convey a sense of serenity. Use the grounding box breathing technique at the start of each flow to find connection and calm. Try to keep these qualities, with the help of the breath, throughout the flow.

PLEASE NOTE
The appendix on page 190 includes a detailed breakdown of each pose, plus variations and modifications. Remember to listen to your body; yoga should never be painful and you can chose to skip any pose that doesn't feel right for you.

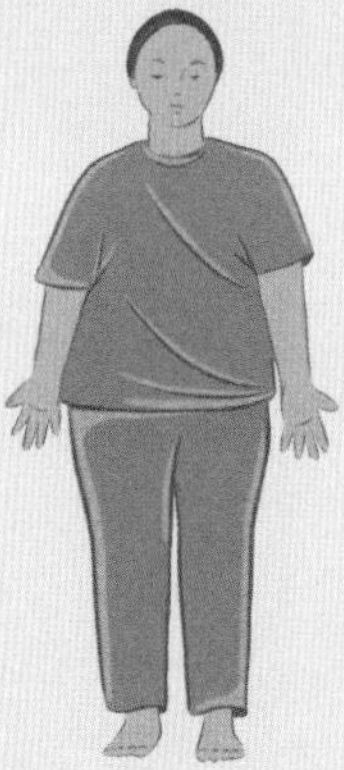

1. STANDING BOX BREATHING

Standing in mountain pose, take 10 rounds of box breathing (see page 116).

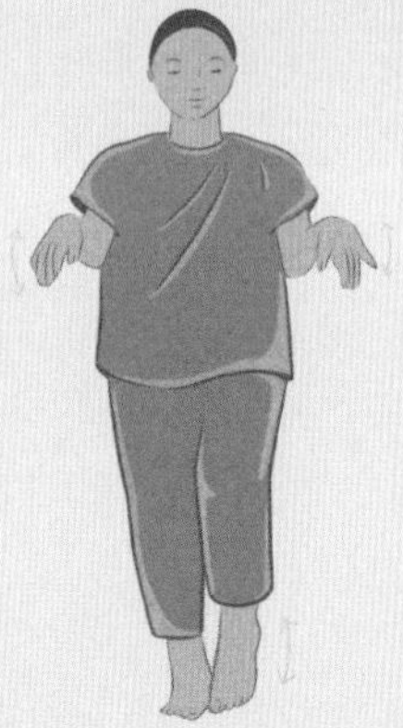

2. FOOT AND WRIST SEQUENCE

Balancing on the right foot, circle the wrists and ankle 5 times in each direction. Repeat on the opposite side.

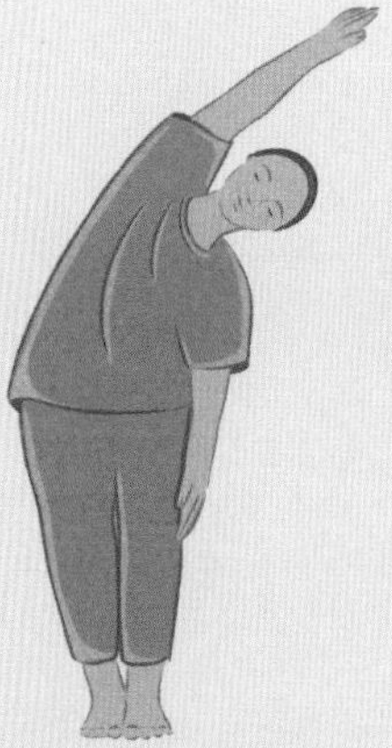

3. STANDING SIDE STRETCH

Inhale lifting the right fingers to the sky and exhale take a side bend to the left. Repeat on the opposite side. Repeat 3 times on each side.

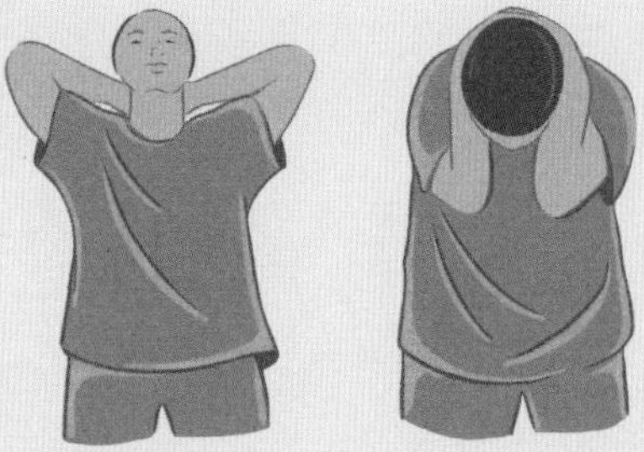

4. STANDING HEART OPENER

Inhale opening the heart and exhale rounding the back. Repeat 5 times.

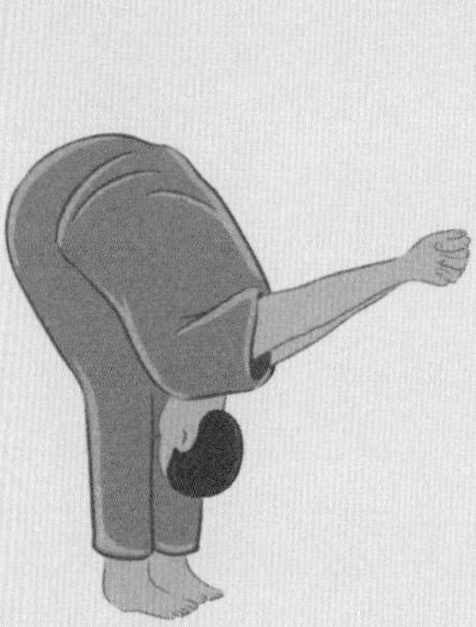

5. STANDING FORWARD BEND WITH LOCK

Exhale and fold the body down into a standing forward bend interlacing the hands behind the back. Hold for 5 breaths.

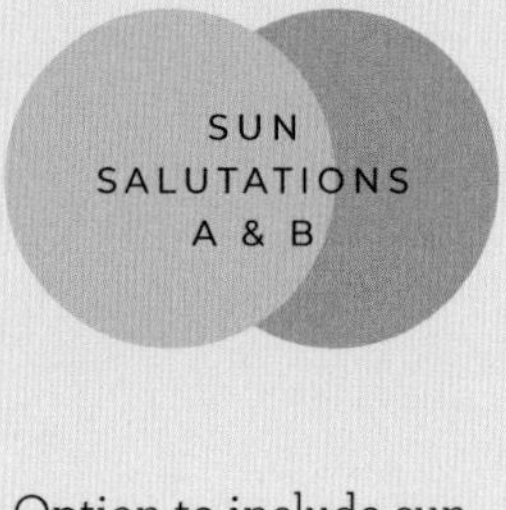

Option to include sun salutations A and B (see pages 16–20).

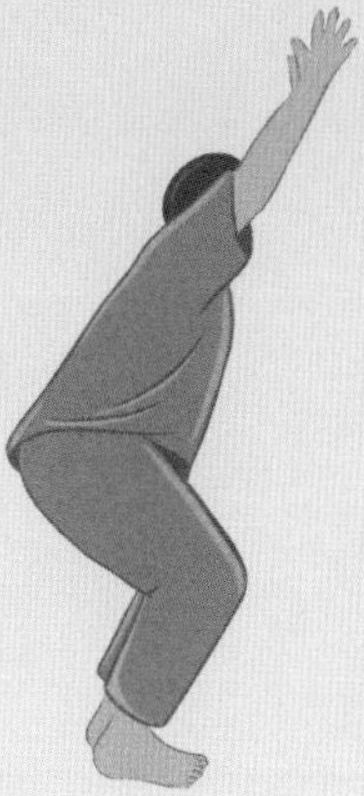

6. CHAIR POSE

Inhale, sweeping into chair pose. Hold for 5 breaths. Option to lift onto tiptoes.

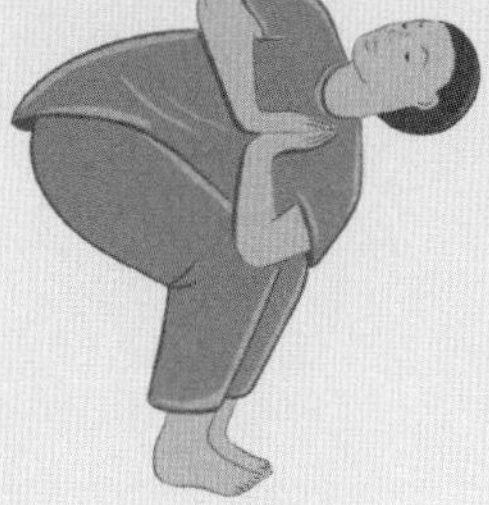

7. TWISTED CHAIR POSE

Bringing the hands into prayer, exhale and twist to the right finding twisted chair. Hold for 3 breaths.

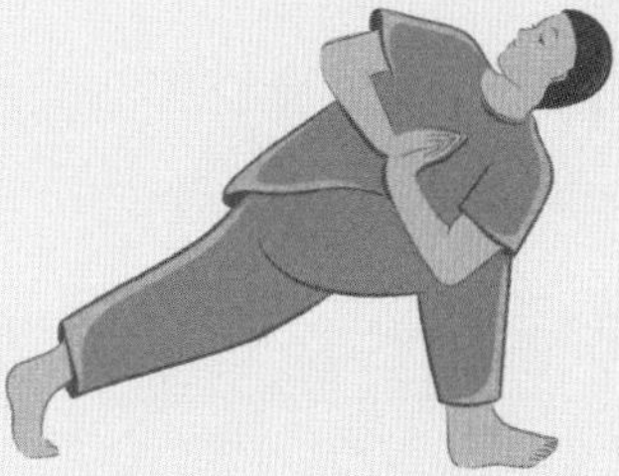

8. TWISTED CRESCENT LUNGE

Exhale as you softly step the left foot back. Hold for 5 breaths.

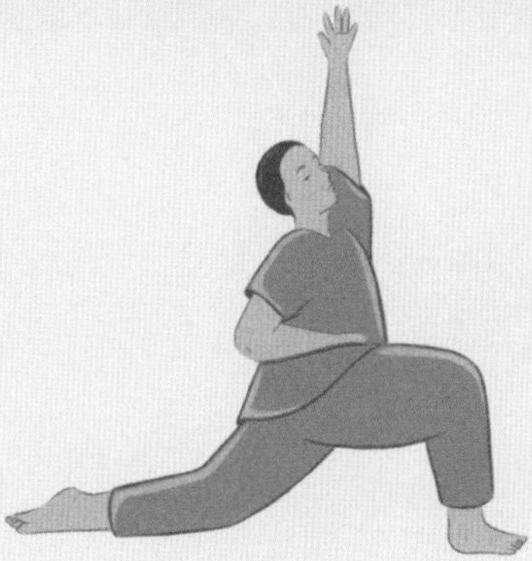

9. LOW LUNGE SIDE STRETCH

Releasing the twist and dropping the back knee, exhale and take a side stretch to the right. Hold for 5 breaths.

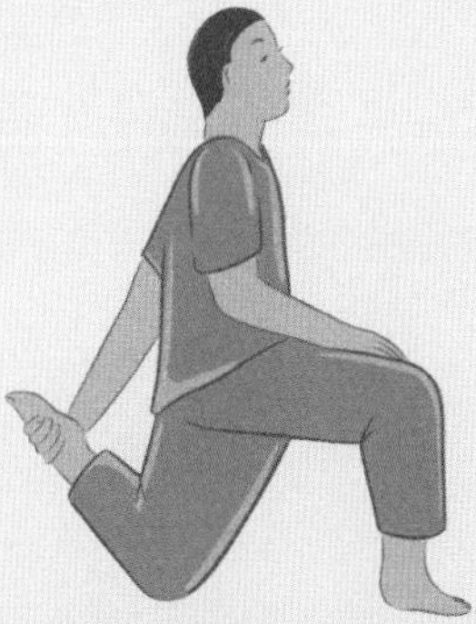

10. LOW LUNGE QUAD STRETCH

Placing the right hand on the thigh, reach the left hand back to take hold of the left ankle. Hold for 5 breaths.

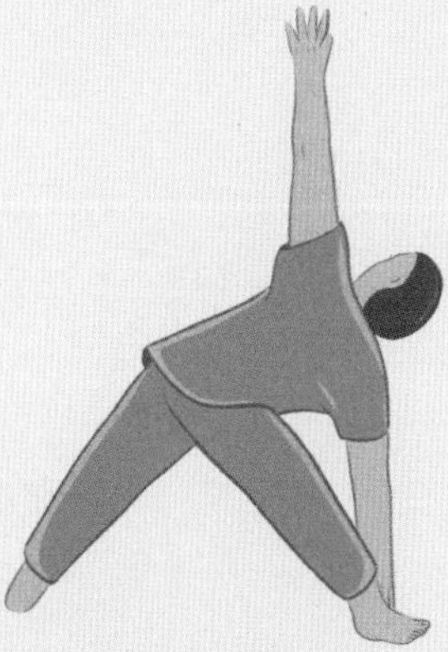

11. TRIANGLE

Release and lift up to stand. Exhale into triangle pose and hold for 5 breaths.

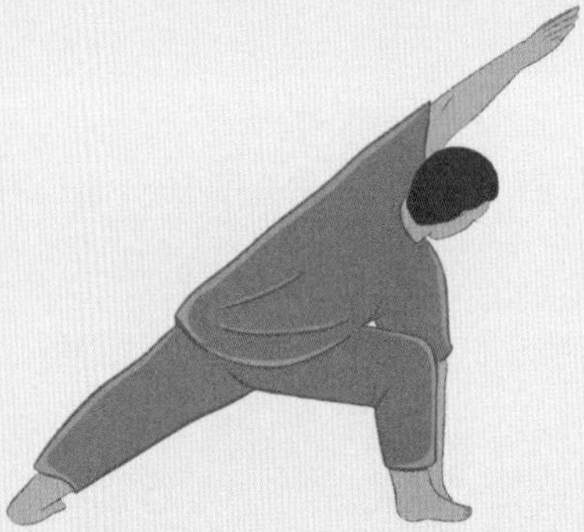

12. EXTENDED SIDE ANGLE POSE

Inhale lifting up, exhale as you bend the front knee and find extended side angle. Hold for 5 breaths.

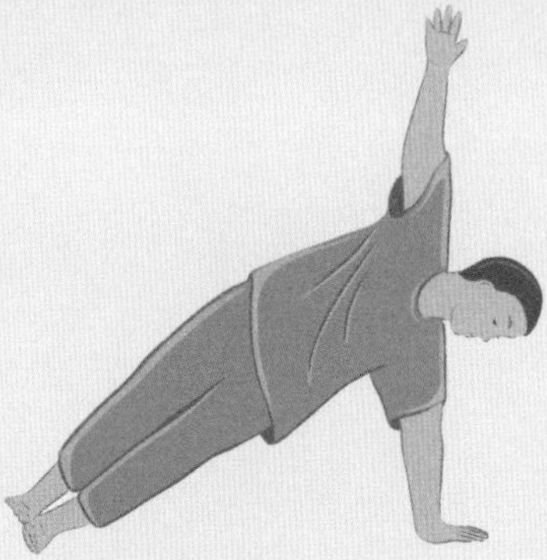

13. SIDE PLANK

Left hand comes down and step the right leg onto the left reaching the right fingers to the sky. Hold for 5 breaths.

REPEAT ON THE LEFT SIDE

STEPS 6–13

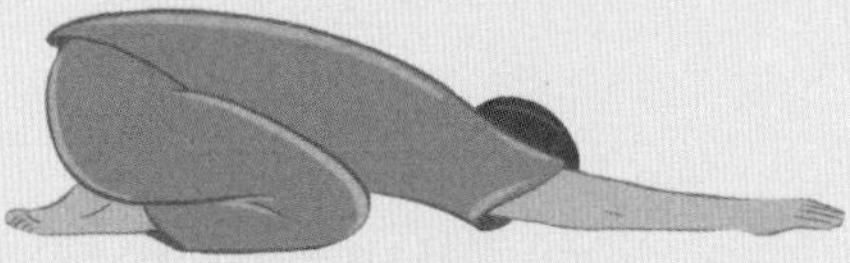

14. CHILD'S POSE

Exhale, melting down into child's pose. Hold for 3 breaths.

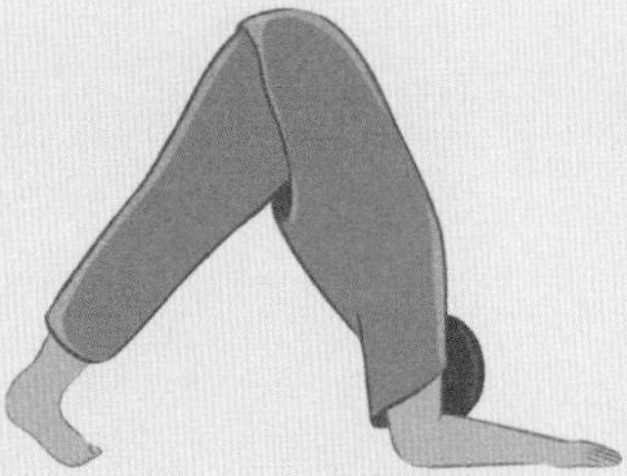

15. DOLPHIN

Coming to tabletop, release the forearms down to the ground and lifting the hips to the sky. Hold for 5 breaths.

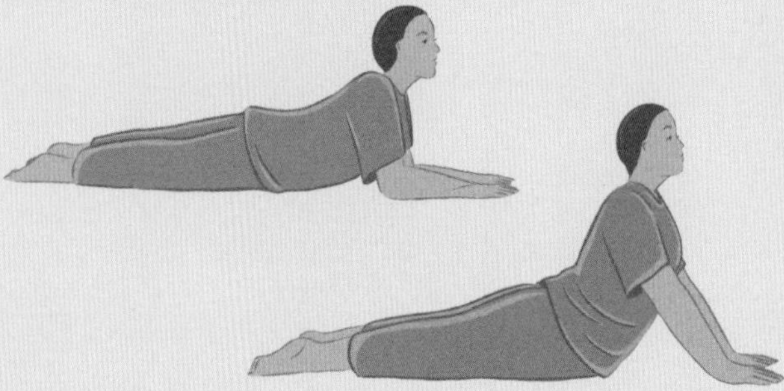

16. SPHINX TO SEAL

Coming onto the belly, find sphinx pose. Inhale to press into the hands and lift the elbows, exhale to release. Repeat ten times.

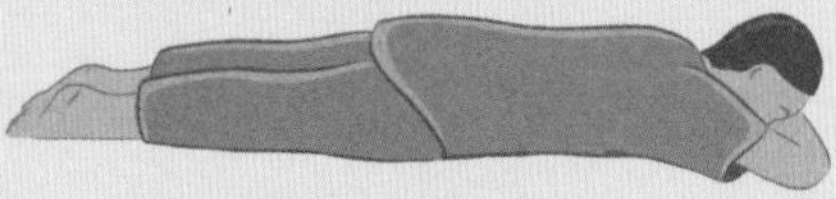

17. LIE ON BELLY

Coming onto the belly, resting the head onto the hands. Release here for 3 breaths.

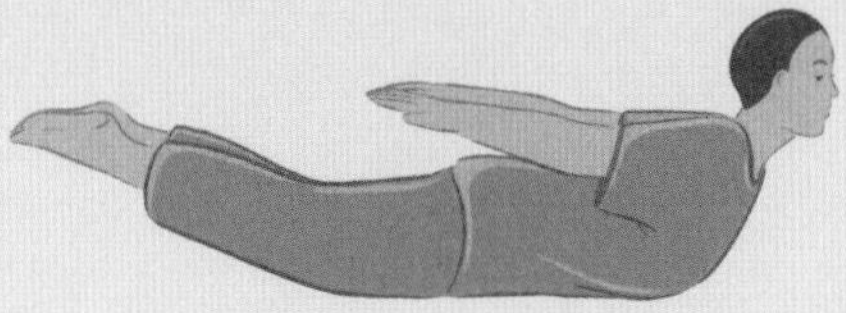

18. LOCUST

Inhale lifting into locust pose.
Hold for 5 breaths.

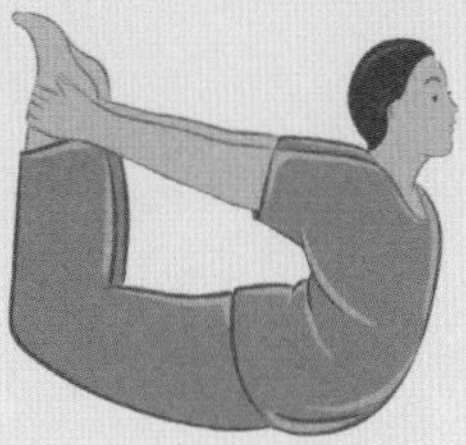

19. BOW POSE

Option to include bow pose
and hold for 5 breaths.

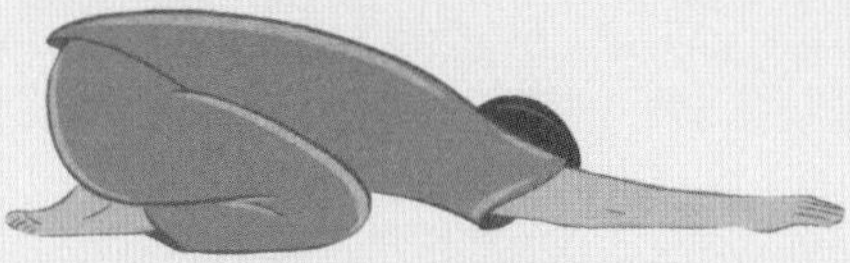

20. CHILD'S POSE

Exhale, melting down into child's pose.
Hold for 5 breaths.

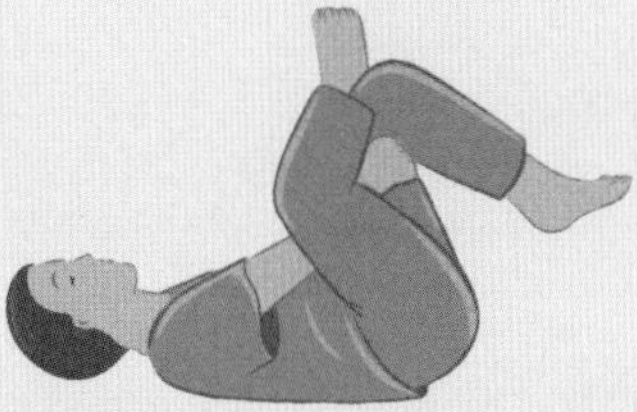

21. RECLINED PIGEON

Coming onto your back, cross the
right foot over the left knee and find
reclined pigeon. Hold for 5 breaths
before repeating on the opposite side.

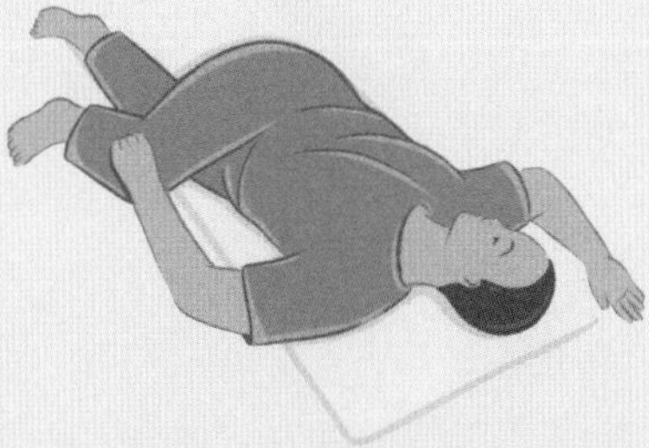

22. SUPINE TWIST

Coming onto your back, hug the right knee in and
come into a supine twist. Hold for 5 breaths before
repeating on the opposite side.

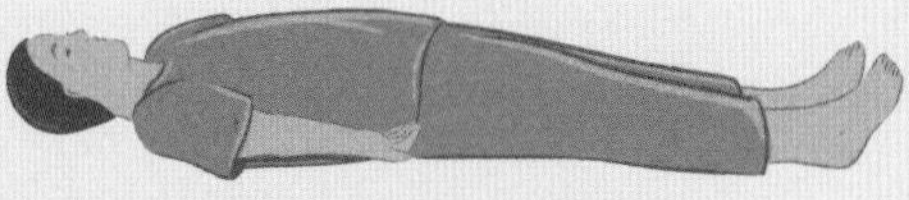

23. SAVASANA

Release and melt into savasana
for 2 minutes or more.

MEDITATION

GRATITUDE MEDITATION

Reflecting the theme of *santosha*, the meditation of the month is a gratitude meditation that will help you foster a sense of appreciation and joy for the life you're living. Research has shown that gratitude meditations can improve mental health by reducing symptoms of anxiety and depression, improving life satisfaction and happiness and boosting resilience and coping skills, among other benefits.

Directions:

1. Come into a comfortable seated position on a chair with an upright spine, somewhere you can be free of distractions.
2. Set a timer for 5 minutes or for as long as you have.
3. Gently close your eyes. If you don't like to close your eyes, you can have them slightly open with the gaze lowered to the floor in front of you to keep your forhead soft.
4. Softly close your lips and let your breath come in through the nose and out through the nose or mouth in its natural rhythm.
5. Before each meditation begins, feel your sitting bones on the chair and your feet on the floor. Imagine roots winding down from these areas, helping you feel secure and grounded.
6. Release control of the breath and bring to mind aspects of your life for which you are grateful. This can be anything from the support of loved ones or moments of joy, to experiences that brought growth or the beauty of nature.
7. As you bring these things to mind, focus on them individually, exploring why you're grateful for them. Consider the feelings associated with these experiences or people and how they have positively impacted your life. Try to recall everything from the sounds, scents, tastes and textures associated with these moments or relationships.
8. Each time your mind starts to wander, gently bring your awareness back to your breath and the present moment.
9. When the timer finishes, sit with your eyes still closed and take a final moment to appreciate the feelings of gratitude you've cultivated. Notice how you feel and any thoughts or feelings that arose.

JOURNAL PROMPTS

Below I have given you eight self-reflection questions linked to this month's cloud theme and the yogic concept of *santosha*. Try answering two questions weekly alongside the daily journal prompts set out on pages 8–9.

- Think about a moment of true happiness where you felt fully content. What were you doing, feeling or experiencing during that time? How can you invite more moments like this into your life?

- Clouds dissipate and change form effortlessly. What worries are you holding onto right now? If you can't do anything to change these worries, can you release any concerns by imagining them drifting away like clouds in the breeze?

- Think about ways in which comparing yourself to others or to societal standards affects your sense of contentment. How can you shift your focus away from comparison and embrace your unique path?

- Clouds will appear different when seen from different viewpoints. Reflect on a situation in which shifting perspective would have changed your understanding. How can you adopt a more flexible perspective going forward?

- As humans we tend to struggle with change and uncertainty. How can you find contentment amid life's inevitable changes and fluctuations?

- Clouds occupy vast spaces in the sky. How can you create space in your life for growth, expansion and new possibilities?

- Think about a challenging experience or setback. How did this moment contribute to your growth and wisdom? How can you find gratitude in the lesson(s) learned?

- Consider areas in your life where you often seek perfection. How does this impact your contentment? How can you embrace imperfection going forwards and find beauty in the imperfect aspects of life?

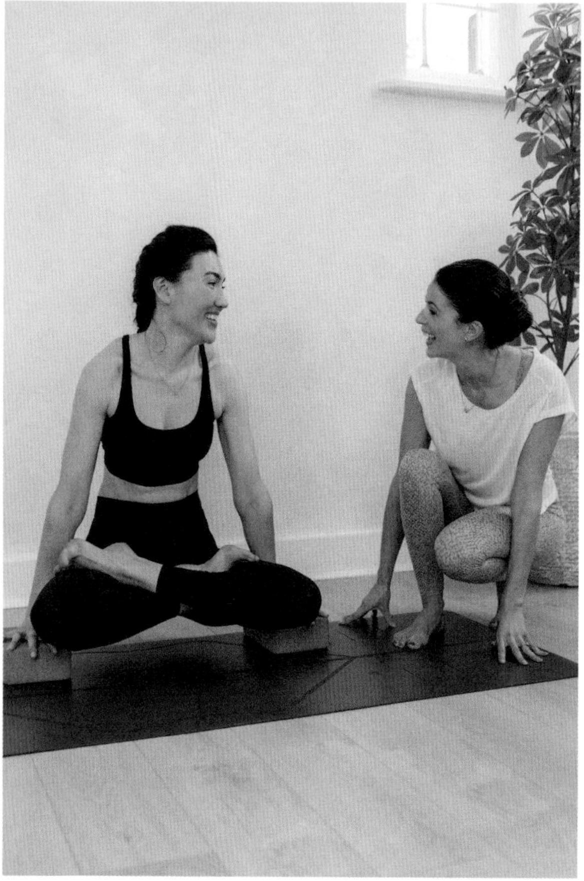
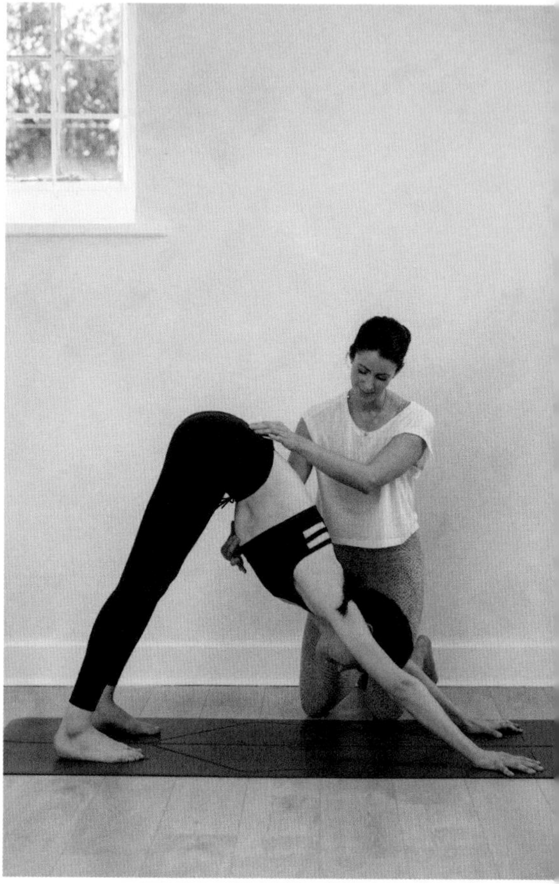
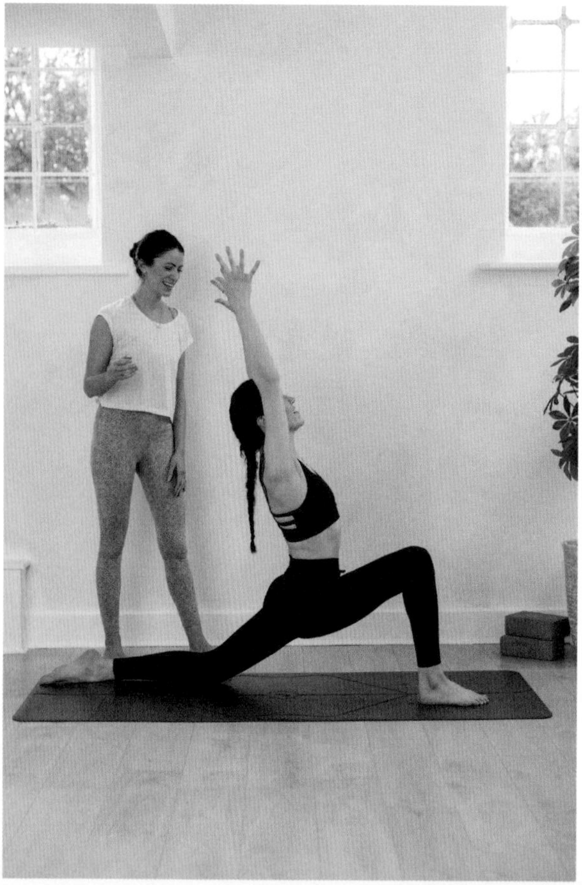
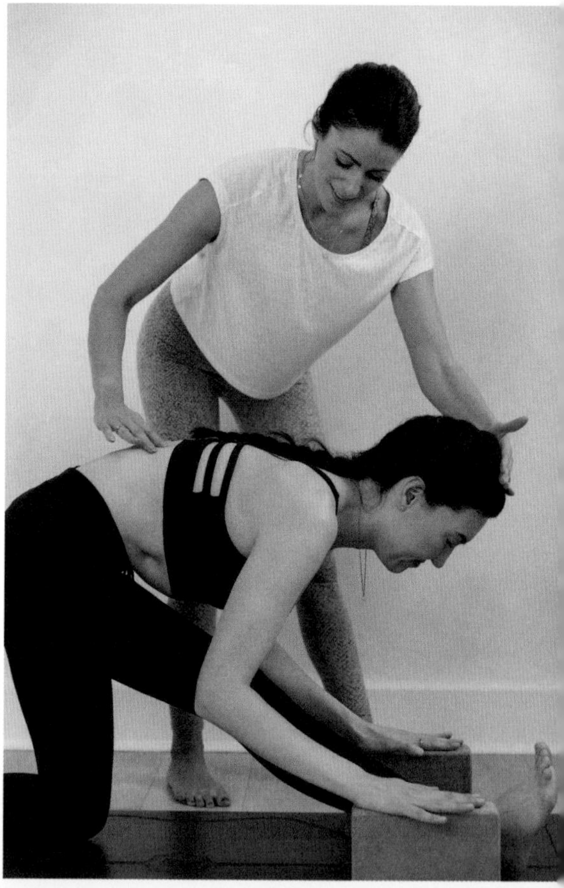

MONTH 8
FIRE

*'THE BEST THING YOU COULD DO
IS MASTER THE CHAOS IN YOU.
YOU ARE NOT THROWN INTO THE FIRE,
YOU ARE THE FIRE.'*

MAMA INDIGO

FIRE

This month is themed around fire and both the signature flow and breathing technique are powerful ones, which we balance with a wonderful meditation called the soft-body meditation. Remember the concept of *sthira-sukha* – the balance of effort and ease – from chapter 4 (see page 72)? It is vital that we cultivate both strength and softness in our yoga journey and listen carefully to what our body needs. If your body requires more restoration, then pick a flow from a previous month or turn to the gentle bedtime flow (see page 13) or seated warm-up flow (see page 10).

We also look at the yogic concept of *tapas* whose root '*tapa*' translates to 'heat' or 'fire'. With *tapas* we practise creating positive change. Think of a yoga pose that you have found challenging to hold so far. Maybe while striving to hold this posture you face physical discomfort, muscle fatigue and mental challenge. The dedication and perseverance required to persist through these difficulties – holding the pose even for a few breaths – represents the principle of *tapas*; embracing the discipline, inner fire and determination needed to overcome obstacles.

As always, a gentle reminder that this is not an invitation to push through pain or to ignore your body's signals that you are trying something you're not ready for. Knowing the difference between *tapas* and pushing yourself past your limits involves mindful awareness. Use your breath as a guide, practise tuning into the sensations and honour your body's limitations.

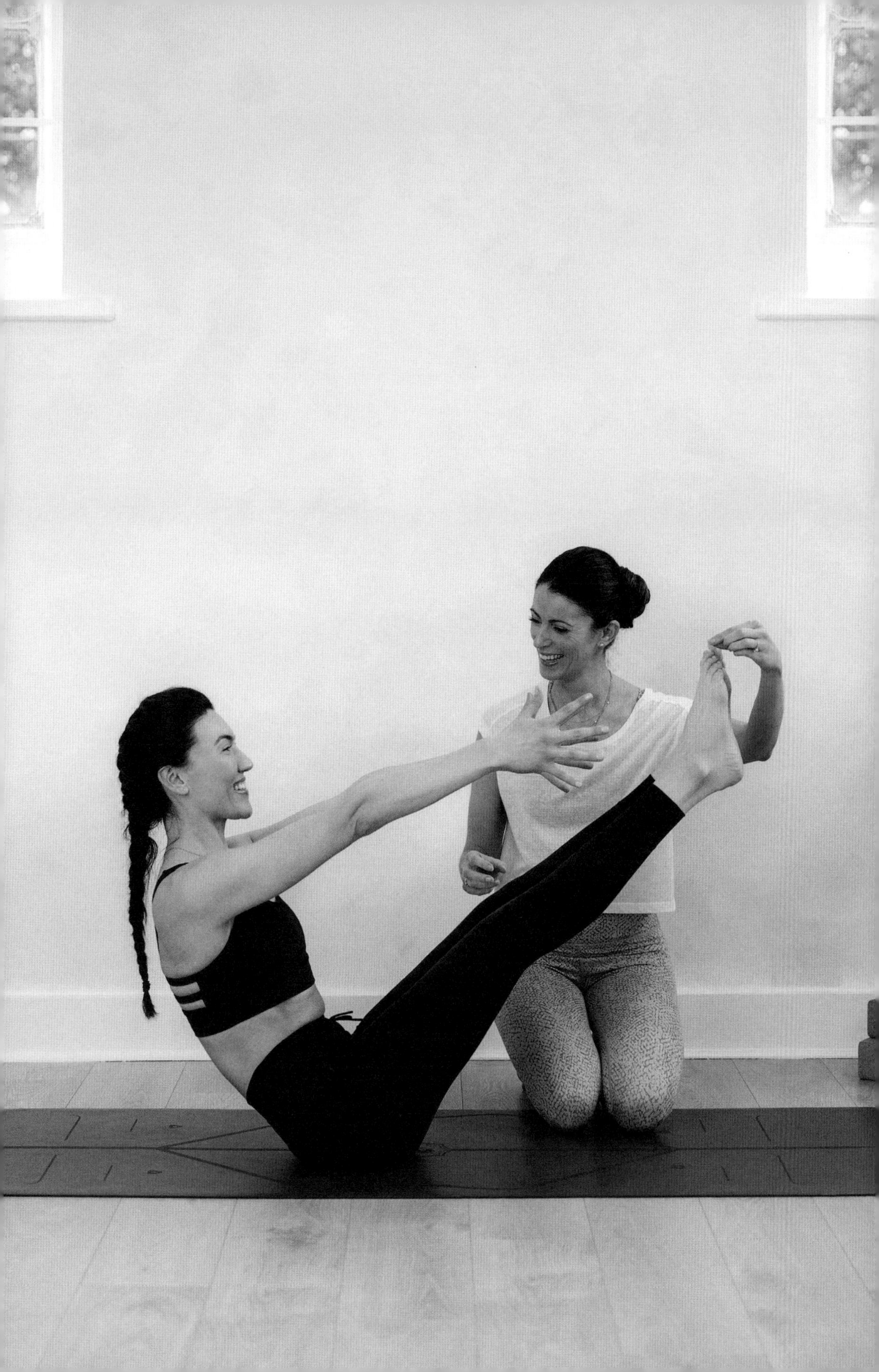

TAPAS (SELF-DISCIPLINE)

DISCIPLINED AND INTENTIONAL EFFORT FUELS PERSONAL GROWTH.

Tapas is the third *niyama* and translates to 'the heat of the practice' or 'self-discipline'. *Tapas* is necessary to 'burn through' negative and unhelpful habits, thoughts and behaviour patterns. It's having the courage to change the things that you can and the dedication and self-discipline to take action towards personal growth. It requires focus and working at the edge of one's comfort zone without pushing towards injury or strain, and it helps us foster resilience, determination and the strength to overcome obstacles.

I have a student whom I have been teaching for many years. She is incredibly strong, but crow pose (*bakasana*, see page 196) became her nemesis. Every time she tried to balance on her hands, she couldn't find the balance point and became frustrated. She didn't give up though and diligently practised techniques to help her conquer the difficult arm balance. One day, while practising, we realised that she was holding her breath every time she tried to balance. She paused, focused on her breath, tried again and she finally achieved a few seconds of balance. Over time my student was able to hold crow pose for longer, feeling a stability she hadn't experienced before – not just physically, she experienced a mental steadiness and focus too.

Tapas isn't just about mastering the pose. It is about the dedication to show up every day, embrace challenges with inner strength and find growth within the process. Progress isn't always linear, it lies in the commitment to keep trying, learning and growing.

Here are some ways we can incorporate *tapas* into our daily lives:

- **On the yoga mat:** Commit to a consistent physical yoga practice. It doesn't need to be daily but work out a schedule that suits you and show up regardless of whether you feel like it, even if it's just 10 minutes. Consistency is the key to cultivating *tapas*.
- **Commitment to goals:** Whatever personal or professional goals you have, stay dedicated and persistent in pursuing them. There are bound to be obstacles along the way, but don't let them get in your way.
- **Learning and growth:** Dedicate time to growth and learning. Expanding your knowledge or developing talents will enable you to grow as a person, look at challenges from different perspectives and make better decisions.
- **Relationships:** Practise *tapas* in your relationships by committing to honest communication, understanding and patience. Practise mindful and active listening – listen fully, don't just listen to speak. Choose your words carefully, being mindful of their impact on the other person.
- **Mindful living:** Dedicate time each day to being fully present, observing your thoughts without attachment, and you will find greater awareness and clarity. Practising meditation and mindfulness are excellent ways to approach mindful living.
- **Time management:** Practise disciplined time management. Organise your schedule, prioritise tasks and stay focused on completing them efficiently (turn off notifications and put your phone away if you need to).

THE BREATH

THE KAPALABHATI BREATH

This month I've chosen a yogic breathing technique that stokes the fire within and is called *kapalabhati,* or skull shining breath. It's an invigorating practice that involves forceful and rapid exhalations alongside a passive inhalation. It typically results in a greater exhalation than normal, so it can be a good breathing technique for people who tend to shallow-breathe.

Kapalabhati generates internal heat and was traditionally used to purify the body and mind while also boosting energy levels and digestion. It helps to strengthen and tone the abdominal muscles and can be a great way to start a dynamic or core-focused practice. The quick activation of the core muscles and compression of the internal organs could have a positive effect on lymph fluid movement and increasing circulation in the abdominal cavity, which may help strengthen the immune system and detoxify the body.

There are a number of contraindications for *kapalabhati* so please note those (see below and right) and if you have any concern about whether this breath is right for you, please speak to your health professional. Some yoga traditions suggest that *kapalabhati* shouldn't be practised during menstruation and others say that it is perfectly fine to do so. I urge you to ask yourself if it is the right technique for you at that time. If the answer is yes, notice how it feels in your body and whether it intensifies any negative symptoms of menstruation.

***Kapalabhati* should not be practised:**

▸ In pregnancy or during menstruation (see note above).

▸ By individuals with high or low blood pressure, heart disease, hernia, gastric ulcer, epilepsy, vertigo, migraine headaches, significant nosebleeds, detached retina, glaucoma, history of stroke, or anyone who has undergone recent abdominal surgery.

▸ If you experience any pain or unusual symptoms with this breathing technique. If this happens, stop immediately.

Directions:

1. Sit in a comfortable seated position with a long spine and take a few slow breaths, tuning in to the breath.
2. Now bring your awareness to the abdominal region. Start to intentionally contract the lower abdominal muscles, pushing the breath out through the nostrils to produce an audible forced and sharp exhale.
3. The emphasis is on the exhalation whereas the inhalation should be passive and automatic. Your abdomen should naturally expand as you inhale. Each active exhale should be vigorous and as short and sharp as possible, the lower abdomen is drawn in as air pushes out. Each inhale is noiseless and effortless as the abdomen relaxes. Aim for an exhalation every 0.5 to 1 seconds.
4. Try 20–50 pumps of air, stop and take three long, slow breaths. Relax the abdominals, watch your breath and tune in to how you feel. When you feel calm, repeat for two more rounds.
5. Afterwards, tune in to all sensations, observing how you are feeling.

WHAT DOES *VINYASA* MEAN?

If you've been to a yoga class before, you may have heard the word *vinyasa*. It means 'to place in a special way' and in the context of *asana* it means, 'linking the postures with the breath'.

However, over the years, the word '*vinyasa*' has been transformed to mean the specific sequence of poses – plank, exhale yoga push-up (*chaturanga*), inhale upward-facing dog and exhale downward-facing dog. You may recognise this from traditional sun salutations (*surya namaskar*, see pages 16–20).

This transformation of the word *vinyasa* to mean the sequence above can be useful to create a more dynamic practice. Adding '*vinyasas*' (*chaturanga* to upward-facing dog to downward-facing dog) between pose sequences can add heat and power and help you build strength and endurance.

Here are three other ways to create more fire and heat in your practice using the idea of a '*vinyasa*':

1. Plank to yoga push-up to upward-facing dog to yoga push-up to downward-facing dog.
2. Three yoga push-ups to upward-facing dog to downward-facing dog.
3. Hold yoga push-up for three breaths to upward-facing dog to downward-facing dog.

If you have more energy and want to add extra spice to your practice, add one or more of these *vinyasa* options between sequences or wherever you feel like it would add value. For this month's flow I have highlighted places where they could be included. Remember to listen to your body and know when this option feels right for you.

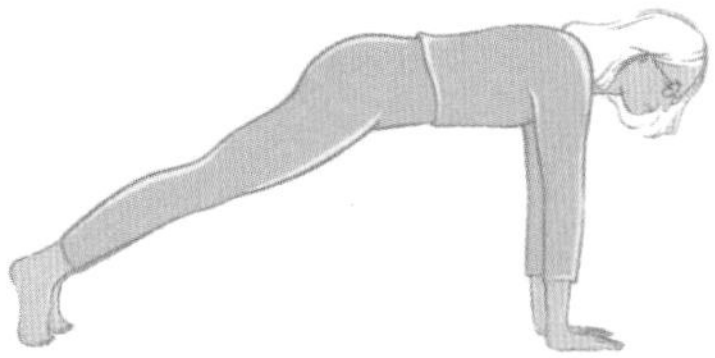

PLANK POSE

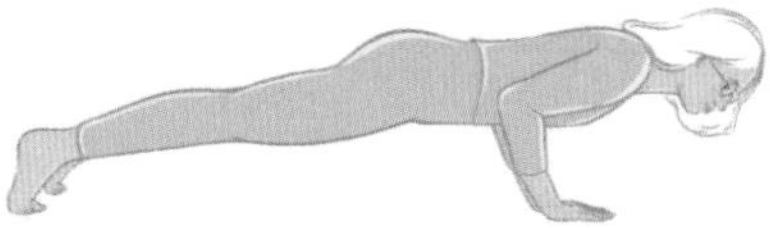

YOGA PUSH-UP

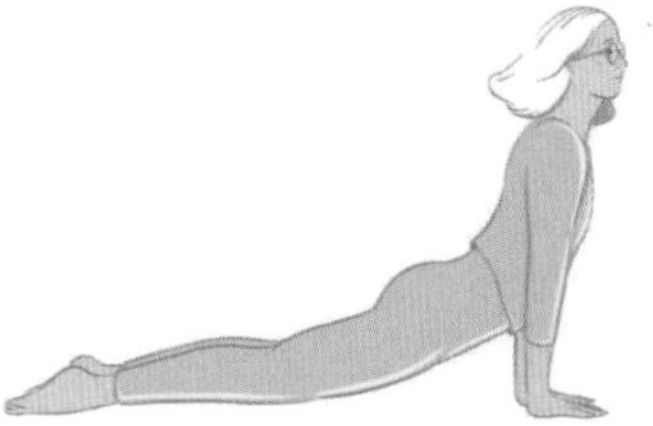

UPWARD-FACING DOG

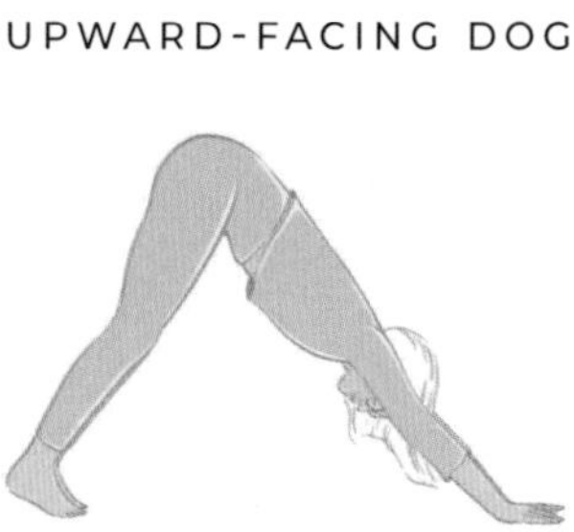

DOWNWARD-FACING DOG

THE FIRE FLOW

The signature flow this month is most definitely fiery. It plays with the theme of fire and as set out on the left, you can add additional *vinyasas* or even sun salutations (see pages 16–20) for extra heat and intensity. Tune in to how the flow feels and use your breath and the sensations within your body as a guide to whether you need more effort or in fact more ease.

This month I introduce our first arm balance of this program: scale pose (*tolasana*). This pose is a helpful arm balance to start with as there is little fear of falling (as there might be in crow pose, *bakasana*). Scale pose will help to strengthen your wrists, arms, shoulder girdle and will fire up your core.

Traditionally this pose is performed with the legs in lotus position, but for many, this isn't an accessible posture (me included). I suggest you either sit in half lotus, if this feels ok with your body, or simply with crossed legs (see page 211). A variation that is extremely helpful for this pose is to place your hands on blocks as this will give you more space to lift your body. Remember that this is an advanced posture and body proportions can make it easier or harder (long arms and a short torso will make this easier than someone with short arms and a long torso). If the pose seems inaccessible to you or causes pain, skip it and come back to it again at a later date.

Aim to practise this flow three or four times per week and if you have more time, feel free to include the seated warm-up flow on page 10 at the start, combine it with the previous months' flows or repeat the flow multiple times.

As you move around your yoga mat, bring some fire qualities with you:

- **Ignite your inner strength:** Mirror the power of fire in poses that build physical strength, such as boat pose and the warriors, and use it to connect with your inner strength and determination.
- **Creating heat:** We have already discussed how fire generates heat, representing purification and transformation. If it feels right for your body, add dynamic sequences like the sun salutations (see pages 16–20) and additional vinyasas into this month's signature sequence to generate more internal heat and invigorate your practice further.
- **Passion and energy:** Allow your heart's energy to radiate like flames by bringing passion and enthusiasm into your practice. How can you find more joy in each posture, what tweaks can you make to the flow to bring more passion?

PLEASE NOTE
The appendix on page 190 includes a detailed breakdown of each pose, plus variations and modifications. Remember to listen to your body; yoga should never be painful and you can chose to skip any pose that doesn't feel right for you.

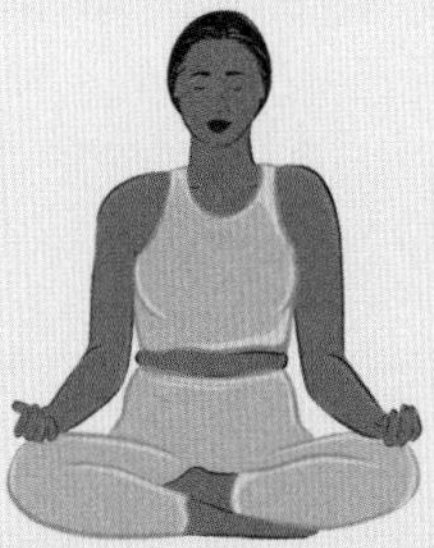

1. SEATED THREE-PART BREATH OR KAPALABHATI

In a seated position, take 10 rounds of the three-part breath (see page 31) or 2–3 rounds of *kapalabhat*i (see page 129).

BEGIN WRIST SEQUENCE

See page 221.

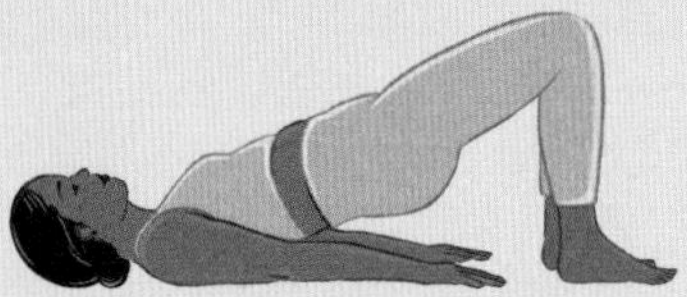

2. BRIDGE

Releasing onto the floor, exhale lifting up into bridge and hold for 5 breaths.

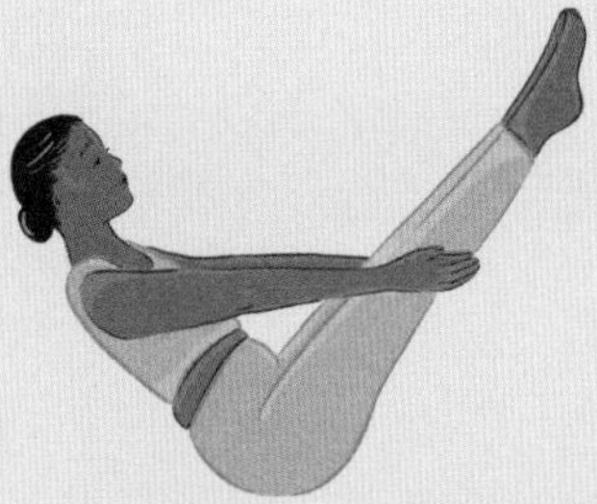

3. BOAT POSE

Come up to sit on the mat. Exhale as you lift into boat pose. Hold for 3 breaths.

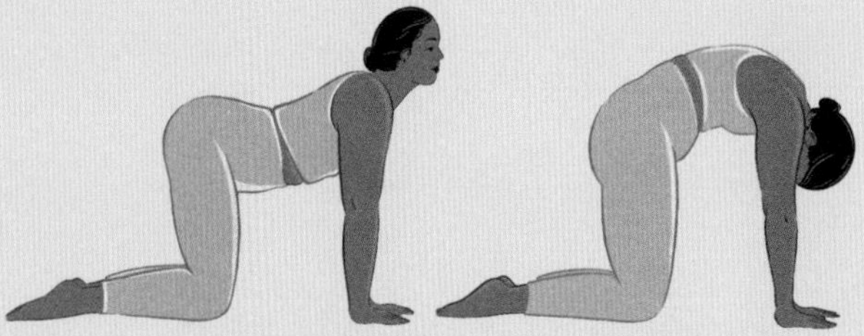

4. CAT AND COW

Coming onto all fours, inhale into cow pose and exhale into cat pose. Repeat 5 times. Option to tuck the toes and hover the knees off the floor.

VINYASA

SUN SALUTATIONS A & B

Option to include a vinyasa (see page 130) and/or sun salutations A and B (see pages 16–20).

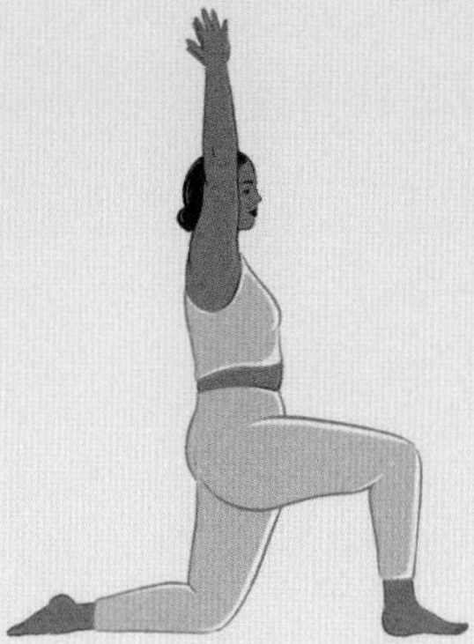

5. LOW LUNGE

Inhale with the right foot forwards into low lunge.

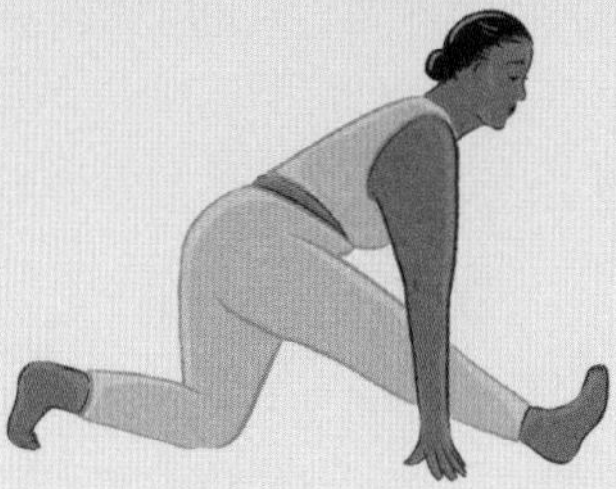

6. HALF SPLIT

Exhale and release to half splits.

REPEAT 5 TIMES

STEPS 5 AND 6

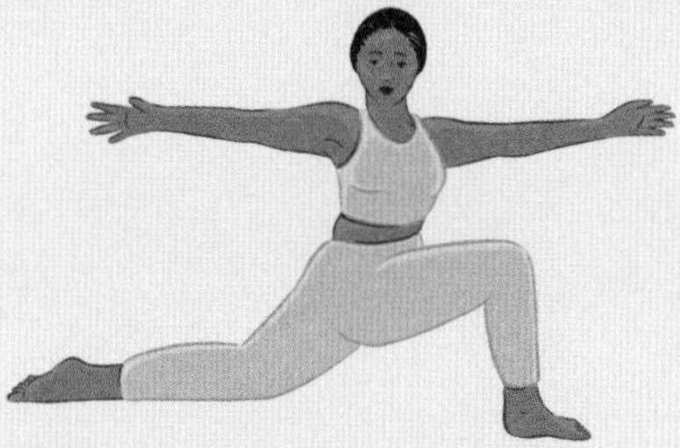

7. LOW LUNGE TWIST

Inhale into low lunge and exhale to find your twist. Hold for 5 breaths.

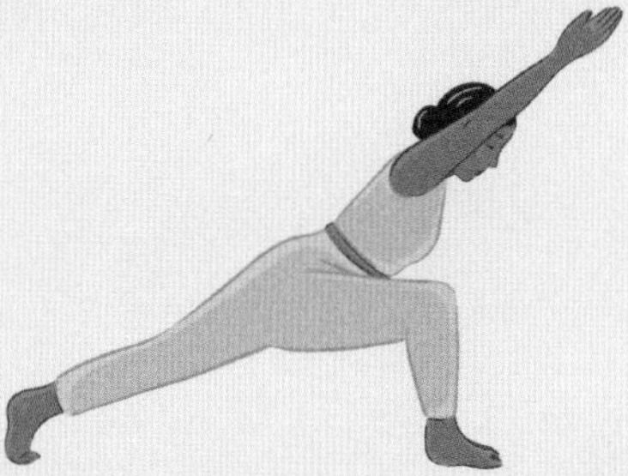

8. HINGED HIGH LUNGE HOLD

Inhale lifting in high lunge and exhale hinging forwards. Hold for 5 breaths.

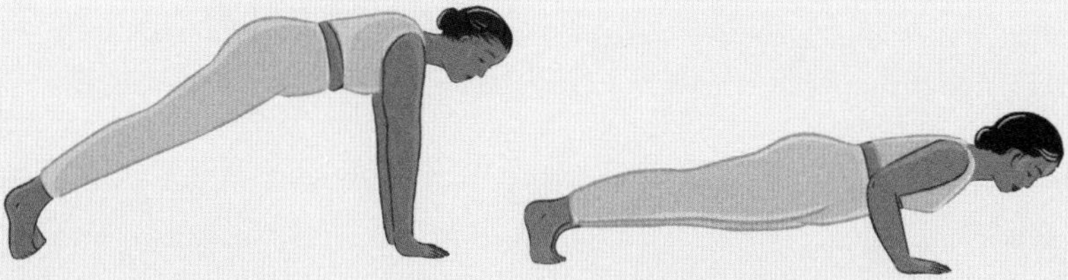

9. YOGA PUSH-UP

From plank pose, exhale into yoga push-up and inhale back to plank. Repeat 5 times.

VINYASA

Option to include a vinyasa (see page 130).

REPEAT ON THE LEFT SIDE

STEPS 5–9

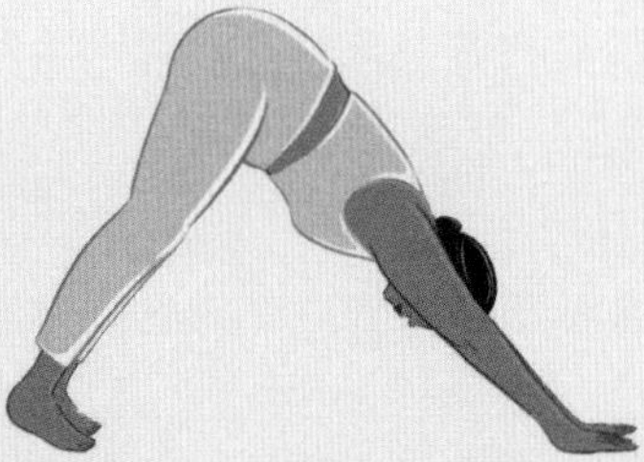

10. DOWNWARD-FACING DOG

Exhale lifting the hips into downward-facing dog and hold for 5 breaths.

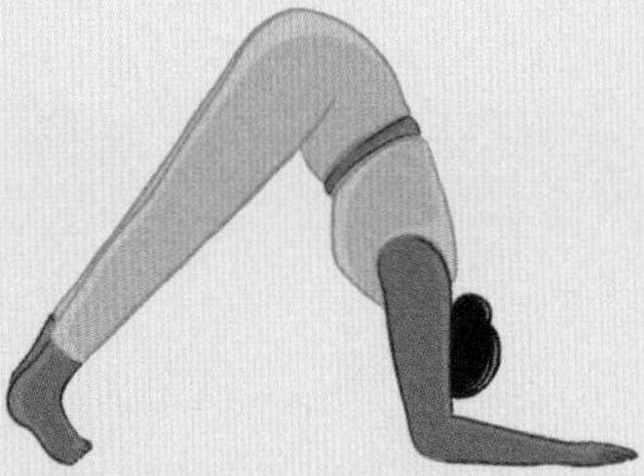

11. DOLPHIN

Release the forearms down to the ground keeping the hips lifted high. Hold for 5 breaths.

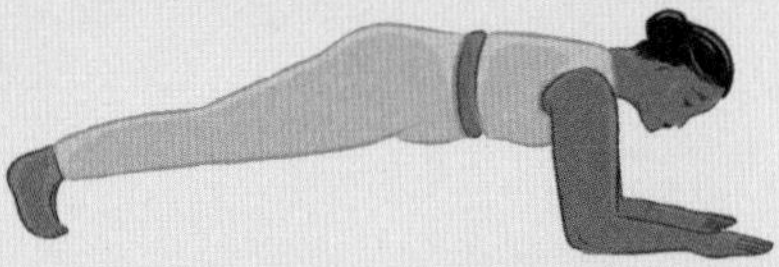

12. FOREARM PLANK

Exhale and step the feet back into forearm plank. Hold for 5 breaths.

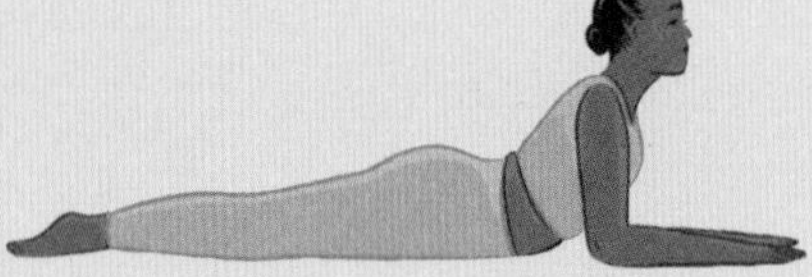

13. SPHINX

Exhale and lower the hips to the floor finding sphinx pose. Hold for 5 breaths.

VINYASA

Option to return to downward-facing dog and include a vinyasa (see page 130).

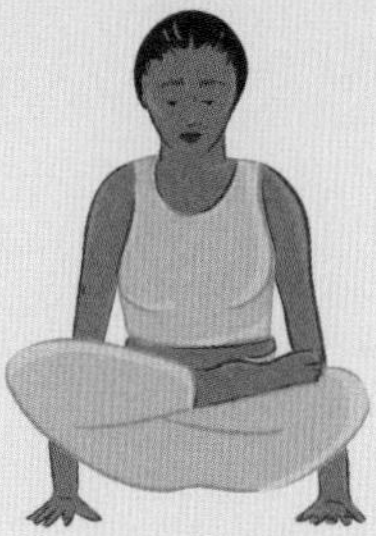

14. SCALE POSE

Coming to a seated position. Exhale as you lift into scale pose. Hold for 1–5 breaths.

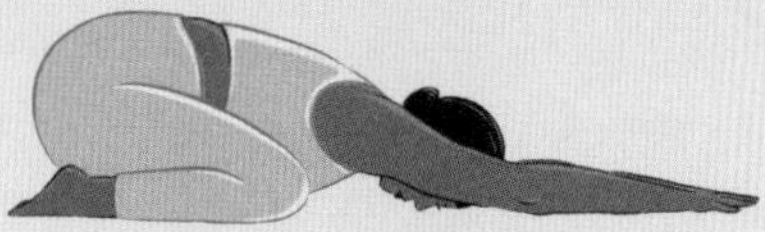

15. CHILD'S POSE

Exhale, melting down into child's pose. Hold for 3 breaths.

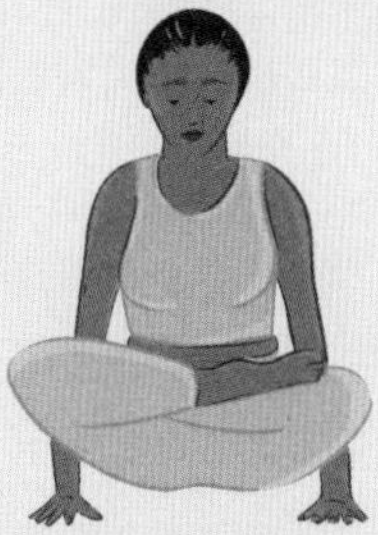

16. SCALE POSE

Option to repeat scale pose for a further 1–5 breaths.

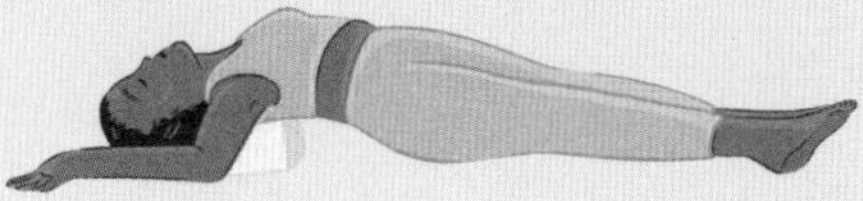

17. RESTORATIVE FISH POSE

Placing a block or cushion under the thoracic spine, melt over the prop and release. Hold for 10 breaths.

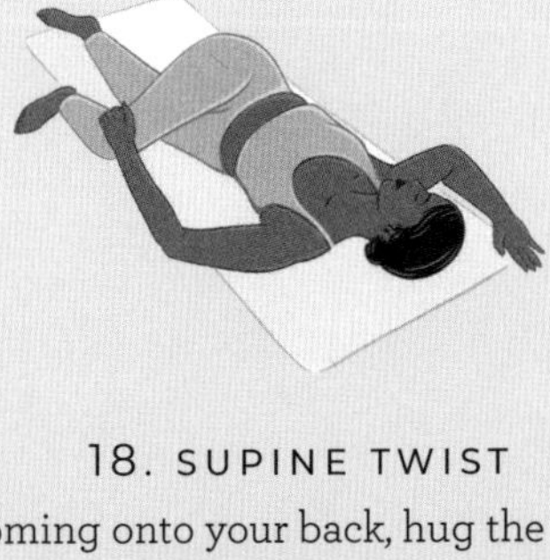

18. SUPINE TWIST

Coming onto your back, hug the right knee in and come into a supine twist. Hold for 5 breaths before repeating on the opposite side.

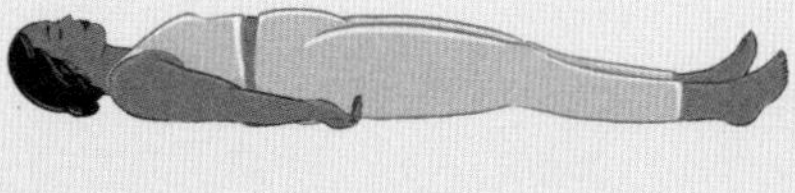

19. SAVASANA

Come back to centre and melt into savasana for 2 minutes or more.

MEDITATION

SOFT BELLY MEDITATION

With so much fire in our practice this month we need to balance it with some softness, so, the meditation I am sharing is one that I call the soft belly meditation. The idea is we start by softening the belly (an area which often holds tension) and then spread that softness through the body. It aims to release tension and promote relaxation and it's a meditation I come back to often.

Directions:

1. Come into a comfortable seated position on a chair with an upright spine, somewhere you can be free from distractions.
2. Set a timer for 5 minutes or for as long as you have.
3. Gently close your eyes. If you don't like to close your eyes, you can have the eyes slightly open with the gaze lowered to the floor in front of you to keep your forehead soft.
4. Softly close your lips and let your breath come in through the nose and out through the nose or mouth in its natural rhythm.
5. Before each meditation begins, feel your sitting bones on the chair and your feet on the floor. Imagine roots winding down from these areas, helping you feel secure and grounded.
6. Now bring your attention to your abdomen. Visualise and feel your belly softening with each out breath. Release all control or hold on this area and imagine each breath massaging any tension away. You can even think the word 'soft' as you inhale, 'belly' as you exhale.
7. Take a slow, mental scan of your body from the toes all the way up to the crown of your head. With each exhale, soften any tension or tightness you are holding.
8. Keep your focus on the breath and the softening sensations. Each time your mind starts to wander, gently bring your awareness back to your belly and the soft breath.
9. When the timer finishes, take a moment with the eyes still closed to sit and notice how you feel and any thoughts or feelings that arose.

JOURNAL PROMPTS

Below I have given you eight self-reflection questions linked to this month's fire theme and the yogic concept of *tapas*. Try answering two questions weekly alongside the daily journal prompts set out on pags 8–9.

- Think about a time when your commitment to a goal ignited a sense of inner fire. How did discipline shape your journey and what did you learn about yourself along the way?

- Reflect on a challenge you're facing at the moment. Can you harness the metaphorical energy of fire and burn away limitations to move forward?

- Write down the daily habits you want in your life. In which of these do you already demonstrate discipline consistently? How could you introduce more discipline to align with your other daily habit goals?

- In what ways can you release negative emotions or old patterns of thinking, symbolically burning them away like fuel for the fire?

- What distractions or habits hinder your discipline? What steps can you take to get rid of these distractions?

- Reflect on a time when you felt afraid to make changes or take a risk. How can you overcome these fears and embrace transformation in the future?

- Write down an example of how discipline has contributed to your achievements in the past. Take time to celebrate the progress made.

- Fire can symbolise both passion and destruction. How can you balance passionate pursuits with responsible and ethical behaviour in your actions?

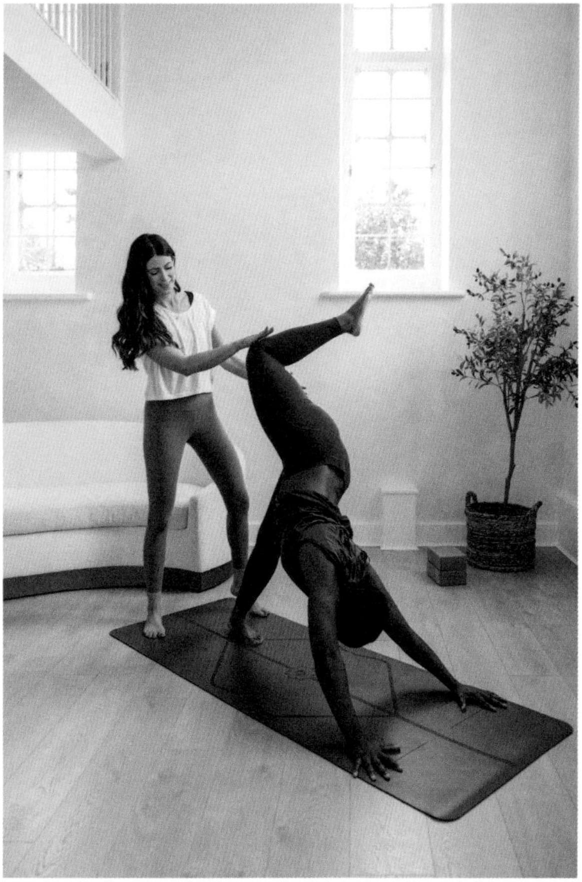
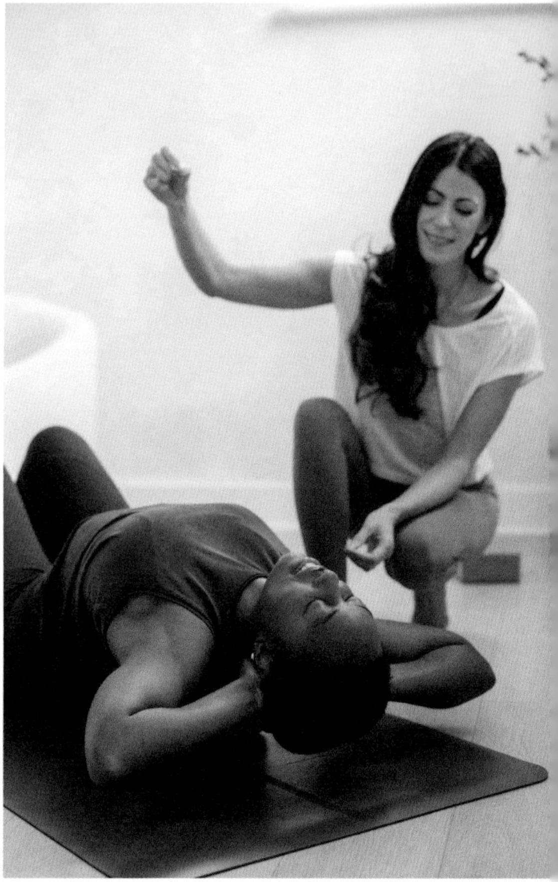
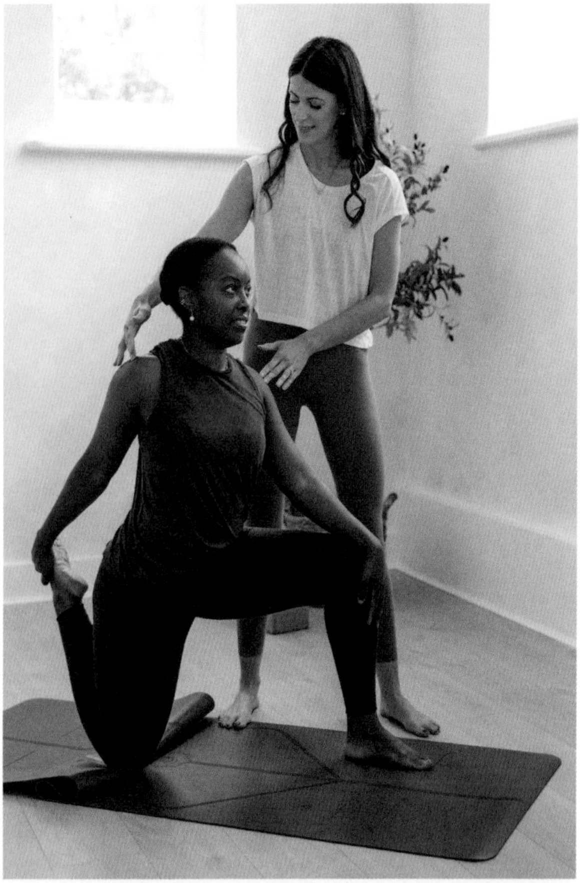
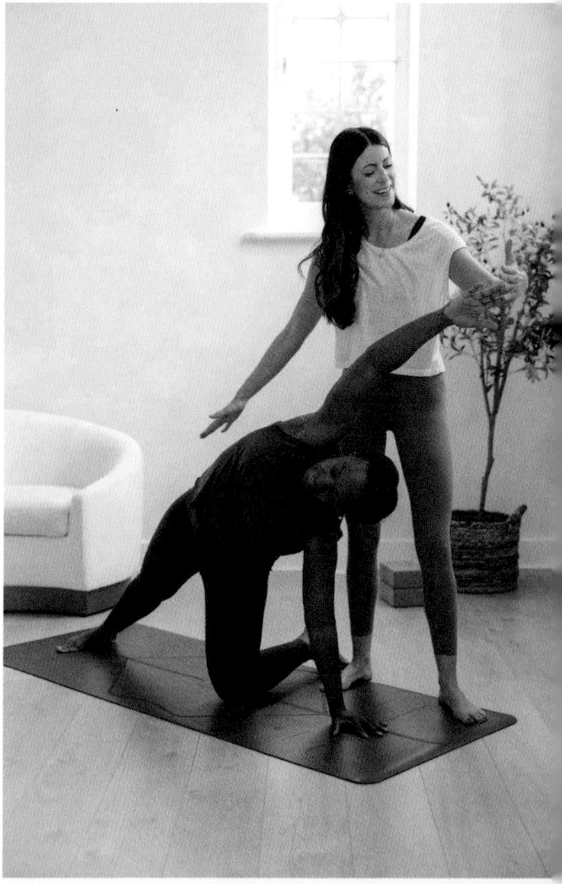

MONTH 9
WILD HEART

'HER HEART WAS WILD,
BUT I DIDN'T WANT TO CATCH IT,
I WANTED TO RUN WITH IT,
TO SET MINE FREE.'

ATTICUS

WILD HEART

A wild heart symbolises a temperament that is untamed and free. We all have an element of a wild heart within us. It embodies a sense of passion, adventure and authenticity and this month we are going to unleash our wild hearts with a yoga flow building towards the pose wild thing. This posture can be used to explore our constraints and limitations and the act of flipping over into it can be a metaphor for breaking free from these self-imposed restrictions. Consider what fears or self-doubts may be holding you back and journey inward in pursuit of courage and connection.

The concept of connection is such a fundamental part of a yoga practice. Internally, it is a pathway for self-discovery, presence and it acts as a bridge between the physical and mental realms. Externally, it helps us recognise the connected nature of all beings and the universe, promoting compassion, empathy and a sense of unity with others.

The heart-opening signature flow is a chance for you to tune in to how you are feeling at this point. What has become easier? What are you shying away from? Consider what fears or self-doubts may be holding you back and journey inward in pursuit of courage and connection. For the parts that you're shying away from, ask yourself why. If it's because they are postures you believe are too challenging, can you find a variation that will help you move forward? (The appendix on page 190 can help.) If you're struggling with the silent practices, can you approach them with an open mind rather than perfection? On some days our minds may wander a lot more than on other days and that's okay – we're not striving for perfection; having the consistency in the practice is what will enable us to reap its long-term benefits. It's also normal to be fearful of journaling and self-reflection as it can make us feel vulnerable and explore emotions that might be painful. Jump into this month's self-study with an open and wild heart and see where it takes you.

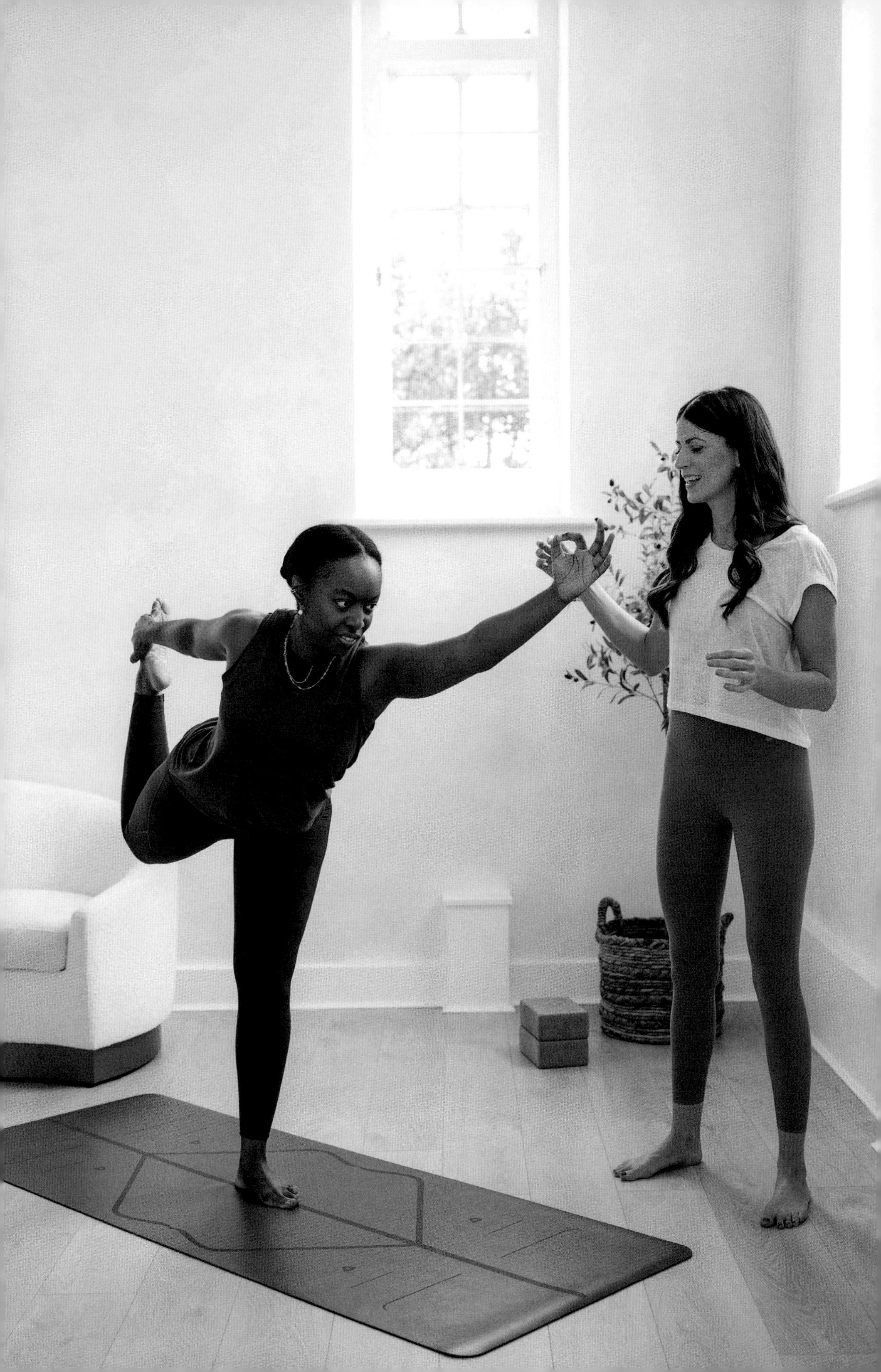

SVADHYAYA (SELF-STUDY)

EXPLORATION AND UNDERSTANDING THROUGH REFLECTION, OBSERVATION AND INTROSPECTION.

The yogic concept we are exploring this month will help you to understand why journaling has been such a key part of your Yoga Happy year. The fourth *niyama* is *svadhyaya,* which translates to 'self-study' or 'self-enquiry'. It's the practice of tuning inwards to explore and reflect deeply on your practice, thoughts, beliefs and behaviour. It's a fundamental aspect of personal growth and self-awareness within yogic philosophy.

Svadhyaya is also about analysing anything that elevates our mind and brings us to our true self. Therefore, it's the study of sacred scriptures and texts to gain insight into one's inner nature and spiritual growth (for example, *The Yoga Sutras of Patañjali, The Hatha Yoga Pradipika* and *The Upanishads*).

Svadhyaya also encompasses the repetition and study of mantras, which were traditionally chosen for you by your teacher. Mantras can be sacred sounds, words or phrases. They are believed to create a sense of balance and harmony as they carry vibrations that resonate in the body and positively impact it, as well as the mind and our energy systems. They have been an integral part of yogic traditions for centuries. Repeating a mantra is a way to anchor the mind to one thought and draw our attention inwards. In chapter 2 we explored a mantra meditation technique (see page 50).

Here are some ways can we incorporate *svadhyaya* into our daily lives:

▸ **On the yoga mat:** Practising *svadhyaya* involves integrating mindfulness, introspection and self-awareness. One way that this can be achieved is through breath observation, noticing how it changes with different poses and movements, helping you create a deeper connection between breath and body. Another way is to begin each practice with an intention or a focus for self-study. This could be something as simple as staying in the moment or an intention of strength.

▸ **Journaling:** Dedicate time to jotting down thoughts, feelings and intentions. Reflect on what is going on in your life. Throughout this book I help you create a journaling habit that will support the concept of self-study.

▸ **Contemplative practices:** Set aside time to read inspirational or philosophical texts. I am not suggesting you inhale as many texts as possible, but instead study them properly and understand them. Reflect on passages that resonate with you and those that don't. Notice what meaning or connection these may have to your life.

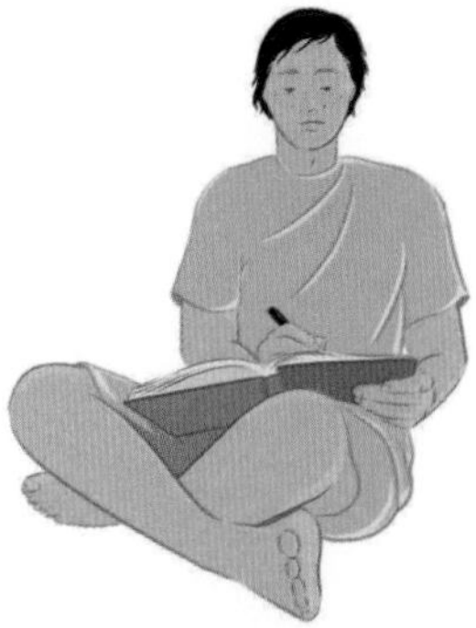

▸ **Evening reflection:** you can do this via journaling. Taking time before bed to look back on your day, any challenges you faced, your actions, interactions and reactions, as well as what you've learned and what went well that day. It can be a really helpful self-study exercise. For example, if a challenge or perhaps a reaction to an event keeps recurring, it's something you know you can focus your attention on addressing.

▸ **Self-expression:** dedicate time to creative pursuits like painting, dancing or any form of self-expression. Notice how these activities make you feel and what they reveal about yourself.

▸ **Feedback:** Reflect on feedback received by others and perhaps even seek it out. Think of constructive criticism as an opportunity for self-improvement and reflection.

THE BREATH

THE 2:1 BREATH

This month we are going to practise the 2:1 breathing technique that some also refer to as 'ratio breathing'. It's a simple breathing exercise that involves extending the exhalation to double the length of the inhalation. It's a method to promote relaxation, calm the nervous system and reduce stress. This breathing technique can help to quieten the noise of life and allow you to connect to your wild heart.

Directions:

1. Come into a comfortable seated position, growing tall through the crown of the head and allowing the spine to be neutral and long.
2. Take a few slow breaths, tuning in and observing the body and mind.
3. Inhale softly and slowly through the nose for a count of four and exhale softly and slowly through the nose for a count of eight.
4. You can increase or decrease the length of the inhale and exhale to suit you, as long as the exhale is double the length of the inhale.
5. Repeat for 10–12 rounds or more.

THE WILD HEART FLOW

In this month's signature flow we open our hearts and find freedom in the body. Weave into each practice the concept of *svadhyaya*, or self-study. What are you feeling in these postures? What do you need to focus on more to find space and ease in your backbends? Lots of the time people think back-bending postures are just about flexibility but we must have strength too.

We delve deeper into back-bending poses this month as we explore dancer pose and wild thing.

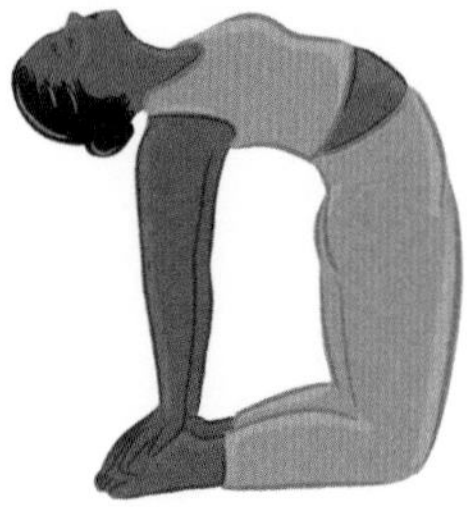

Here are some tips that may help you find comfort and freedom in your back-bending postures:

1. **Spinal extension:** With all backbends think about finding as much length through the spine as possible. Imagine someone is drawing the crown of your head upwards by a piece of string, away from the tailbone to lengthen the spine. This will help you avoid hinging only in certain points of the spine, such as the lower back or lumbar spine.
2. **Watch the neck:** Instead of allowing the neck to drop back, which can cause hyperextension of the cervical spine, slightly nod the chin down to engage the deep neck flexors. This should help you make the curve of the spine more uniform, forming it less from the cervical spine (the neck) and more from the thoracic spine (the upper back).
3. **Engage the glutes:** Our gluteus maximus (the biggest butt muscle) is a hip extender and helps to stabilise the pelvis and spine. In backbends we want both hip extension and stabilisation, so gently squeeze the glutes.
4. **Imagine a piece of string:** That string is attached to the middle of your chest and it is pulling you up towards the ceiling and allowing you to breathe fully and freely as you keep the spine long.

5. **Use your breath as a guide:** Aim for a smooth, even breath in back-bending postures. If the breath becomes restricted, that is your message to gently ease out slightly to help you find more space.
6. **Listen to your body:** I've said this many times already but please remember that all bodies are different. Be mindful of your body's signals and respect its limitations. If you feel pain or discomfort beyond the normal stretching sensation, ease out of the pose or modify it accordingly (further guidance in the appendix on page 190). Also notice how you feel after the practice to help inform how you may modify or progress a pose next time.
7. **Balance strength and flexibility:** Backbends are not just about flexibility. Take dancer pose as an example; you need strength and stability in the core and standing leg to keep you balanced, as well as strength in the back to create the arch in the spine and hold it. Alongside this you need flexibility in the quadriceps and hip flexors of the lifted leg and in the shoulders, chest and abdomen to allow the front body to open.

Aim to practise this flow 3–4 times per week and if you have more time, feel free to include the seated warm-up flow on page 10 at the start, combine it with the previous months' flows or repeat the flow multiple times.

As you move around your yoga mat, bring some wild-heart-themed qualities with you:

▸ **Courage:** Your wild heart is unafraid of embracing the unknown and stepping beyond your comfort zones. This doesn't mean pushing yourself into something you're not ready for but trying something new with an open and curious mind.

▸ **Creative:** Explore postures in your own unique way, finding creativity and self-expression within each pose. Maybe it's an arm circle in side plank or a cat and cow type of flow in low lunge – connect with what feels good for you and your body in that moment. And remember that variations and modifications are always available for every posture, empowering you to find what feels authentic and freeing for your body.

▸ **Breathe for freedom:** The breath is a source of freedom and liberation. Slow, expansive breaths on the yoga mat will allow you to connect with your inner wildness, finding freedom in each inhale and release in each exhale.

PLEASE NOTE

The appendix on page 190 includes a detailed breakdown of each pose, plus variations and modifications. Remember to listen to your body; yoga should never be painful and you can chose to skip any pose that doesn't feel right for you.

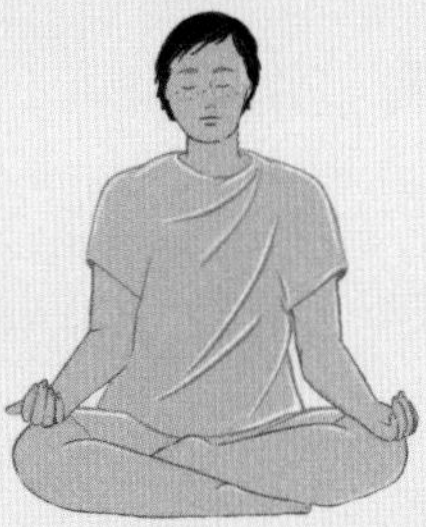

1. SEATED 2:1 BREATHING

In a seated position, take 10 rounds of 2:1 breathing (see page 143).

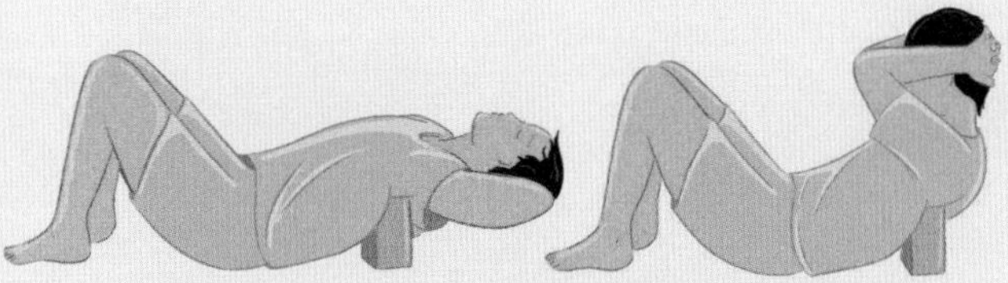

2. RESTORATIVE FISH CAT AND COW

From restorative fish pose, hands interlaced behind head, inhale to open the chest, then exhale to gently round. Repeat 5 times.

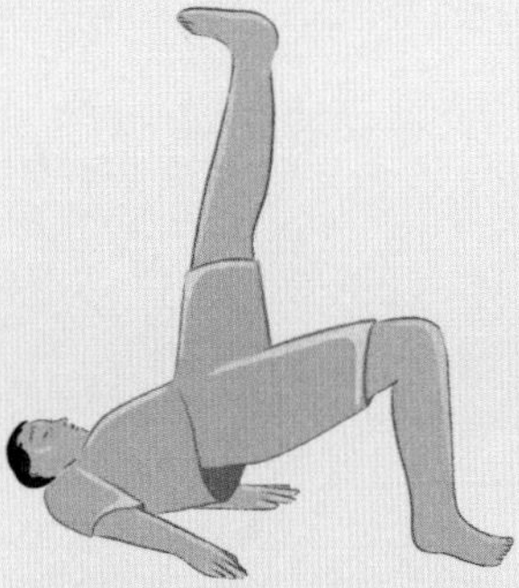

3. BRIDGE ONE LEGGED LIFTS

From a lying down position, place the right foot onto the floor and lift the left leg to the sky. Exhale to lift the hips into bridge and inhale to lower. Repeat 10 times on both sides.

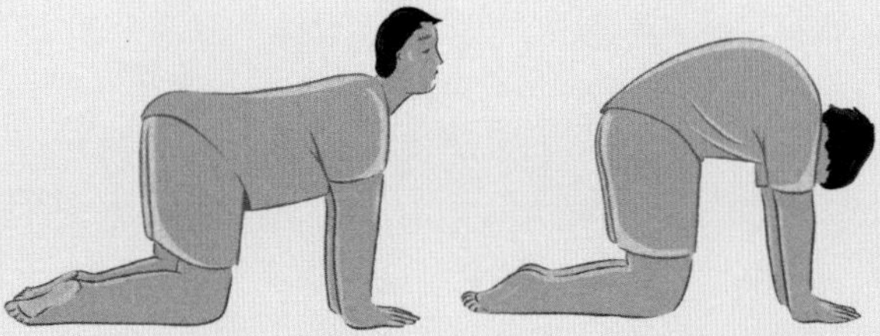

4. CAT AND COW

Coming onto all fours, inhale into cow pose and exhale into cat pose. Repeat 5 times.

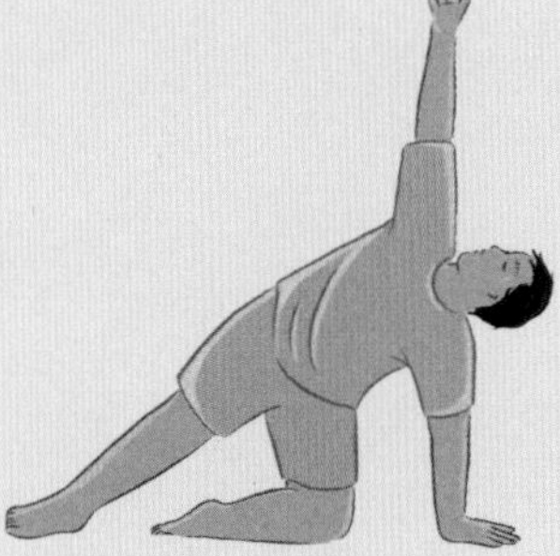

5. SIDE PLANK KNEE DOWN

Opening the body to the right, lifting the right fingertips to the sky. Hold for 5 breaths.

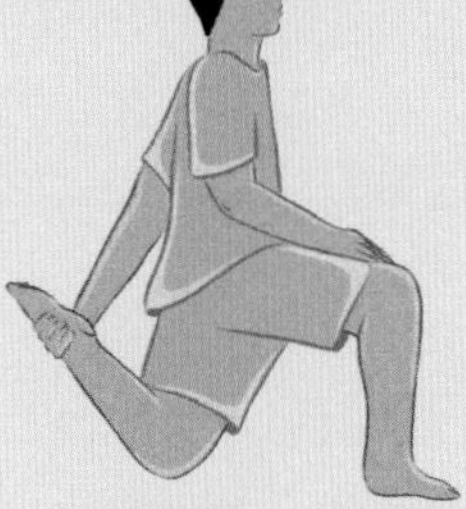

6. LOW LUNGE QUAD STRETCH

Step the right foot forward and find a low lunge quad stretch. Hold for 5 breaths.

REPEAT ON THE LEFT SIDE

STEPS 5 AND 6

SUN SALUTATIONS A & B

Option to include sun salutations A and B (see pages 16–20).

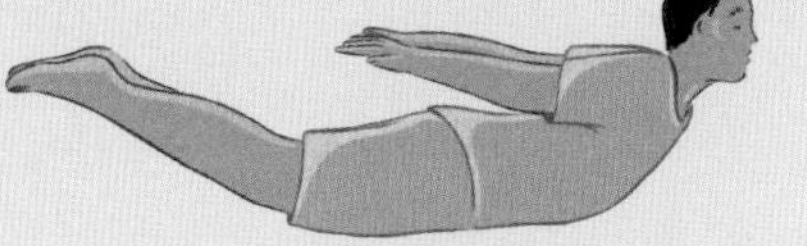

7. LOCUST

Coming onto the belly, inhale and lift into locust pose. Hold for 5 breaths.

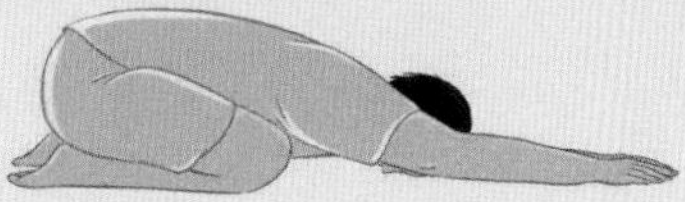

8. CHILD'S POSE

Exhale, pushing the hips back and melting into child's pose. Hold for 5 breaths.

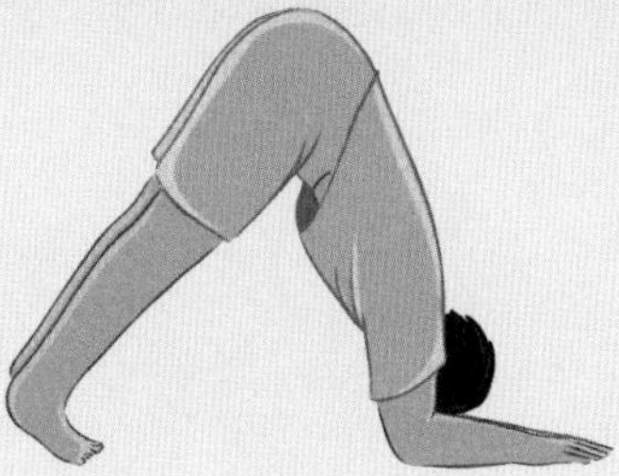

9. DOLPHIN

Coming to tabletop, release the forearms down to the ground and lift the hips to the sky. Hold for 5 breaths.

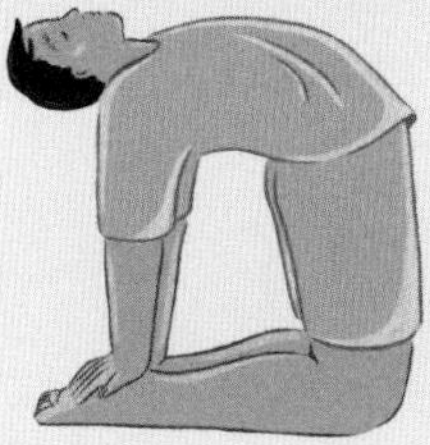

10. CAMEL

Coming onto the knees, inhale and lift the chest into camel pose. Hold for 3–5 breaths.

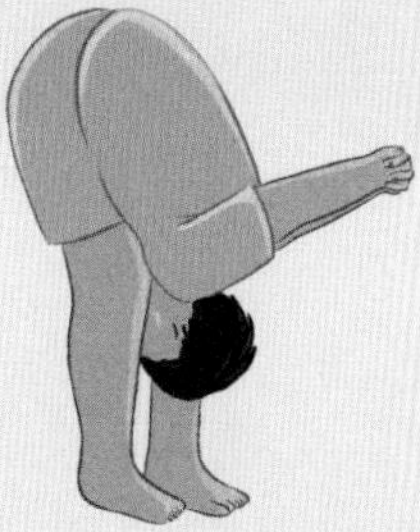

11. STANDING FORWARD BEND WITH LOCK

Coming to stand, exhale and fold forward interlacing the hands behind the back. Hold for 5 breaths.

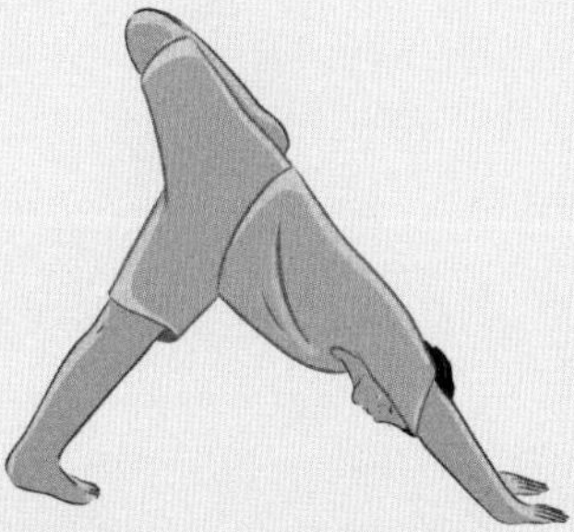

12. DOWNWARD-FACING DOG HIP OPENER

Exhale, releasing the hands and stepping to downward-facing dog. Reach the right leg up and back and bend the knee to open the hip. Hold for 5 breaths.

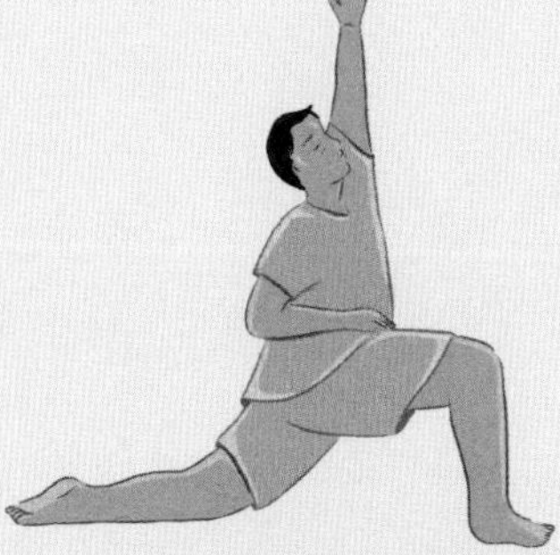

13. LOW LUNGE SIDE STRETCH

Step the right foot forward, inhale the left fingers to the sky and exhale taking a side stretch to the right. Hold for 5 breaths.

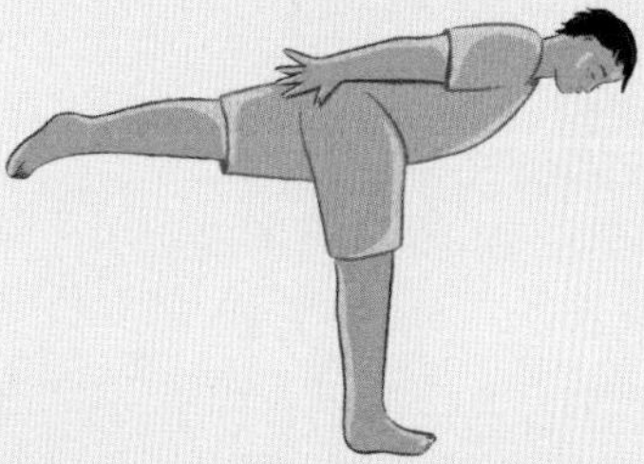

14. WARRIOR III

Lift into high lunge, exhale shifting the weight forwards lifting into warrior III. Hold for 3 breaths.

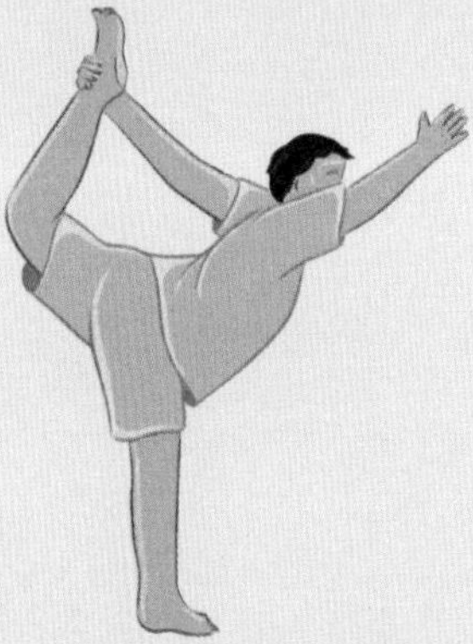

15. DANCER

Inhale to stand, take hold of the left foot behind you with the left hand and exhale to dancer. Hold for 5 breaths.

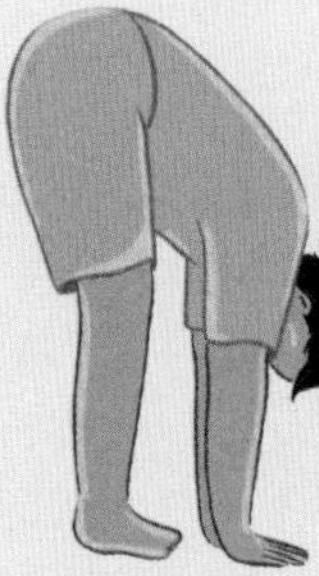

16. STANDING FORWARD FOLD

Exhale to release the foot and fold the body forwards. Hold for 5 breaths.

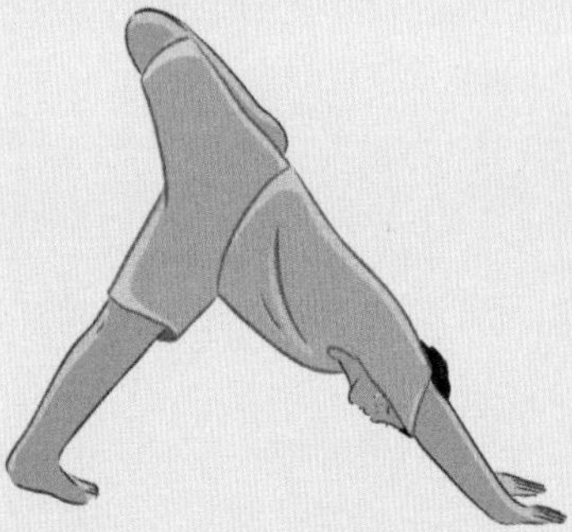

17. DOWNWARD-FACING DOG HIP OPENER

Exhale stepping back and lifting the hips. Reach the right leg up and back and bend the knee to open the hip. Hold for 1 breath.

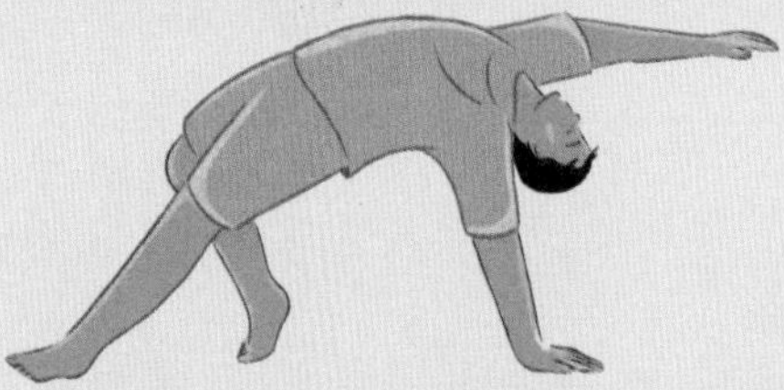

18. WILD THING

Option to flip your dog over into wild thing. Hold for 3–5 breaths.

REPEAT ON THE LEFT SIDE

STEPS 12–18

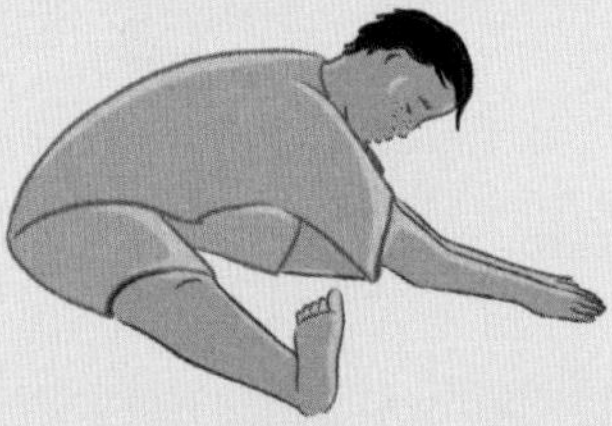

19. WIDE ANGLE SEATED FORWARD BEND

Coming to sit on the floor, the legs wide. Inhale to lengthen and open the chest, exhale to fold between the legs. Hold for 5 breaths.

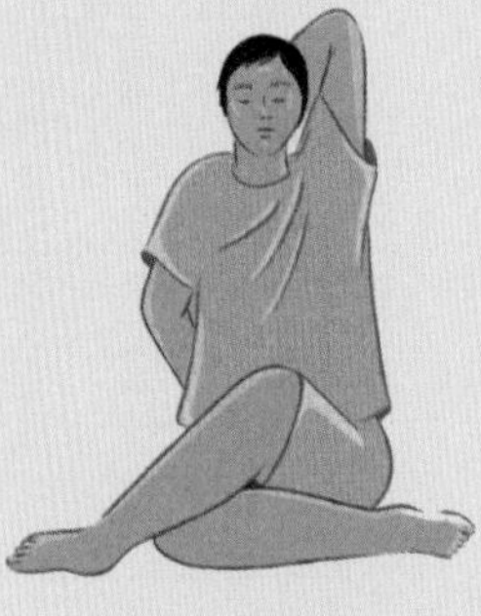

20. COW FACE

Cross the left leg on top of the right, finding cow face pose. Hold for 5 breaths. Repeat on the opposite side.

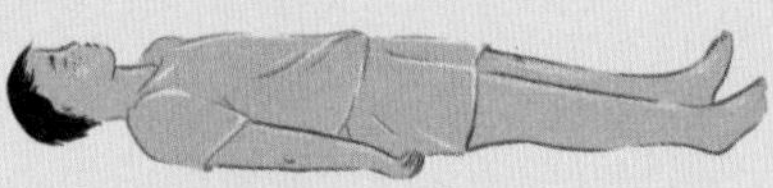

21. SAVASANA

Lie back and melt into savasana for 2 minutes or more.

MEDITATION

LOVING-KINDNESS MEDITATION

To fit with our wild heart theme of love, this month's signature meditation is a loving-kindness or '*metta*' meditation. This meditation helps us to cultivate compassion, which is an important component of mindfulness. We need to develop the ability to show ourselves, others and the world love and kindness. It can help to improve our happiness, confidence and emotional well-being. It can allow us to respond more positively to unpleasant and negative events and emotions and it can help us feel more connected and less alone.

The meditation is based around the following affirmations/mantras:

- May all beings be safe and free from suffering.
- May all beings be peaceful.
- May all beings be filled with loving kindness.
- May all beings accept themselves just as they are.

Directions:

1. Come into a comfortable seated position with an upright spine, somewhere you can be free of distractions.
2. Set a timer for 5 minutes or for as long as you have.
3. Gently close your eyes. If you don't like to close your eyes, you can have the eyes slightly open with the gaze lowered to the floor in front of you to keep your forehead soft.
4. Softly close your lips and let your breath come in through the nose and out through the nose or mouth in its natural rhythm.
5. Now start to silently bring yourself feelings of kindness, similar to those you would give to a loved one. We all have the same feelings of inadequacy, we can all make mistakes, we are all human. Start to slowly and silently repeat to yourself two to three times (or more): 'May I be safe and free from suffering; may I be peaceful; may I be filled with loving-kindness; may I accept myself just as I am.'
6. Now bring to mind a loved one. Silently share this kindness and compassion with them two to three times (or more): 'May you be safe and free from suffering: may you be peaceful; may you be filled with loving kindness; may you accept yourself just as you are.'
7. Now bring to mind someone whom you perhaps find a little more difficult – whom you don't get on with as well. Silently share this kindness and compassion with them two to three times (or more): 'May you be safe and free from suffering: may you be peaceful; may you be filled with loving kindness; may you accept yourself just as you are.'
8. Now bring to mind all beings, everywhere and share this loving kindness with everyone. Silently repeat two to three times (or more): 'May all beings be safe and free from suffering; may all beings be peaceful; may all beings be filled with loving-kindness; may all beings accept themselves just as they are.'
9. Each time your mind starts to wander, gently bring your awareness back to the present moment.
10. When the timer finishes, take a moment with the eyes still closed to sit and notice how you feel and any thoughts or feelings that arose.

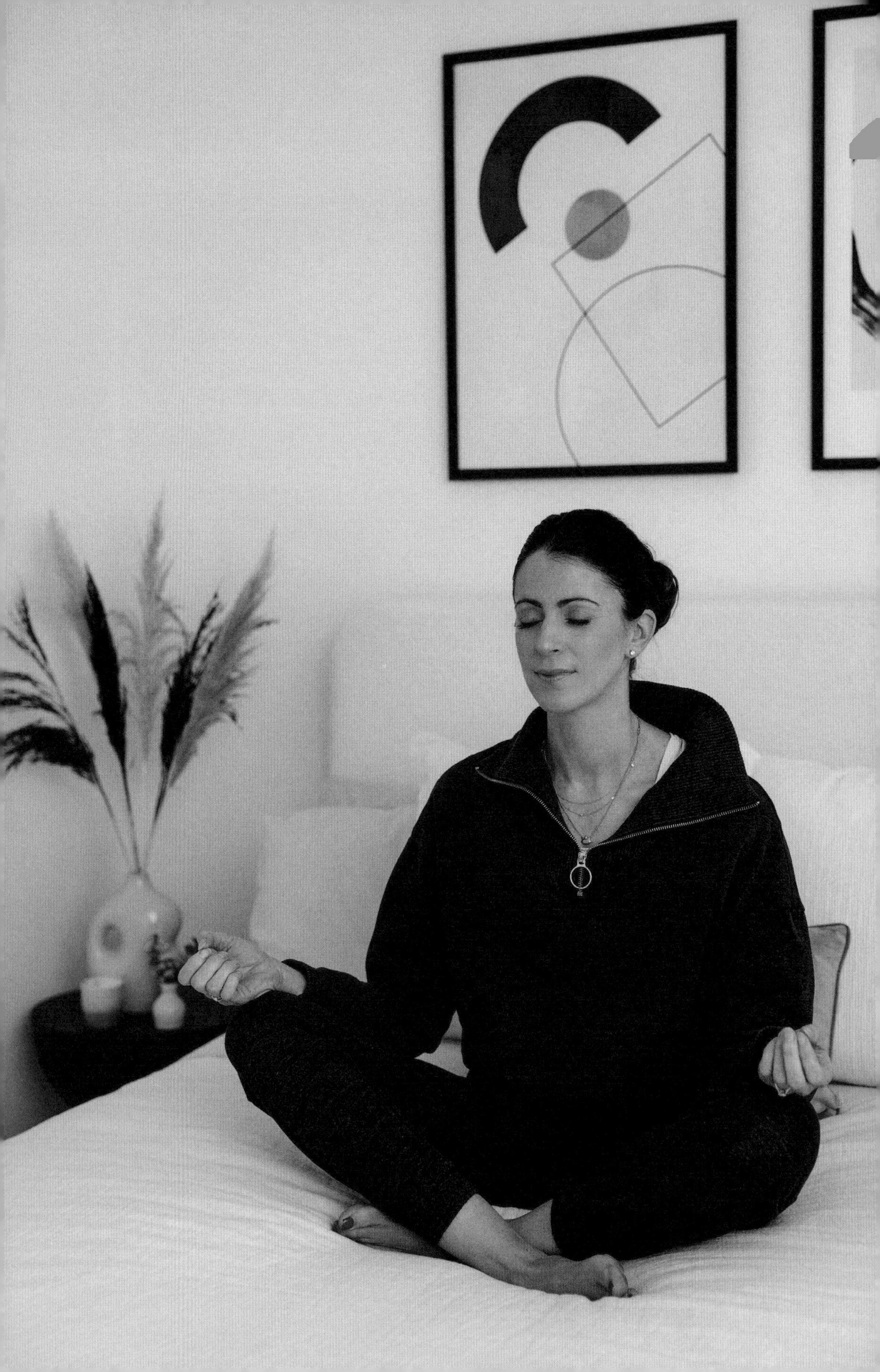

JOURNAL PROMPTS

Below I have given you eight self-reflection questions linked to this month's wild heart theme and the yogic concept of *svadhyaya*. Try answering two questions weekly alongside the daily journal prompts set out on pages 8–9.

- What activities or practices bring you a sense of freedom, joy and uninhibited expression and how can you include these in your life more frequently?

- What core beliefs and values shape your decisions and the way you behave? Are these beliefs serving your growth and well-being or do you need to let some go?

- How do you maintain harmony between your wild heart and the other aspects of your life (like relationships, work and responsibilities)? Do you need better balance and how could you achieve it?

- What areas of your life do you feel resistance towards? Is this resistance revealing something about your fears or growth areas?

- Reflect on a time when your wild heart pushed you to take a risk or make a bold decision. What did you learn from that experience?

- Are there any recurring patterns or habits you have noticed in your thoughts, emotions or behaviours? How do these impact your life?

- Reflect on a time where your wild heart helped you navigate change or adversity. How did it contribute to your resilience and can you harness this going forwards?

- What new insights or lessons have you gained from reflecting on your past experiences and actions from your daily journaling prompts?

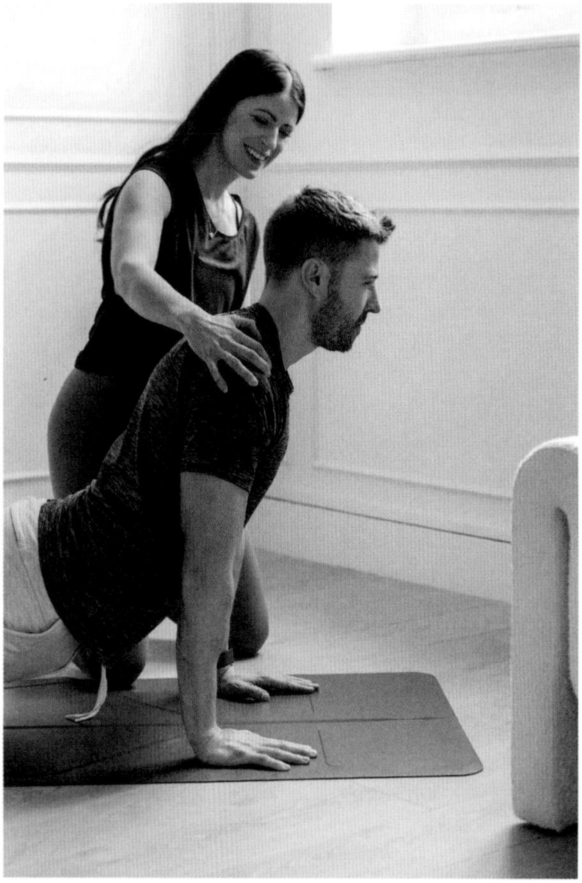
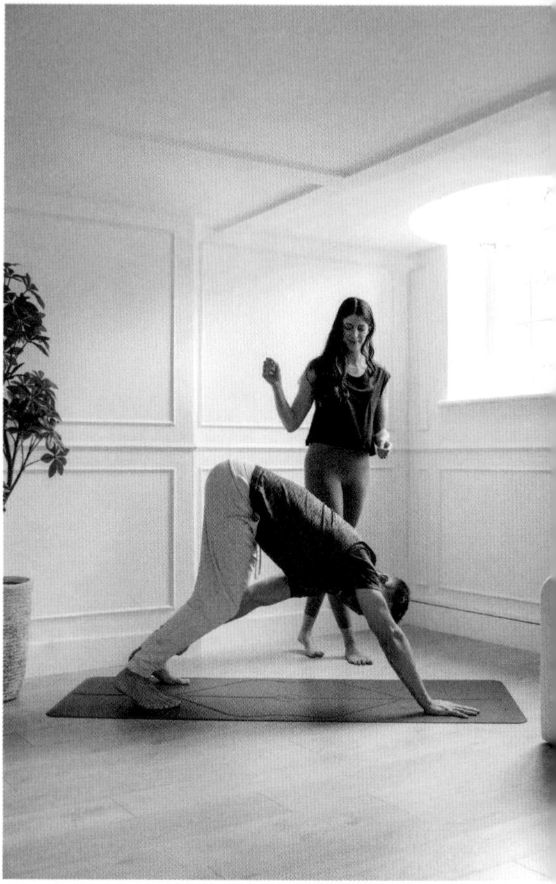
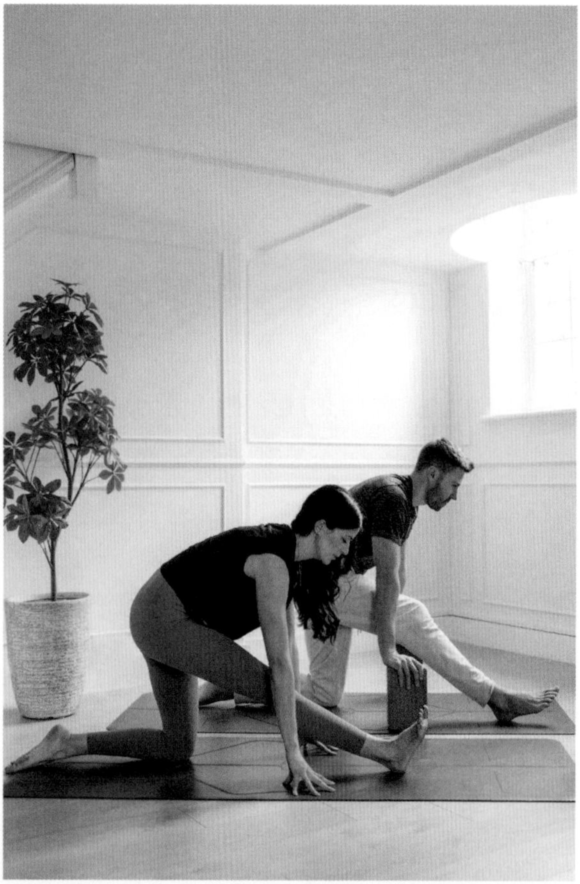
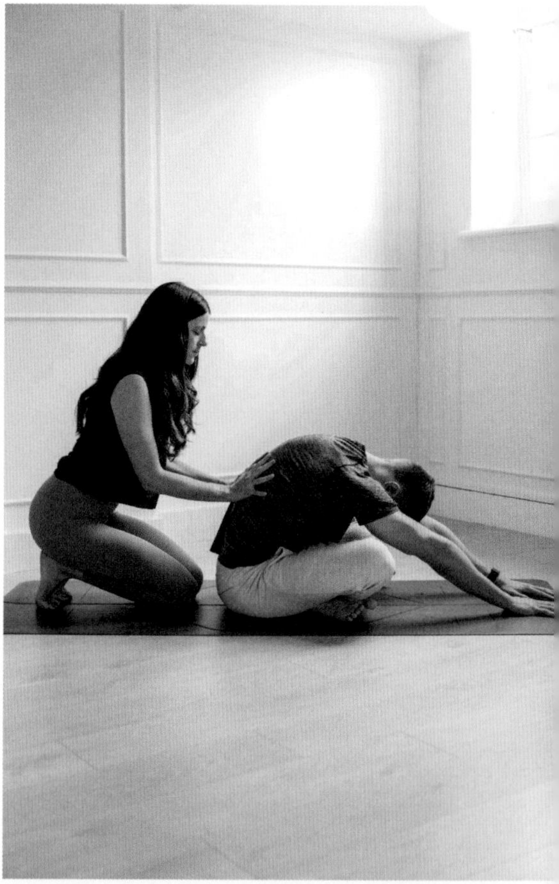

MONTH 10
BAMBOO

'WHAT WE ARE WAITING FOR IS NOT AS IMPORTANT AS WHAT HAPPENS TO US WHILE WE ARE WAITING. TRUST THE PROCESS.'

MANDY HALE

BAMBOO

Bamboo represents integrity, growth and resilience. Like grass, its roots grow horizontally in an intricate way: they weave themselves around other roots to create an extensive and interconnected root network. The structure of the bamboo itself allows the roots to bend and flex while maintaining strength. This means that when strong winds come, the roots and structure stop the bamboo from being uprooted or breaking. When we have strong roots (like those the *yamas* and *niyamas* teach us) we have a solid foundation in life to weather the storm.

This month we come to our final niyama, *ishvara pranidhana,* which invites us to surrender and let go. As humans, we struggle with the idea of surrendering for many reasons, such as fear of the unknown, a desire to control life and a misconception that surrender means weakness. However, a key part of navigating life's challenges is to let go and trust the process, so that is what we will practise on and off the mat over the next four weeks.

The flow this month is a flexibility flow working on forward folding postures. Remember that you need to balance flexibility with strength (*sthira-sukha,* see page 72) and combining flows from previous months with this month's sequence will complement the signature class. Please also remember that yoga isn't about what the posture looks like. Close your eyes if you need to (safely!) and tune in to the sensations of each pose asking yourself, 'Do I need to vary this posture to make it more appropriate for me in this moment?'.

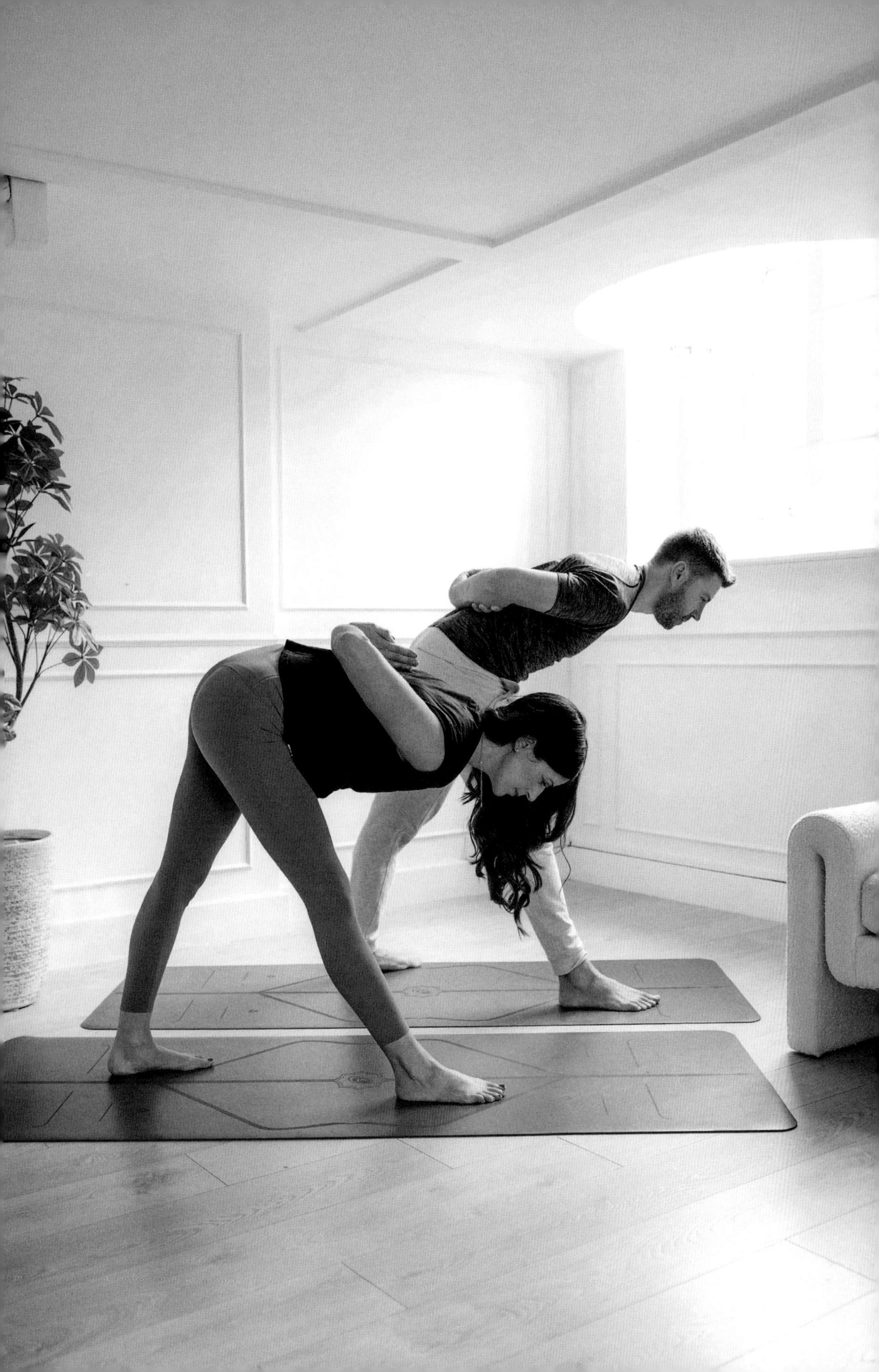

ISHVARA PRANIDHANA (SURRENDER)

OPEN HEARTED SURRENDER TO A HIGHER POWER.

The fifth and final *niyama* is *ishvara pranidhana,* which is a philosophical concept rooted in surrendering to a higher power. It's the practice of letting go of the ego's desire for control and acknowledging a connection with something greater than oneself. *Ishvara pranidhana* invites us to embrace a flexibility in life similar to that of the resilient bamboo. Having faith in a higher power rids us of the fear of the unknown and helps us cultivate resilience and inner peace, which are both essential for navigating the complexities of our modern world. It isn't a passive resignation or submission, but an active acknowledgement of a force beyond personal limitations.

For those that are religious, this concept can seem easier to grasp as it aligns with the concept of God or a divine presence. But for those who aren't religious, you can think of the higher power as the sanctity of life, a universal energy or a transcendent force. It rids us of the burden of trying to dictate every outcome. Instead, it allows us to trust the natural flow of life, accepting both joys and challenges. It promotes mindfulness, allowing us to be present with each moment without excessive worry about the past or future.

We are all wrapped in changing layers created by societal, cultural or personal constructs. With *ishvara pranidhana* we recognise the shared inner light among all beings. *Ishvara pranidhana* encourages empathy, compassion and understanding due to the interconnectedness and common humanity beyond external differences.

Here are some ways can we incorporate *ishvara pranidhana* in our daily lives:

▸ **On the yoga mat:** *Savasana* can help you embody aspects of *ishvara pranidhana.* When you end your practice and find *savasana,* surrender the body and breath fully and let go of all control, releasing the urge to change anything or do anything. Cultivate the qualities of faith, trust and receptivity. Observe sensations, thoughts and emotions without attachment or judgement. Surrender your weight to the earth and trust it is supported in order to open yourself to a deeper experience of 'rest'.

▸ **Stress and anxiety:** In the fast-paced world we live in, stress and anxiety are prevalent. *Ishvara pranidhana* offers us a reminder to let go of the burden of controlling every outcome and surrender to the current of life. For example, next time you are in the car, stuck in an unexpected traffic jam with no other route to take, breathe through the anxiety or frustration and try to let go of the feeling of stress. There is nothing you can do in this moment; the attachment to the frustration is the part causing you suffering, so practise letting go.

▸ **Attachments:** Linked to the point above, attachment to possessions, status or outcomes can cause suffering (more on this in chapter 11). Try and find fulfilment beyond materialism. Know that external elements don't define your essence and assess what are the important things in your life that truly bring you joy and contentment.

▸ **Gratitude:** Cultivate gratitude and trust in the universe or a higher power. Find blessings and moments of sunshine through the clouds when you are facing challenging times. I always find nature to be a good source of gratitude when life feels heavy.

▸ **Mindfulness:** A reminder to focus on presence in daily activities. Whether it's eating, walking, working, playing with your children, consciously immerse yourself in what you're doing, and let go of all distractions and worries.

▸ **Self-inquiry:** Reflect on personal beliefs or desires that seem part of your identity. Are they rooted in the ego taking control? Can you consciously surrender them, allowing deeper alignment with a higher truth?

THE BREATH

THE BHRAMARI BREATH

The signature breathing technique for this month is the *bhramari pranayama*. *Bhramari* is a large black Indian bee and this breath is also known as 'humming bee breath' due to the sound made on the exhale. It can be a powerful tool to help relieve frustration, anxiety and anger – helping us act rather than react. The steady humming sound produced while exhaling helps to quieten the mind and encourages the surrendering of attachments to thoughts.

Humming also stimulates the vagus nerve which is a key component of the parasympathetic nervous system (our 'rest-and-digest' system). Activation of the vagus nerve triggers the relaxation response, reducing heart rate, lowering blood pressure and promoting a sense of calm.

Directions:

1. Come into a comfortable seated position, growing tall through the crown of the head and allowing the spine to be neutral and long.
2. You can use the fingers to gently close the ears or alternatively rest the hands on the thighs.
3. Take a few slow breaths, tuning in and observing the body and mind.
4. Inhale softly and slowly through the nose, feeling the expansion of the abdomen and chest.
5. To exhale, slowly hum the breath out through closed lips making a steady, low-pitched sound, similar to that of a buzzing bee. See if you can feel the resonance of the sound through your head and throat.
6. Repeat for 10–12 rounds or more.

THE BAMBOO FLOW

This month's signature flow is themed around surrender and includes a collection of forward folding postures that require flexibility in the hips, lower back and hamstrings. Props like blocks can be helpful for poses like half splits and pyramid pose, but you can also modify these postures by bending the front leg or placing your hands to your heart rather than on the floor.

With deep stretches, I always tell my students to *take them slowly*. Go into a stretch at say 30% of your maximum stretch, connect with the breath and slow your exhales. This helps to tell your body it is safe. Then gradually deepen the stretch with each exhale, tuning into the sensations and being mindful not to push your body too far.

The reason this is helpful is because we have something called a stretch reflex. This is an automatic, involuntary response that occurs when a muscle is rapidly stretched. Sensory receptors in the muscles (called muscle spindles) send signals to the brain to contract the muscle, protecting it from overstretching or tearing. Going slowly into deep stretches allows the body to adapt and respond to the stretch reflex, which reduces the likelihood of triggering an intense reflexive muscle contraction.

Slowing the breath and making slow deliberate movements during yoga stretches can activate the parasympathetic nervous system. This signals to the body that it is safe and that there is no immediate threat, meaning the muscles can relax and lengthen.

Aim to practise this flow three or four times per week and if you have more time, feel free to include the seated warm-up flow on page 10 at the start, combine it with the previous months' flows or repeat the flow multiple times.

As you move around your yoga mat, bring some bamboo qualities with you:

▸ **Flexibility and strength:** Embodying the balance between flexibility and strength in postures mirrors the qualities of bamboo. Yoga has the misconception that it's only about being bendy, but we balance that with strength.

▸ **Graceful movement:** The swaying of bamboo in the wind is like a dance. Bring fluidity and grace into your movements and transitions.

▸ **Resilience:** Bamboo withstands the pressures of nature without breaking. Cultivate mental resilience in your practice, persevering through its challenges by believing in yourself.

PLEASE NOTE
The appendix on page 190 includes a detailed breakdown of each pose, plus variations and modifications. Remember to listen to your body; yoga should never be painful and you can chose to skip any pose that doesn't feel right for you.

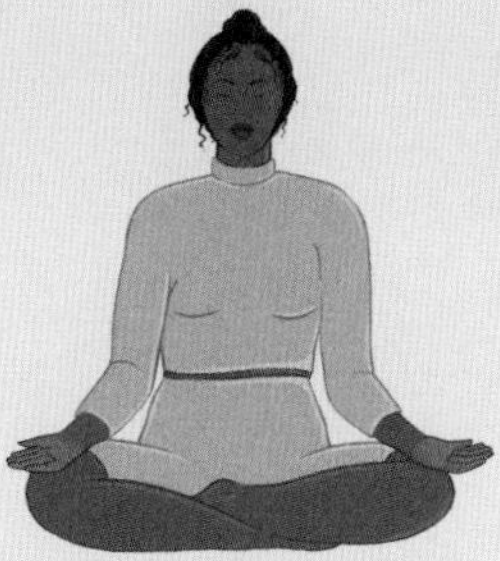

1. SEATED HUMMING BEE BREATH

In a seated position, take 10 rounds of the humming bee breath (see page 157).

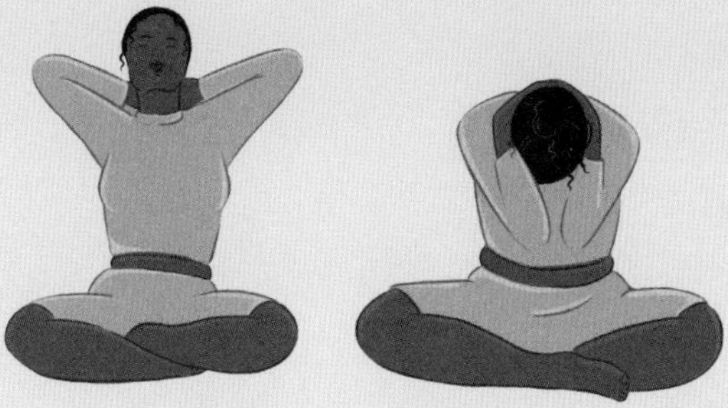

2. SEATED HEART OPENER

Interlacing the hands behind the head, inhale to open the chest, exhale to round in. Repeat 5 times.

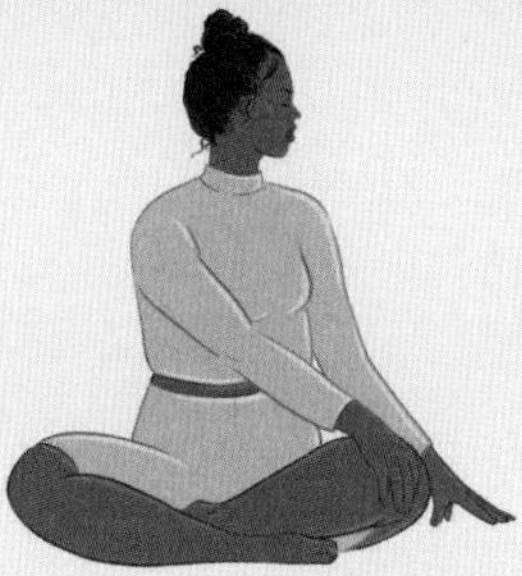

3. SEATED TWISTS

Twist and hold for 5 breaths on each side.

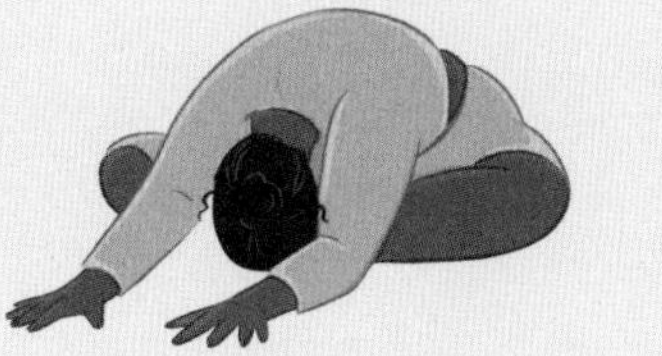

4. SEATED FOLD

Fold forward over the legs and hold for 5 breaths.

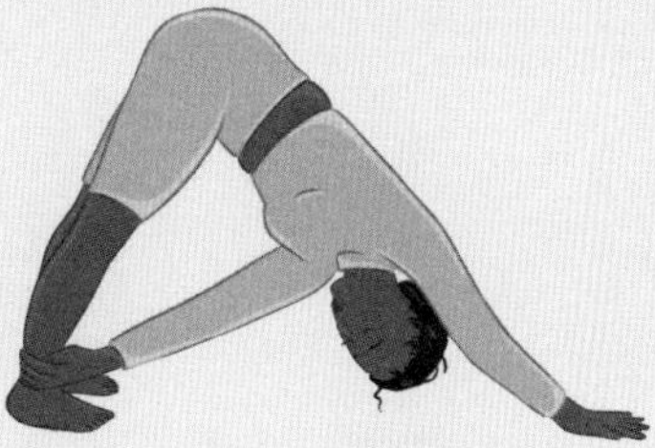

5. DOWNWARD-FACING DOG TWISTS

From downward-facing dog, reach the left hand to the right ankle, shin or thigh and take a twist. Hold for 5 breaths before repeating on the opposite side.

SUN SALUTATIONS A & B

Option to include sun salutations A and B (see pages 16–20).

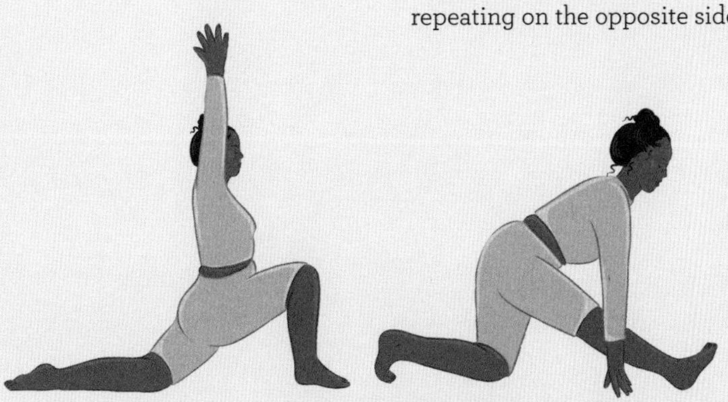

6. LOW LUNGE TO HALF SPLIT

Inhale with the right foot forwards into low lunge. Exhale and release to half splits. Repeat 5 times.

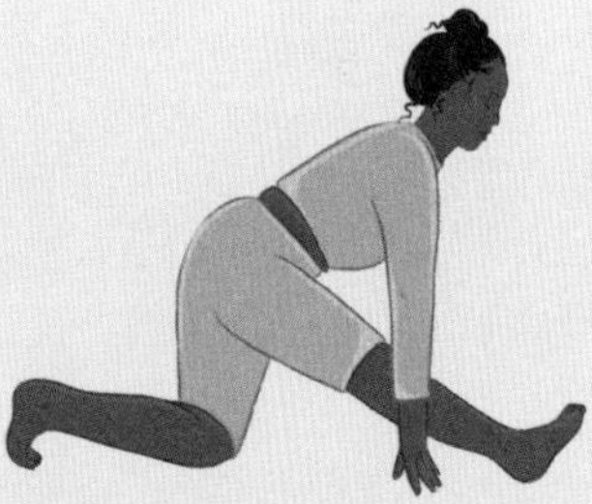

7. HALF SPLIT

Hold half split for a further 5 breaths.

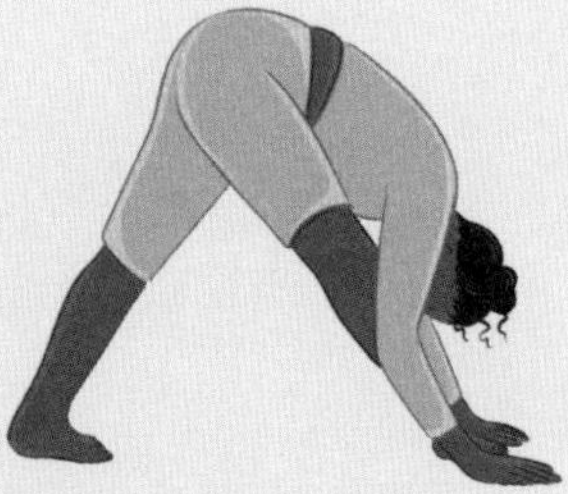

8. PYRAMID

Inhale and lift to standing, exhale and find pyramid pose. Hold for 5 breaths.

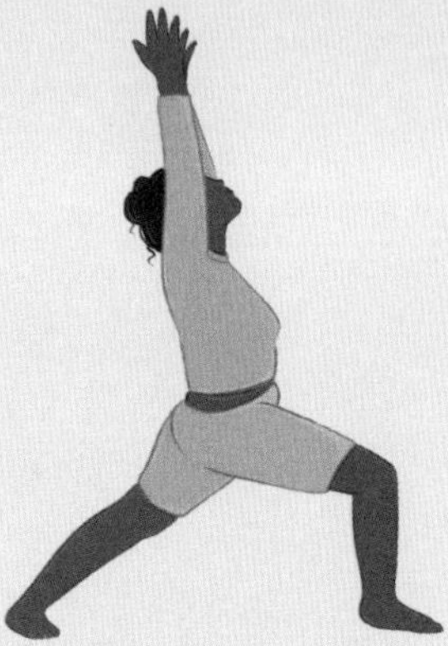

9. WARRIOR I

Inhale into warrior I or high lunge, option to come onto back toes, exhale and twist, finding twisted crescent lunge. Hold for 5 breaths.

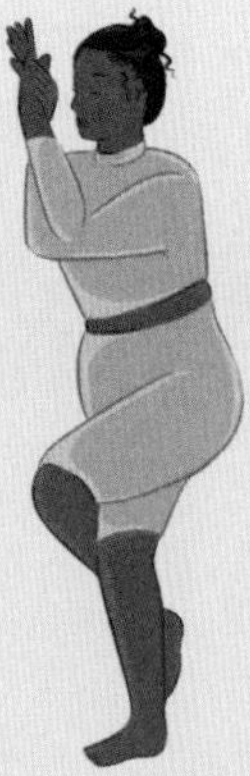

10. EAGLE

Step to the front of the mat and exhale wrapping the body into eagle pose. Hold for 5 breaths.

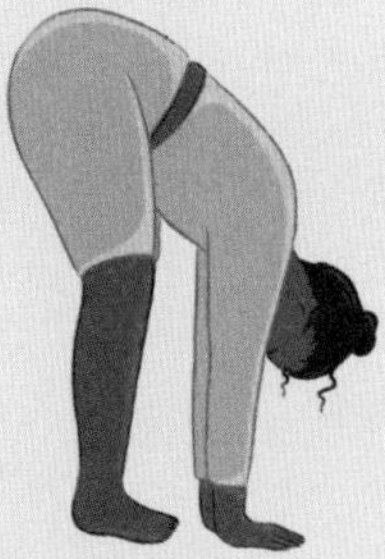

11. STANDING FORWARD BEND

Inhale to unravel, exhale and fold the body down into a standing forward bend. Hold for 5 breaths.

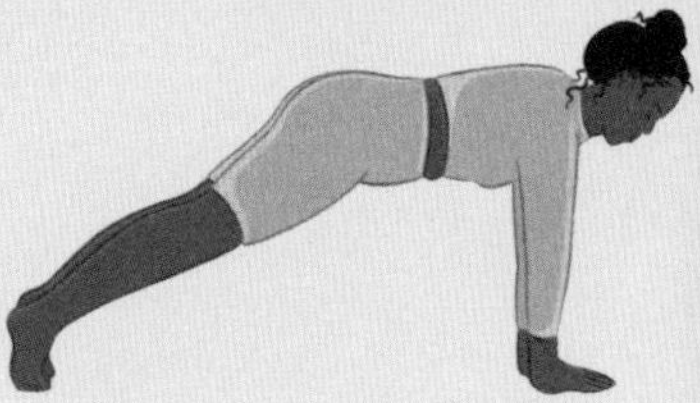

12. PLANK

Plant the hands and step back to plank. Hold for 5 breaths.

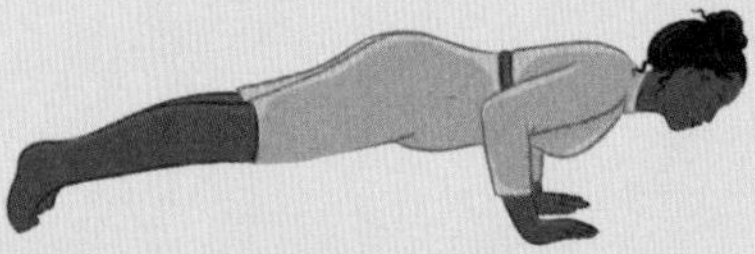

13. YOGA PUSH-UP

Exhale as you lower through yoga push-up.

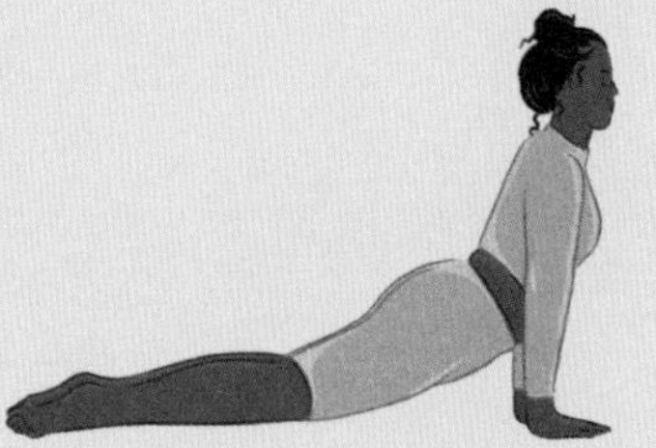

14. UPWARD-FACING DOG

Inhale to upward-facing dog and hold for a further 5 breaths.

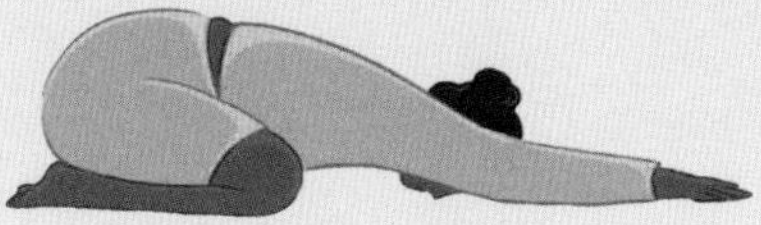

REPEAT
ON THE
LEFT SIDE

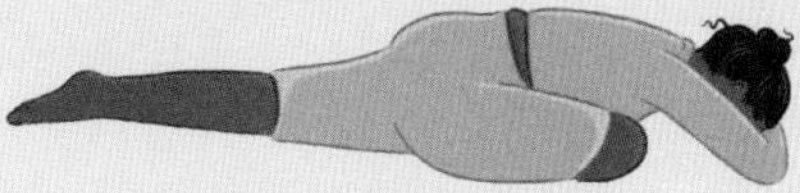

15. CHILD'S POSE

Exhale, dropping the knees and melting back into child's pose. Hold for 5 breaths.

STEPS 6–15

16. PIGEON

Placing the right shin across the front of the mat, find pigeon pose. Hold for 5 breaths.

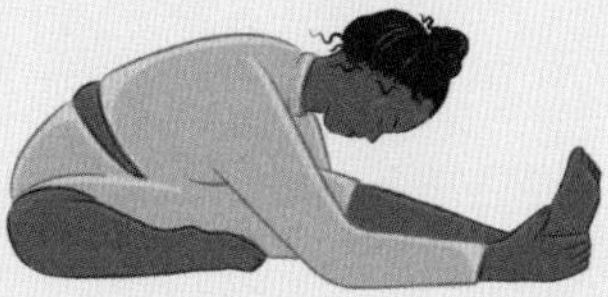

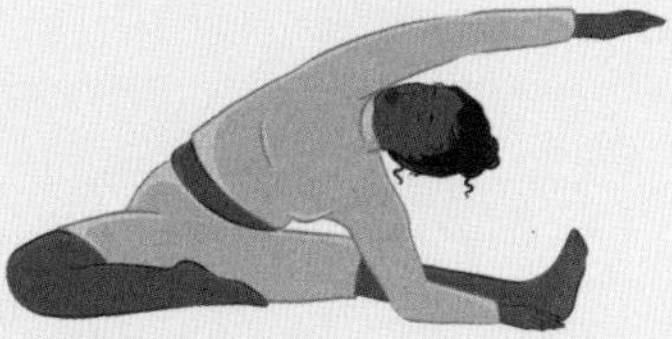

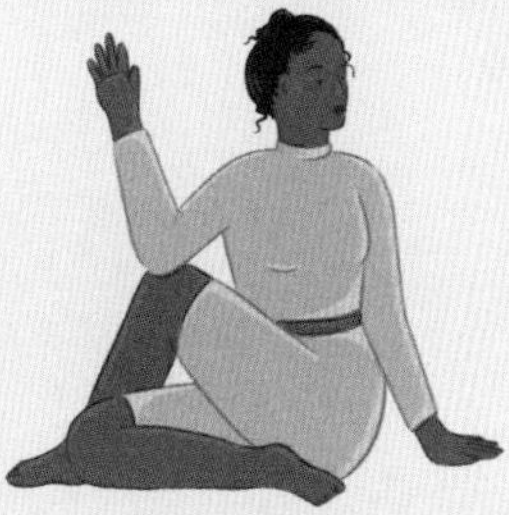

17. HEAD TO KNEE FORWARD FOLD

Swing the left leg forwards. Inhale to lengthen, exhale to fold. Hold for 5 breaths.

18. REVOLVED HEAD TO KNEE

Inhale to centre, exhale and revolve into a side stretch. Hold for 5 breaths.

19. HALF LORD OF THE FISHES

Step the left foot over the right thigh, inhale to lengthen and exhale twist. Hold for 5 breaths.

REPEAT
ON THE
LEFT SIDE

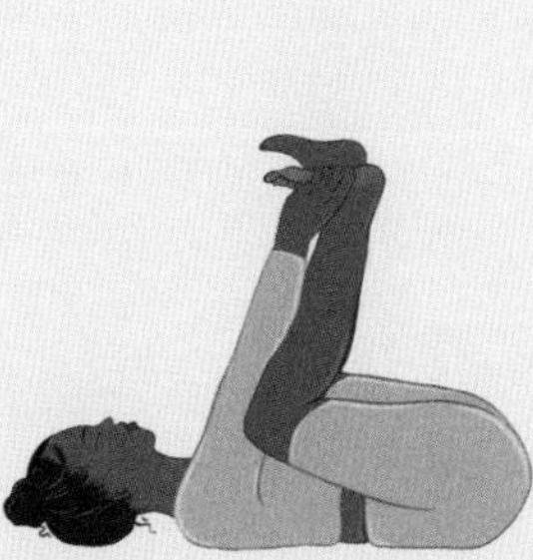

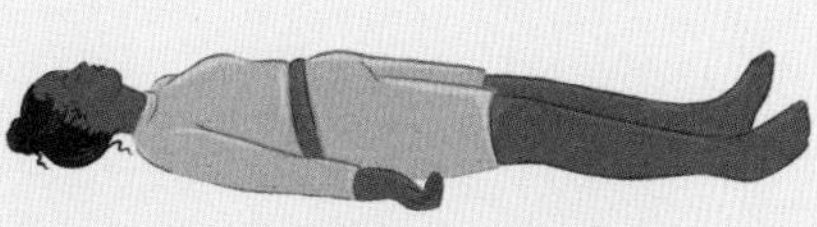

STEPS 16–19

20. HAPPY BABY

Coming onto the back, take hold of both feet and exhale into happy baby. Hold for 5 breaths.

21. SAVASANA

Release softly and melt into savasana for 2 minutes or more.

MEDITATION

MEDITATION FOR SURRENDER

To fit with our theme of *ishvara pranidhana*, this month's signature meditation is a meditation for surrender. This meditation will help you let go of control, release attachments and embrace the rhythm of life. It will also help you feel more grounded and calm by surrendering the need to control every aspect of life.

Directions:

1. Come into a comfortable seated position on a chair with an upright spine, somewhere you can be free of distractions.
2. Set a timer for 5 minutes or for as long as you have.
3. Gently close your eyes. If you don't like to close your eyes, you can have the eyes slightly open with the gaze lowered to the floor in front of you to keep your forehead soft.
4. Softly close your lips and let your breath come in through the nose and out through the nose or mouth in its natural rhythm.
5. Before each meditation begins, feel your sitting bones on the chair and your feet on the floor. Imagine roots winding down from these areas, helping you feel secure and grounded.
6. With each exhale, have a feeling of letting go and fully releasing all control.
7. If a mantra resonates with you, repeat the following affirmation: 'I surrender to the flow of life,' or simply say, 'let go', or any other mantra that feels right for you.
8. Picture yourself surrounded by a warm, comforting light. As you are enveloped in this light, visualise yourself releasing any worries, fears or attachments. Imagine them floating away and surrendering to the supportive light.
9. Allow yourself to feel a sense of peace and acceptance, embracing the feeling of letting go and trusting that things will happen as they should.
10. When the timer finishes, take a moment with the eyes still closed to sit and notice how you feel and any thoughts or feelings that arose.

JOURNAL PROMPTS

Below I have given you eight self-reflection questions linked to this month's bamboo theme and the yogic concept of *ishvara pranidhana*. Try answering two questions weekly alongside the daily journal prompts set out on pages 8–9.

▸ What areas of your life require more flexibility? How might embracing this flexibility bring positive change?

▸ How comfortable are you with the idea of surrendering control? Reflect on a time when surrendering control led to positive outcomes.

▸ Are there any attachments you find difficult to release or surrender? How might holding onto them impact your well-being?

▸ Bamboo is simple yet strong. Think about ways to simplify your life or mindset that will contribute towards your inner strength.

▸ How present do you feel in everyday life? What practices or habits can help you cultivate more mindful awareness and presence?

▸ Bamboo often grows in clusters, which support each other as they grow. Reflect on the relationships you have in your life and how they support your personal growth.

▸ Consider a challenging situation you've faced or are facing. How did / does your perspective change when you let go of trying to control the outcome?

▸ Bamboo is the perfect example of the yogic concept of *sthira-sukha* (the balance between effort and ease) due to its durability and flexibility. Think about the balance between stability and adaptability in your life and where the balance may be lacking.

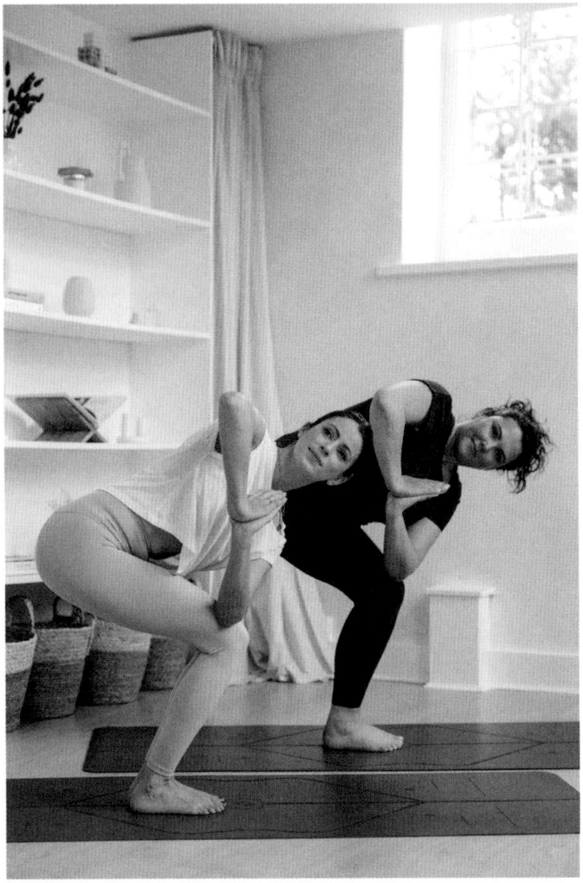
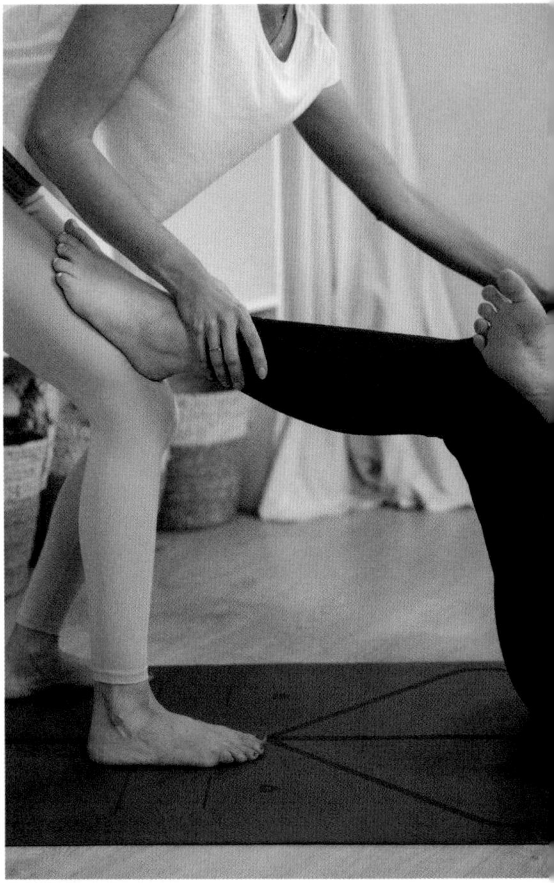
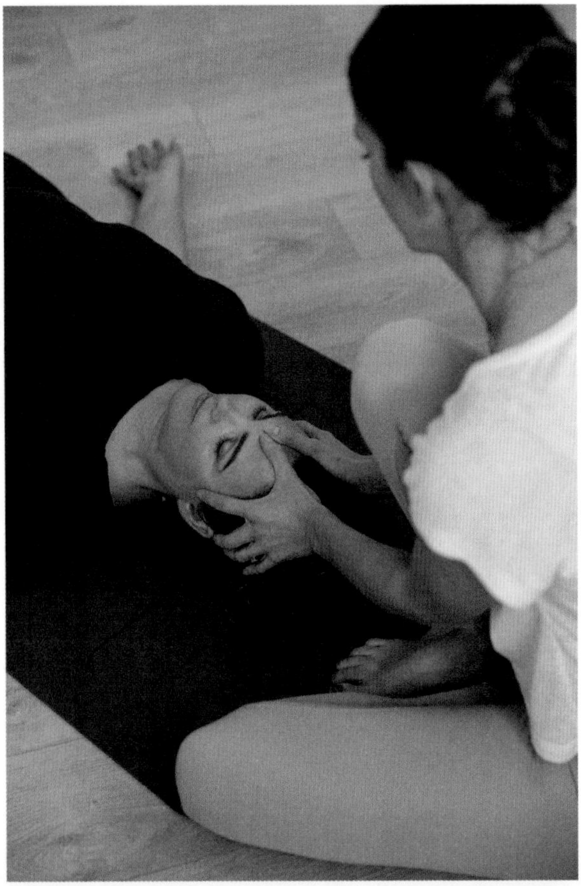
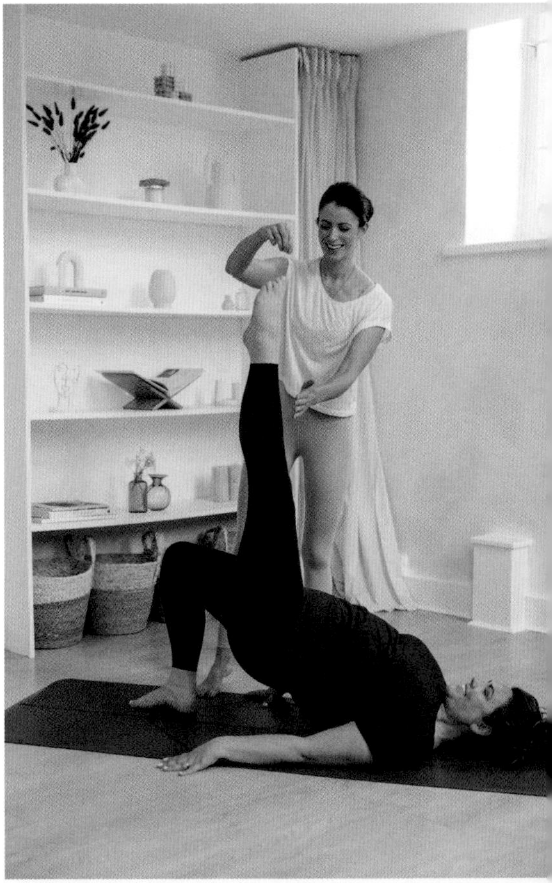

MONTH 11
BOULDER

'ATTACHMENT CONSTRAINS OUR VISION SO THAT WE ARE NOT ABLE TO SEE THINGS FROM A WIDER PERSPECTIVE.'

DALAI LAMA

BOULDER

This month is designed to help you identify and release some boulders from your life. By boulders I mean attachments and obstacles that cloud the mind, contribute to your suffering and are stopping you from feeling free. The signature yoga flow is centred in awareness and attachment. We will explore the arm balance crow pose (*kakasana*) for the first time with a clean slate and fresh narrative (no, 'I could never do this,' please).

I will also introduce you to the yogic concept of the *kleshas*, which are five obstacles that, in short, can mess with how we see things. They offer insight into what's causing us to suffer and be dissatisfied in life. Through understanding and awareness, we can work towards reducing their influence and find greater contentment. This month's journaling questions will help you work towards this too.

As you settle into your practice this month, consider the significance of the boulder. It symbolises not only the weight of any obstacles in your path but also the solidity of your commitment to transformation. Observe how in certain postures and movements, you can break the mould. You can disrupt your established patterns by adding variations within these poses and find growth and liberation in change.

For this month's breathing technique, we return to the equal ratio breathing from chapter 4 but with a small tweak. I have introduced you to 10 different mindfulness and meditation techniques and this month gives you the freedom of choice. It's time to begin developing the practice of tuning in to what will serve you best on each given day.

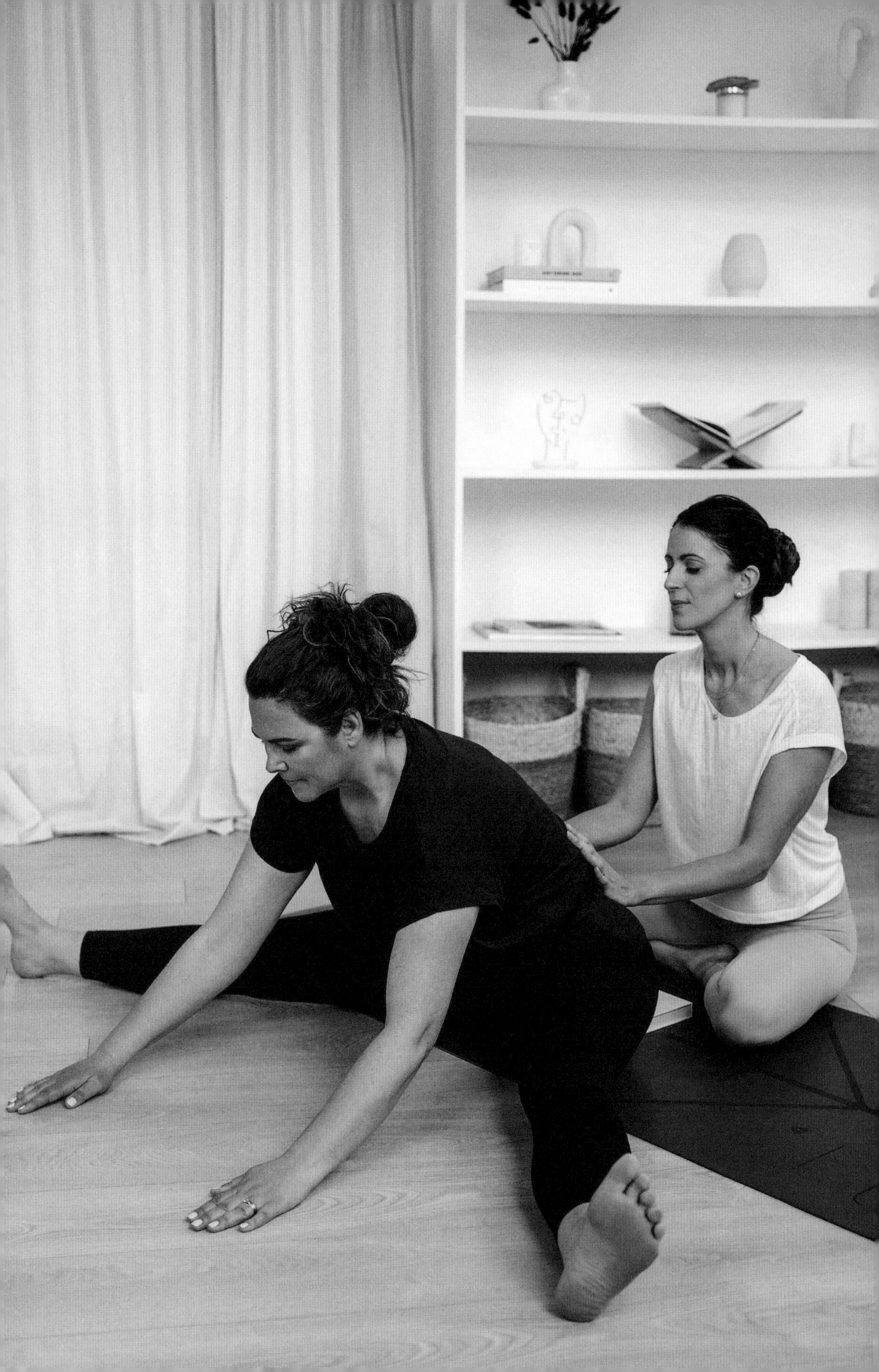

THE *KLESHAS*

MENTAL OBSTACLES HINDERING OUR PATH TO INNER PEACE AND CLARITY.

In *The Yoga Sutras of Patañjali*, there are five obstacles of the mind that hide our true self and cause us suffering; these are known as the *kleshas*. They are:

1. ***Avidya*:** Ignorance and not seeing things clearly. This is considered to be the root cause of all suffering. Think of this like a big rock, covering the clear path of a river. It prevents us from seeing things as they truly are. It clouds our understanding and it makes navigating through life's challenges more difficult.
2. ***Asmita*:** Egotism or insecurity. This can be thought of as a massive boulder separating the river into smaller streams. This creates a sense of separateness and making us believe that we are different (better or worse) from everyone and everything around us and therefore blocking that natural flow of interconnectedness.
3. ***Raga*:** Attachment to the pleasurable parts of life. Imagine heavy rocks clinging to the riverbed making it hard for the river to flow smoothly. Similarly, clinging to attachments makes it hard for us to move forward and experience new things.
4. ***Dvesa*:** Resistance to things we don't like. The giant sharp rocks in the riverbed that we try to avoid are *dvesa* – a strong dislike or avoidance of certain things. It creates suffering and again keeps us from moving forwards.
5. ***Abhinivesa*:** Attachment to life, fearing death. Think of this like a massive boulder at the bend in the river. It stops the natural flow, creating resistance to changes, meaning we are afraid to let go.

Just as removing the boulders would allow the river to run freely, overcoming these *kleshas* clears the mind's path and enables a smoother, more peaceful journey in life.

Here are some ways can we incorporate each *klesha* into our daily lives:

▸ ***Avidya* (ignorance):** How often do you judge or come to a conclusion about something without knowing all the details? Question assumptions before jumping to conclusions and practise mindfulness and self-reflection to avoid lack of awareness or misunderstanding.

▸ ***Asmita* (ego):** ego arises when we overly identify with our self-image or achievements. Be aware of this and practise humility, thinking about how as beings, we are all connected and acknowledge that individual accomplishments don't define our true essence.

▸ ***Raga* (attachment):** Practise enjoying experiences in the moment and not fixating on holding onto them permanently. Find contentment and gratitude for what you have while embracing change.

▸ ***Dvesa* (aversion):** Gradually expose yourself to situations or ideas that trigger aversion in you, for example, the visit to the dentist you have been putting off. Soften the resistance and realise it was the resistance that was causing you to suffer. Embrace discomfort as a means to overcome strong dislikes.

▸ ***Abhinivesa* (fear of loss):** Focus on building inner strength and resilience to allow you to navigate transitions with ease. Acknowledge and accept that change is a non-negotiable part of life rather than resisting it.

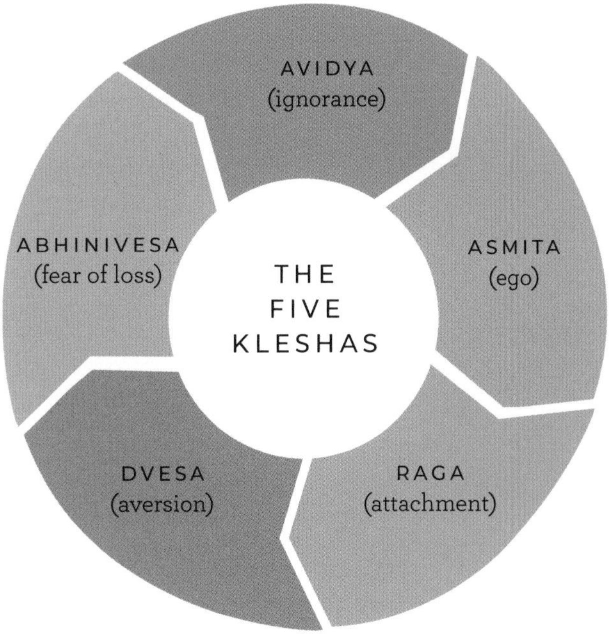

THE BREATH

THE SAMA VRITTI VARIATION

With the signature breathing technique for this month we go back to the technique introduced in chapter 4, *sama vritti* or equal ratio breathing (see page 74). You may remember that this technique can help calm the mind, improve focus and bring our nervous system back into balance.

Instead of practising *sama vritti* to a count of four, shift the length of the inhale and exhale by one each time. I call this the 'climb the mountain approach'. For example, start with a count of four and work up to a count of eight or ten. You can alternatively create a 'wave' whereby you start with four, work up to ten and then go back down to four.

Try both the mountain and wave techniques and notice how they make you feel, then use that information to inform which variety you choose and when. You may find that the climbing the mountain variation leaves you feeling calmer and lowers your energy whereas the wave method leaves you feeling more energetic.

Directions:

1. Come into a comfortable seated position, growing tall through the crown of the head and allowing the spine to be neutral and long.
2. Take a few breaths, tuning in and observing the body and mind.
3. Inhale softly and slowly through the nose for a count of 4 and exhale softly and slowly through the nose for a count of 4. Repeat this a few times to prepare.
4. Now inhale softly and slowly through the nose for a count of 5 and exhale softly and slowly through the nose for a count of 5.
5. Repeat the step above but add one count each time until you reach a count of 8–10 (or whatever limit feels right for you).
6. Choose either to stay at a lengthened count for a few more rounds or to wave the practice back to a count of 4 by decreasing the count each time, reversing the process above.

THE BOULDER FLOW

This month's signature flow works up to the arm balance, crow pose (*kakasana*). This is an infamous yoga posture in which you balance the knees on the elbows or backs of the arms. There are many variations of crow; a starting point is to lift one foot and have one foot grounded. Stay curious and play around with sensation. Visualise yourself lifting into the pose. Perhaps the full expression of the pose won't happen today but believe you can do it one day.

Four tips that I think are really helpful for students learning crow pose include:

1. **Don't look down:** Your gaze should be slightly forward in front of the hands – if you look down you will tend to fall.
2. **Lose the fear:** Grab cushions to place underneath you so that you learn how to fall safely. Once you lose the fear of falling, crow pose becomes so much easier.
3. **No floppy feet:** Point the toes and hug the inner thighs inwards, towards the centre, spreading energy through the legs.
4. **Find your spider fingers:** Just as your toes stop you from falling forwards, your fingers help you to balance. Practise shifting your weight forwards and gripping the floor with the fingers to find balance.

PLEASE NOTE

The appendix on page 190 includes a detailed breakdown of each pose, plus variations and modifications. Remember to listen to your body; yoga should never be painful and you can chose to skip any pose that doesn't feel right for you.

As we near the end of your Yoga Happy year, it's useful to think about the idea of self-practice and self-exploration. Come to the mat with an idea of breaking the mould or letting go of attachments. Can you add movement to the postures you've started to become familiar with and notice what your body needs more or less of? Can you tweak the flows to make them more appropriate for what you need, for example, lift and lower of the leg in side plank? Change things up and notice how it challenges you to tune in to how the body feels.

Aim to practise this flow three or four times per week and if you have more time, include the seated warm-up flow on page 10 at the start, combine it with the previous months' flows or repeat the flow multiple times.

As you move around your yoga mat, bring some boulder-themed qualities with you:

▸ **Grounding energy:** Let a boulder's steadfast presence inspire you to connect deeply with the earth. Feel supported in every pose. Focusing on the foundations (the parts of the body touching the floor) and finding stability there, can foster a sense of safety and solidity in your practice.

▸ **Presence and stillness:** Be present in each posture, anchoring your attention to the breath and the sensations in your body. Allow yourself to find a sense of calm amidst movement. Notice how the stillness in side plank or crow feels very different from the stillness in child's pose.

▸ **Adaptability:** While seemingly unchanging, boulders adapt to their environment slowly over time. Listen to your body, modify poses when you need to and adapt your practice to suit your needs, change and growth.

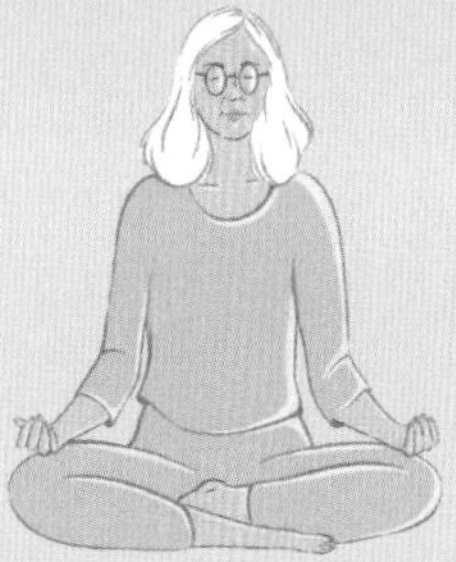

1. SEATED SAMA VRITTI

In a seated position, take 10 rounds of *sama vritti* variation (see page 170).

BEGIN WRIST SEQUENCE

See page 221.

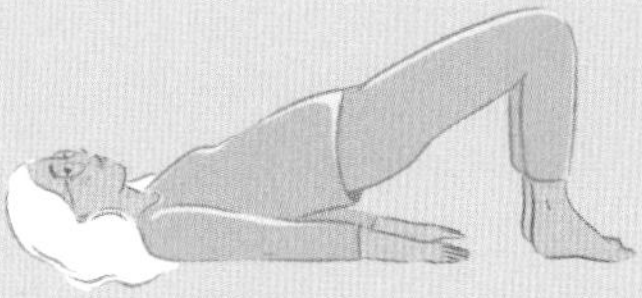

2. BRIDGE

Bringing the feet onto the floor, exhale to lift the hips into bridge. Hold for 5 breaths.

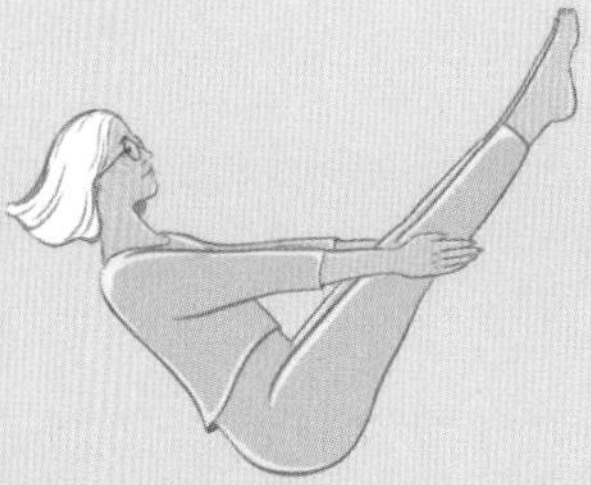

3. BOAT

Come up to sit on the mat. Exhale as you lift into boat pose. Hold for 3 breaths.

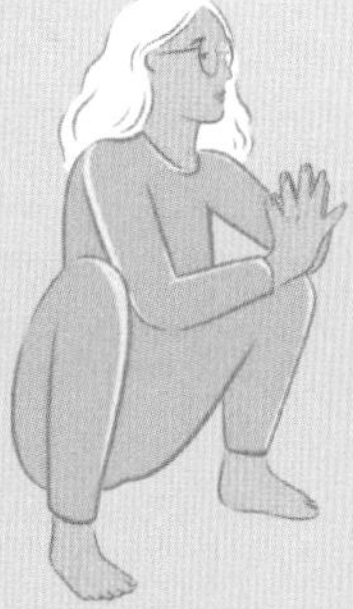

4. YOGI SQUAT

Plant the feet and shift forward into a yogi squat. Hold for 5 breaths.

SUN SALUTATIONS A & B

Option to include sun salutations A and B (see pages 16–20).

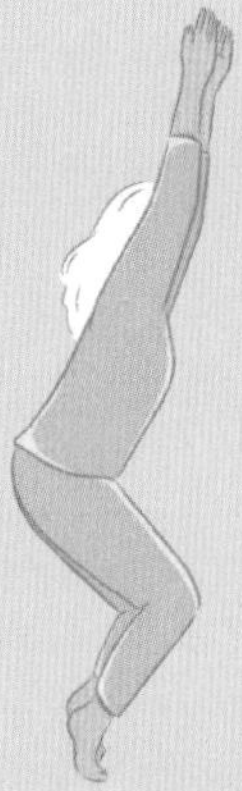

5. CHAIR ON TIPTOES

Inhale, sweeping into chair pose. Hold for 5 breaths. Option to lift onto tiptoes.

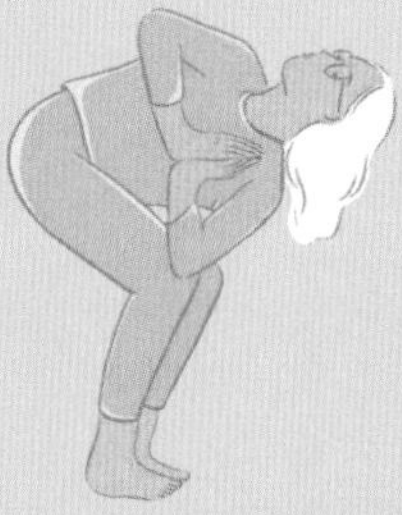

6. TWISTED CHAIR

Bringing the hands into prayer, exhale and twist to the right finding twisted chair. Hold for 3 breaths.

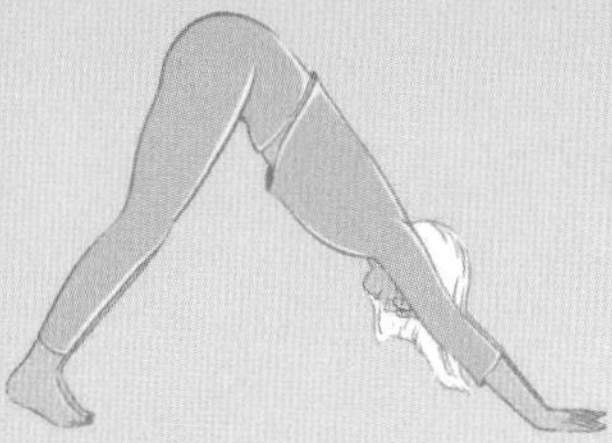

7. DOWNWARD-FACING DOG

Exhale, planting the hands and stepping back into downward-facing dog. Hold for 5 breaths.

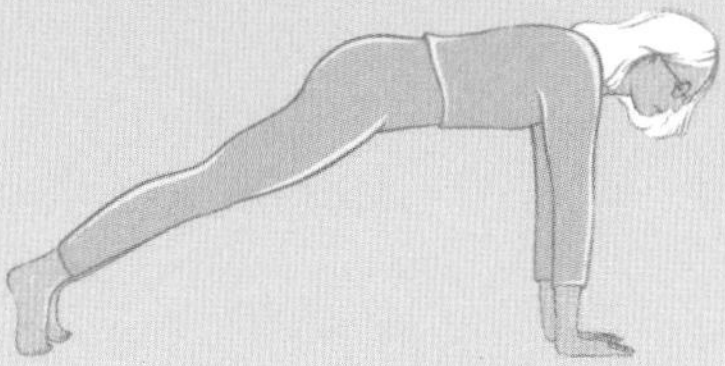

8. PLANK

Shift the shoulders forward and find plank pose. Hold for 5 breaths.

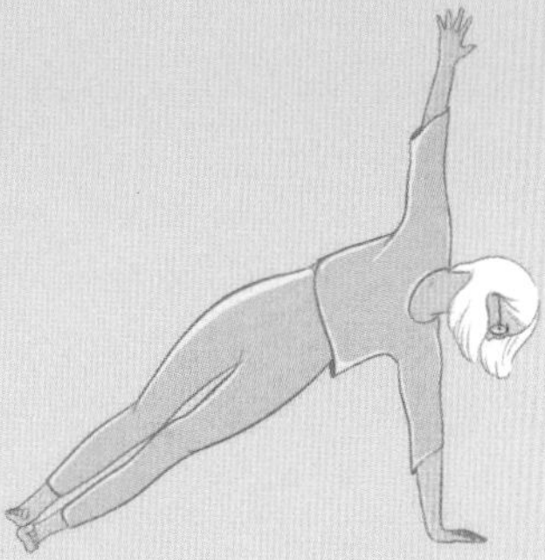

9. SIDE PLANK

Inhale the right fingers to the sky opening into side plank. Hold for 5 breaths.

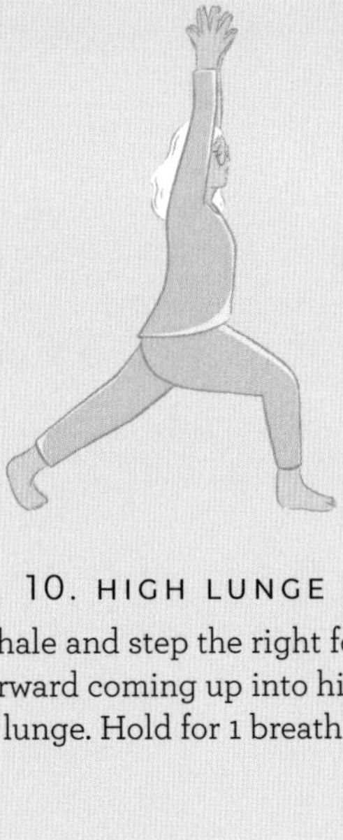

10. HIGH LUNGE

Inhale and step the right foot forward coming up into high lunge. Hold for 1 breath.

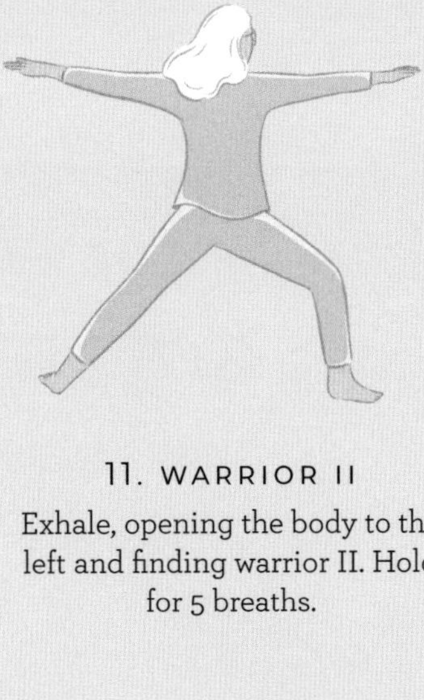

11. WARRIOR II

Exhale, opening the body to the left and finding warrior II. Hold for 5 breaths.

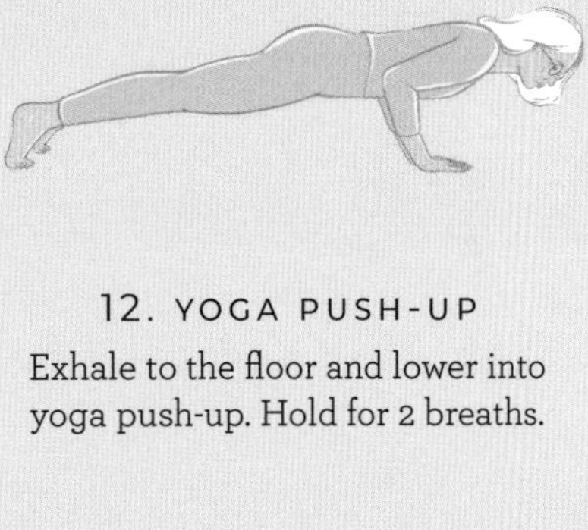

12. YOGA PUSH-UP

Exhale to the floor and lower into yoga push-up. Hold for 2 breaths.

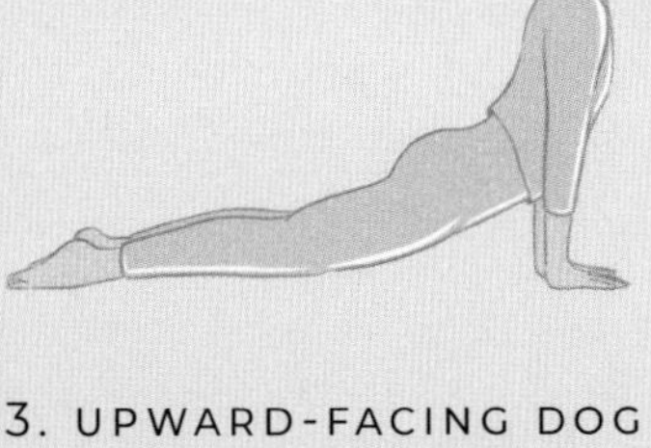

13. UPWARD-FACING DOG

Inhale into upward-facing dog. Hold for 2 breaths.

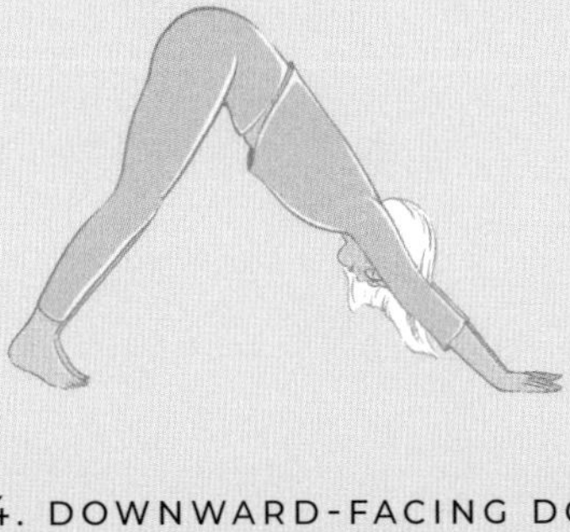

14. DOWNWARD-FACING DOG

Exhale, lifting the hips into downward-facing dog and hold for 5 breaths.

REPEAT ON THE LEFT SIDE

STEPS 5–14

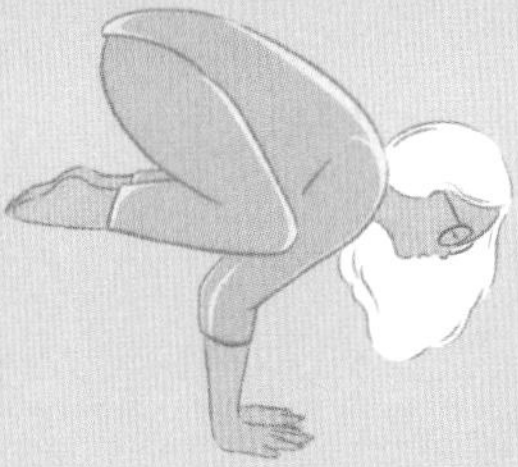

15. CROW POSE

Coming into yogi squat, exhale and lift into crow pose. Hold for 1– 5 breaths.

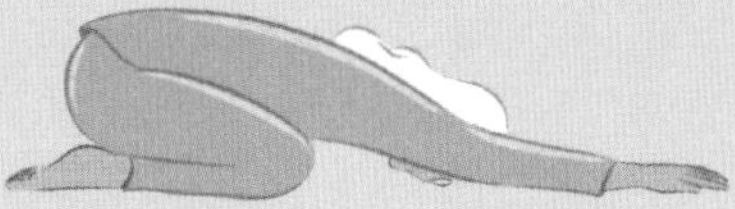

16. CHILD'S POSE

Exhale, melting down into child's pose. Hold for 1– 3 breaths.

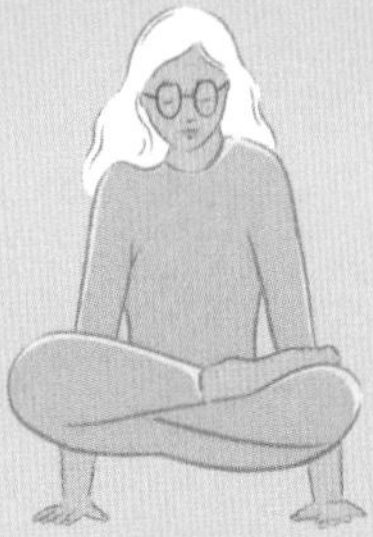

17. SCALE POSE

Coming to a seated position. exhale as you lift into scale pose. Hold for 1–5 breaths.

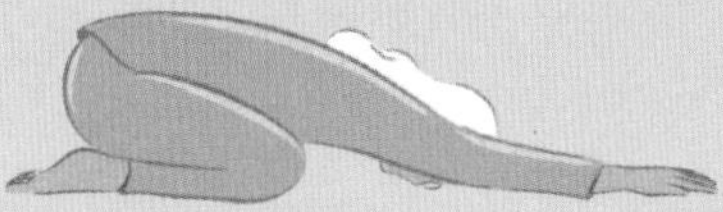

18. CHILD'S POSE

Exhale, melting down into child's pose. Hold for 5 breaths.

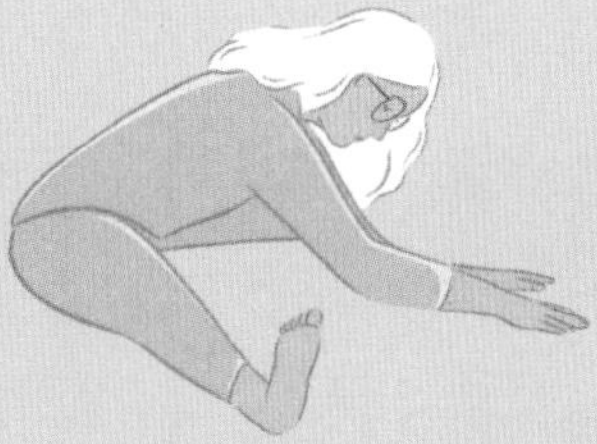

19. WIDE-ANGLE SEATED FORWARD BEND

Coming to sit on the floor, with the legs wide. Inhale to lengthen and open the chest, exhale to fold between the legs. Hold for 5 breaths.

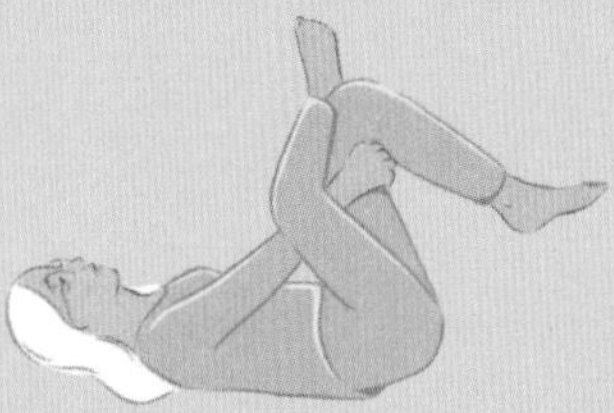

20. RECLINED PIGEON

Coming onto your back, cross the right foot over the left knee and find reclined pigeon. Hold for 5 breaths before repeating on the opposite side.

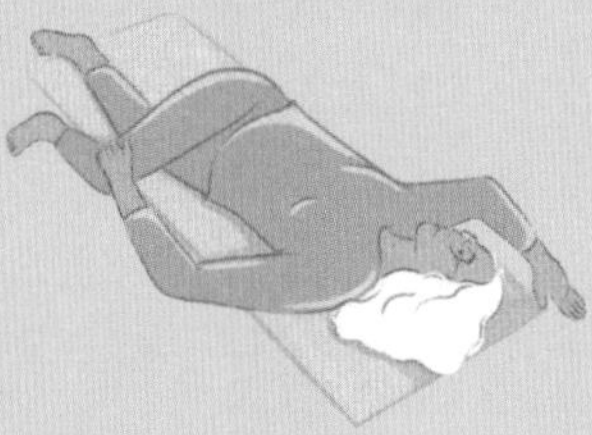

21. SUPINE TWIST

Hug the right knee in and come into a supine twist. Hold for 5 breaths before repeating on the opposite side.

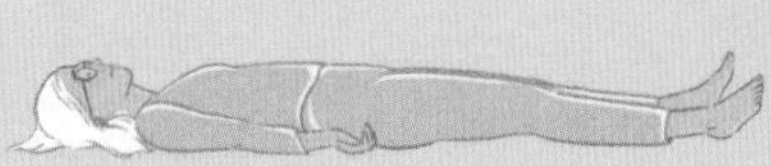

22. SAVASANA

Come back to centre and melt into savasana for 2 minutes or more.

MINDFULNESS AND MEDITATION

Over the course of the previous 10 months, I shared different meditation and mindfulness practices. This month, instead of providing another, I invite you to listen to your body and mind and decide which of those practices is right for you in the moment. Perhaps it is the simple breathing meditation or maybe you need to get outside with a walking meditation. Only you know which practice will support you best.

1. Breathing meditation (see page 36)
2. Mantra meditation (see page 50)
3. Walking meditation (see page 66)
4. Quit the autopilot (see page 79)
5. Body scan meditation (see page 94)
6. Mindful cleaning (see page 108)
7. Gratitude meditation (see page 122)
8. Soft belly meditation (see page 136)
9. Loving-kindness meditation (see page 149)
10. Meditation for surrender (see page 162)

JOURNAL PROMPTS

Below I have given you eight self-reflection questions linked to this month's boulder theme and the *kleshas*. Try answering two questions weekly alongside the daily journal prompts set out on pages 8–9.

▸ Reflect on a time when you acted from a place of ignorance or misunderstanding. How did this lack of awareness impact your thoughts or decisions? What steps can you take to cultivate greater awareness in similar situations in the future?

▸ Think of a time where you felt a strong need to prove yourself or defend your identity and how it made you act and feel. Consider how letting go of the need for validation or comparison might help you in future similar situations.

▸ Which attachments do you find it challenging to let go of and why? Do these things bring true contentment or can you practise non-attachment?

▸ What experiences do you resist or avoid and how does it impact your well-being or growth? What can you do differently?

▸ Think about a change you're facing that makes you uncomfortable or scared. How does the fear of this change affect your thoughts or actions? Consider how accepting the idea of change could help you navigate things more openly.

▸ What routines, habits or rituals help you feel grounded? How do these practices contribute to your overall well-being or sense of stability in life?

▸ Reflect on a previous challenging experience. How did you weather the storm and what lessons did you learn from the experience?

▸ Consider the people that provide stability and support in your life, much like how a boulder relies on its surroundings. How do these support systems contribute to your sense of security and resilience?

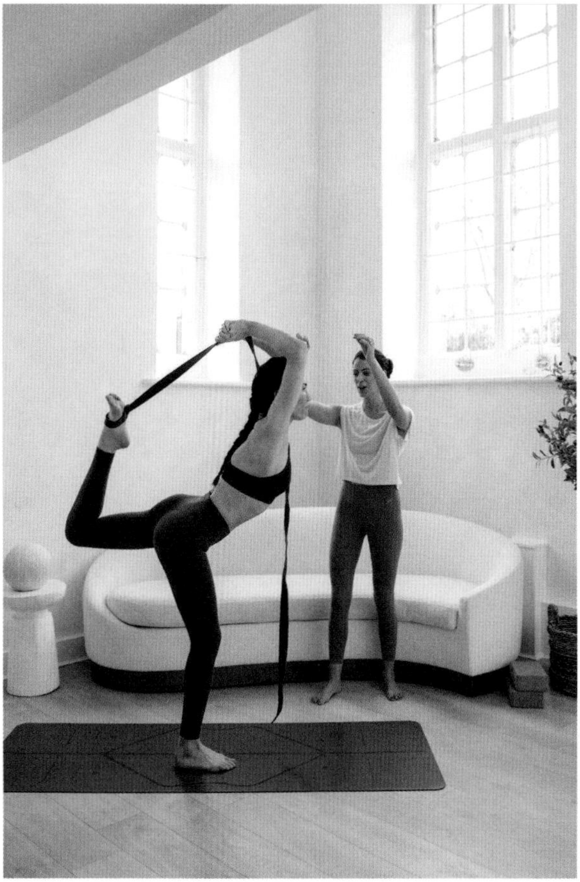
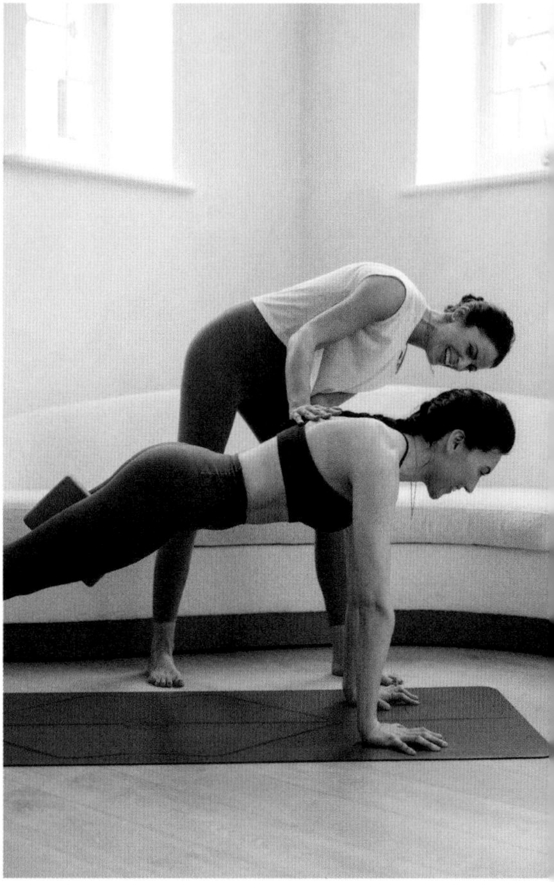
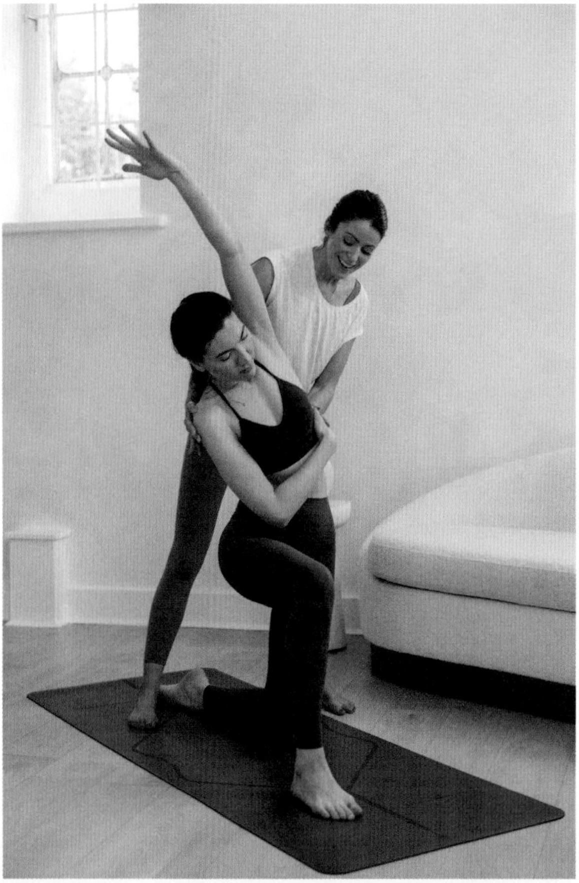
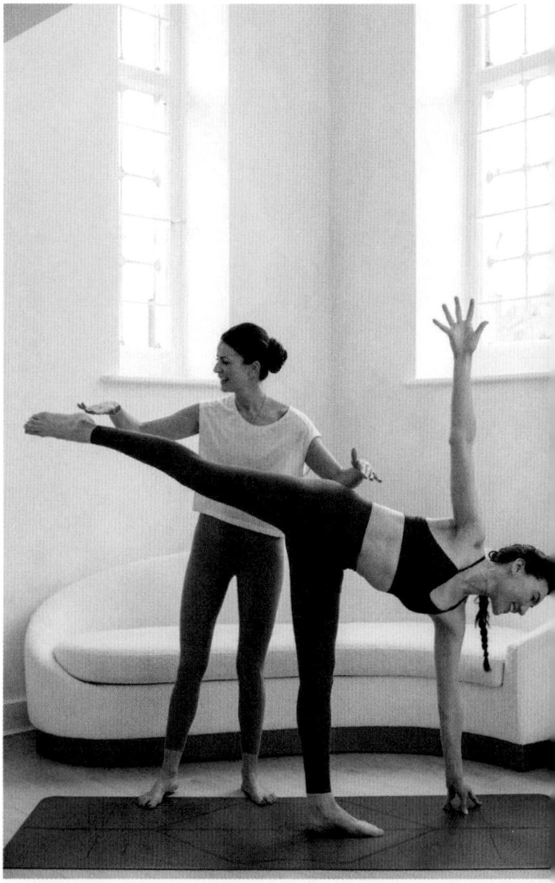

MONTH 12
BUFFALO

'COWS RUN AWAY FROM THE STORM WHILE THE BUFFALO CHARGES TOWARD IT – AND GETS THROUGH IT QUICKER. WHENEVER I'M CONFRONTED WITH A TOUGH CHALLENGE, I DO NOT PROLONG THE TORMENT, I BECOME THE BUFFALO.'

WILMA MANKILLER

BUFFALO

For the final month of *The Yoga Happy Year* we are going to work on harnessing our inner buffalo, the animal that represents freedom and strength. When a storm is approaching, buffalos run directly into it to allow them to get through it quicker, while cows tend to run away from it. This is a good metaphor for life. We all experience storms at one point or another, whether it's from obstacles at work, a family disagreement or unforeseen challenges. It is natural, like the cow, to want to avoid these storms but by doing so we are just pushing back the inevitable – and usually causing suffering in the meantime. Let's start to harness our inner buffalo, facing challenges head on and approaching them with courage and strength.

By now you will have experienced how yoga helps us not just in the physical body, but also by nourishing our mind and soul. It dissolves self-imposed boundaries and/or limiting belief systems engrained in us and broadens our perceptions. It allows us to look outside of ourselves and find connection, perhaps to a higher power or simply to the universe as a whole. This connection is vital in living a strong and joyful life filled with purpose.

This month I'm sharing one last element of yogic philosophy with you – the three fundamental qualities of nature known as the *gunas: sattva, rajas* and *tamas.* They represent key qualities or energies that shape all aspects of life. Understanding how these *gunas* manifest in our thoughts, actions and emotions can offer insight into our inner workings.

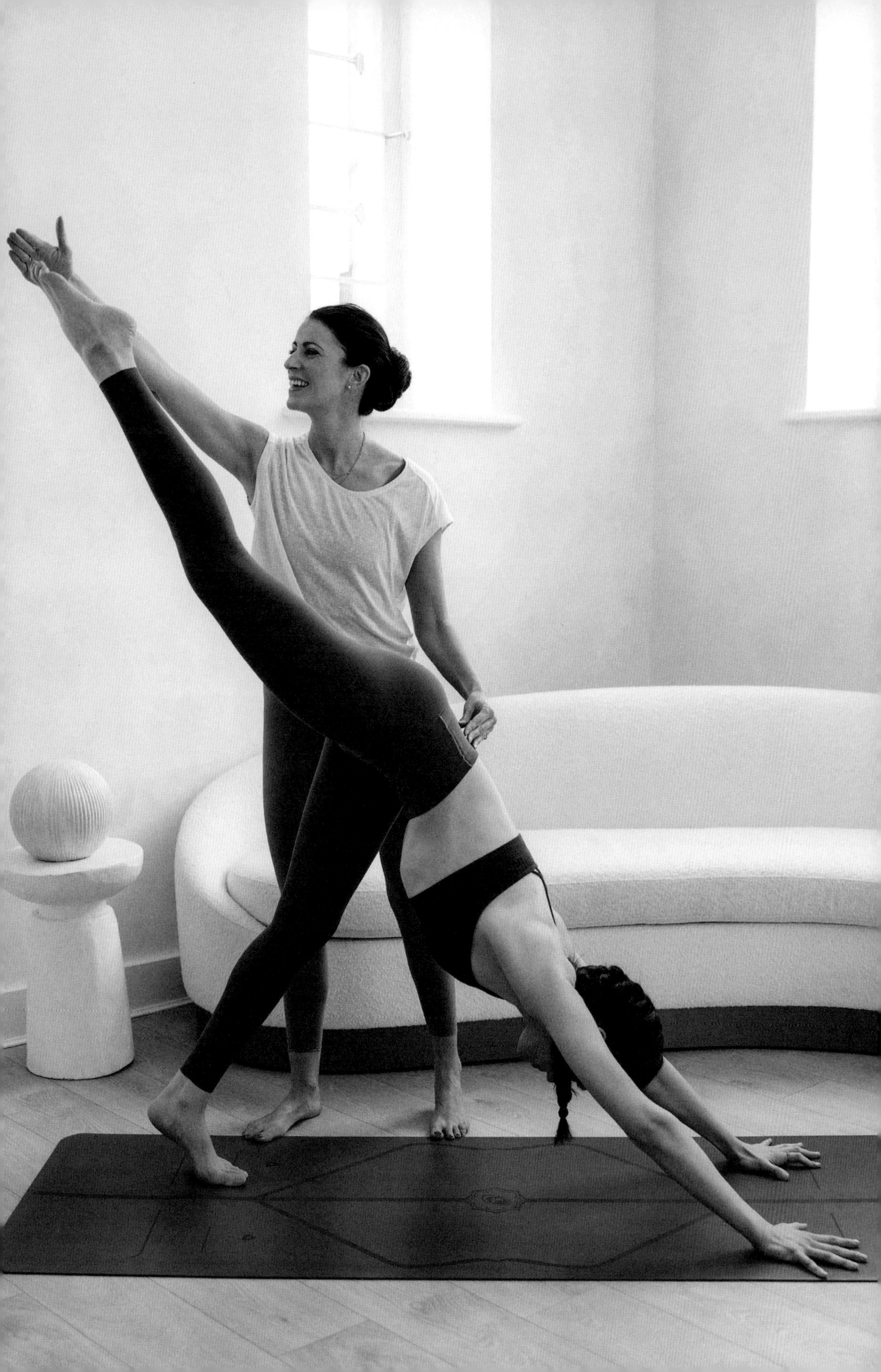

THE *GUNAS*

OUR MINDS INFLUENCE OUR ACTIONS, GUIDING US TOWARDS BALANCE OR IMBALANCE IN LIFE.

The word *gunas* translates to 'qualities' or 'attributes'. They exist in differing levels within individuals and the world around us, influencing thoughts, behaviours and experiences. For example, in humans, a person experiencing inner peace and clarity during meditation embodies *sattva*. Whereas, in the natural world, swamps and polluted areas reflect *tamasic* qualities due to their stagnant nature.

The three *gunas* are:

1. ***Sattva*:** The quality of purity, harmony and balance. It is associated with clear perception and constructive action. It embodies goodness and brings clarity and wisdom. When *sattva guna* is predominant in one's mental and emotional state, actions and/or behaviours, individuals exhibit calm, compassion and joy. Their actions tend to be selfless and motivated by a desire to help others and contribute positively in life. Practices such as meditation, mindfulness, *asana*, acts of selfless service and a diet of fresh, whole foods help cultivate *sattva* and support a *sattvic* lifestyle.

2. ***Rajas*:** The quality of activity, passion and restlessness. *Rajas* is dynamic, representing action, desire and ambition. It fuels movement and change, but excessive *rajas* can lead to attachment, stress, overactivity and competitiveness. To help balance *rajas*, *pranayama* is helpful, as is being mindful in action and preventing excessive activity or restlessness.

3. ***Tamas*:** The quality of inertia, darkness and stagnation. It represents heaviness and is associated with lethargy, ignorance and delusion. A *tamas* predominance may make one feel sluggish, lazy, negative and resistant to change, however it is worth noting that *tamas* is a necessary quality for sleep and rest. To help balance *tamas* requires practices that counteract its qualities of lethargy and stagnation, such as physical activity, engaging in creative pursuits and mindfulness practices.

By consciously navigating the interplay of these *gunas*, we can foster greater harmony and alignment in our lives. Going back to our theme of the buffalo, we can find reflections of the *gunas* in the buffalo's different states: *sattva* in its calm demeanour among other buffalos, *rajas* in its energetic or assertive moments and *tamas* in its sluggish or resistant phases.

Here are some ways can we incorporate the *gunas* in our daily lives:

1. **Self-reflection:** During the day we have different mental states - times when we feel calm and balanced (*sattva*), when we are driven by activity and desires (*rajas*) and times where we are feeling more sluggish or dull (*tamas*). Observe yourself throughout a day noticing each of these states. Recognising helps us to understand our tendencies and allow us to make conscious choices.

2. **Practise moderation:** Be disciplined with the amount of time spent working, manage time efficiently and ensure that you incorporate periods of stillness and relaxation to balance out high-energy activities. Avoid over-stimulating habits or excessive busyness. *Rajas* is essential for action, but if we don't allow time to pause and rest, we can leave ourselves stressed.

3. **Break the sluggish cycle:** Introduce movement and practices into your routine to help combat lethargy and avoid excessive sleep or inertia. Engage in physical exercise, breathing techniques or activities that uplift and energise you.

4. **Non-attachment and balance:** Seek a lifestyle that embraces the positive aspects of all three *gunas* but refrain from becoming overly attached to any one of them. Adjust routines, habits and environments to seek balance.

THE BREATH

This month, you get to choose the breathing technique that best suits what you need. I have shared 10 different breathing techniques in this book and I invite you to choose the one that's right for you each day. Here is a summary of the different techniques and the main quality they may evoke for you:

1. Three-part breath (see page 31) – grounding
2. *Ujjayi* breath (see page 46) – energy
3. Golden thread (see page 60) – focus and calm
4. *Sama vritti* (see page 74) – calm or balance
5. *Sitali* and *sitkari* (see page 130) - cooling
6. *Nadi shodhana* (see page 88) - balance
7. Box breath (see page 116) – calm and regulation
8. *Kapalabhati* (see page 129) – heat and energy
9. 2:1 breath (see page 143) – calm and relaxation
10. *Bhramari* (see page 157) – calm and stress-reduction

THE BUFFALO FLOW

Our last signature flow comes back to the theme of effort and ease (*sthira-sukha*, see page 72). Enjoy the blend of softness and strength, inhaling peace, exhaling power. As in previous months, ask yourself how you can adapt this flow to include more of what you need in that moment. For example, if you need more power bring in 'power *vinyasas*' throughout (see page 130). If you're searching for softness and freedom, choose a gentle cat and cow instead of a plank. I have included some challenges in this month's flow but it's completely up to you whether you practise them or not.

In Native American cultures, buffalos are considered sacred and are often seen as a symbol of abundance and strength. Let the last theme of the year act as a reminder of the sacredness of your body and how it houses the divine essence of your true self. Continue to treat your body with love (*ahimsa*) and truly listen to what it's telling you, not what you think it needs.

Aim to practise this flow three or four times per week and if you have more time, feel free to add the seated warm-up flow on page 10 at the start, combine it with the previous months' flows or repeat the flow multiple times.

As you move around your yoga mat, bring some buffalo qualities with you:

- **Connection to the earth:** Buffalos are grounded animals. Learn from this and channel this connection to the earth as you practise to feel rooted, connected and present during each pose and transition.
- **Facing challenges head on:** I explained at the start of this chapter how buffalos run straight into and through a storm. If you do substitute the flow or postures this month, be mindful of what you're avoiding. Can you face the flows and postures you find challenging head on, always seeking adjustments where needed? We often shy away from the movements our body finds hard but perhaps actually needs. Find your inner buffalo to tackle the challenge.
- **Strength and stability:** Ground yourself firmly, maintain strong foundations and cultivate inner and outer strength.

PLEASE NOTE

The appendix on page 190 includes a detailed breakdown of each pose, plus variations and modifications. Remember to listen to your body; yoga should never be painful and you can chose to skip any pose that doesn't feel right for you.

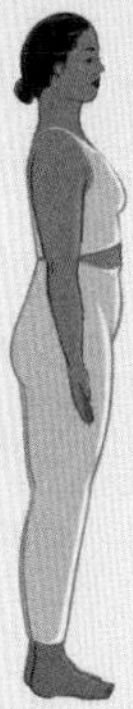

1. STANDING BREATH OF CHOICE

From standing, take 10 rounds of a breathing technique of your choice (see page 182).

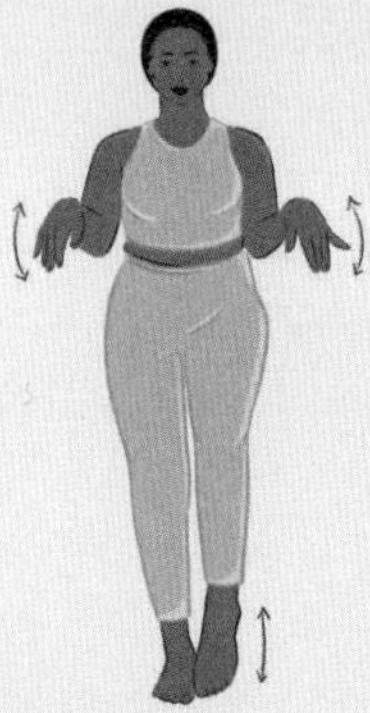

2. FOOT AND WRIST SEQUENCE

Balancing on the right foot, circle the wrists and ankle 5 times in each direction. Repeat on the opposite side.

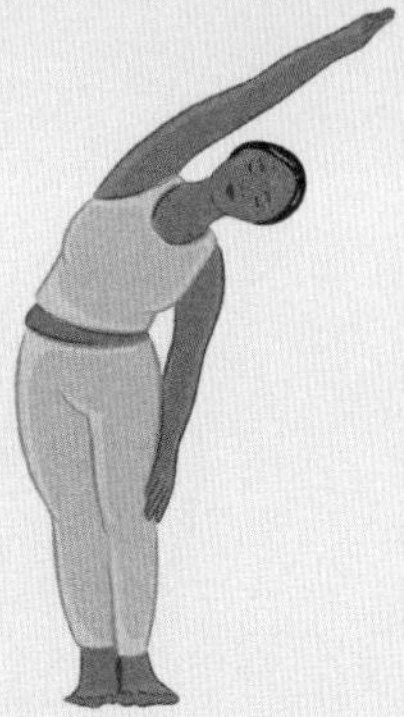

3. STANDING SIDE STRETCH

Inhale, lifting the right fingers to the sky and exhale, taking a side bend to the left. Repeat on the opposite side. Repeat 3 times each side.

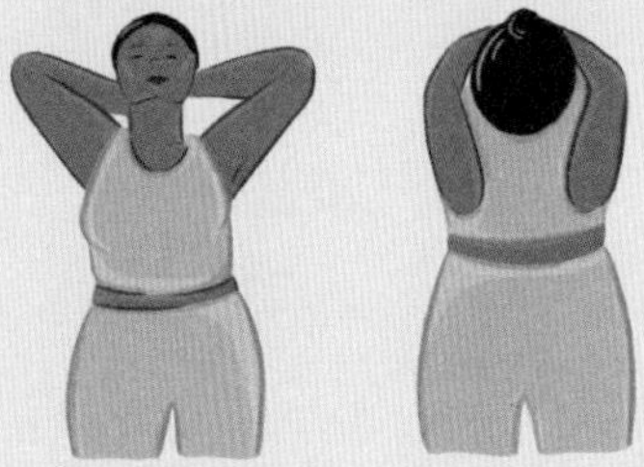

4. STANDING HEART OPENER

Inhale, opening the heart and exhale rounding the back. Repeat 5 times.

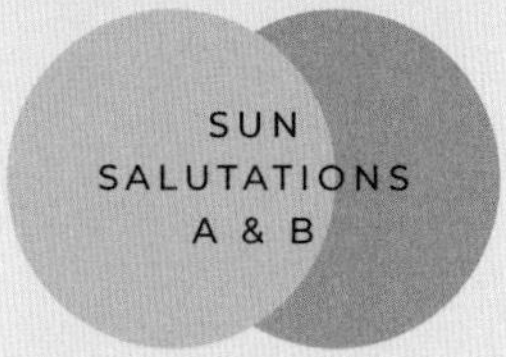

Option to include sun salutations A and B (see pages 16–20).

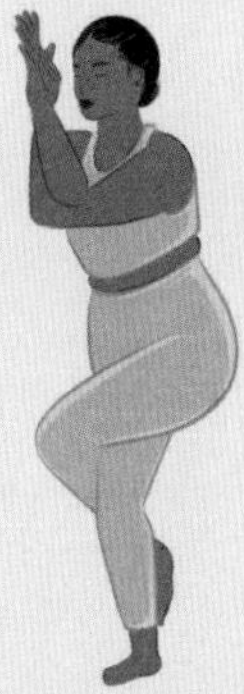

5. EAGLE

Inhale, lifting the left foot, exhale and wrap the body into eagle pose. Hold for 5 breaths.

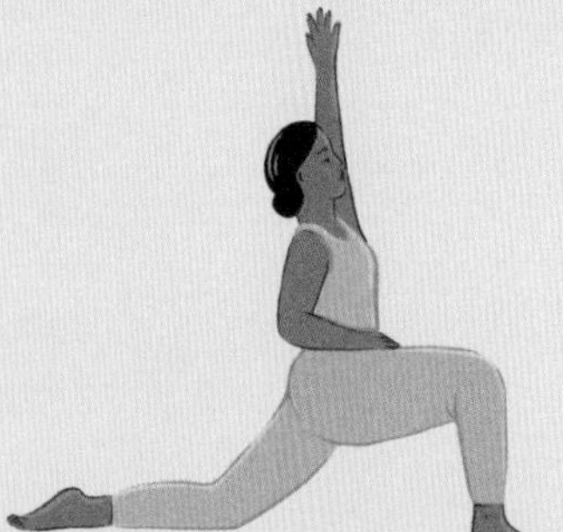

6. LOW LUNGE SIDE STRETCH

Unravel and step the left foot back, finding low lunge side stretch. Hold for 5 breaths.

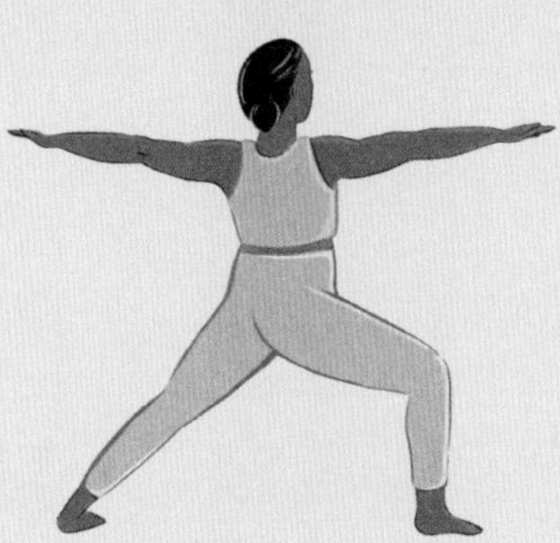

7. WARRIOR II

Exhale opening into warrior II. Hold for 5 breaths. Option to lift the front heel.

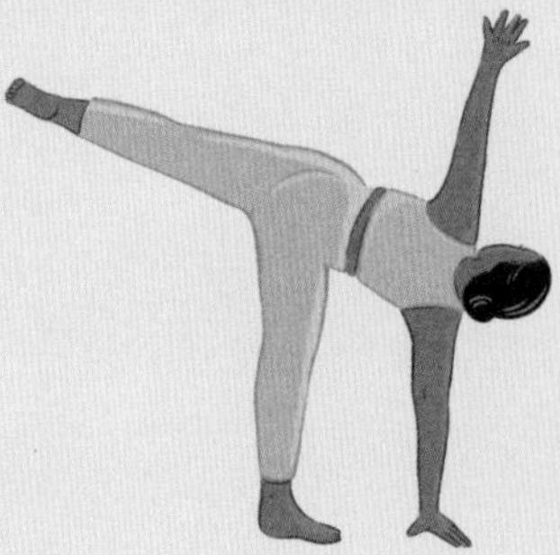

8. HALF-MOON

Inhale to lengthen forward, exhale to lift into half moon. Hold for 5 breaths. Option to pulse the back leg up and down.

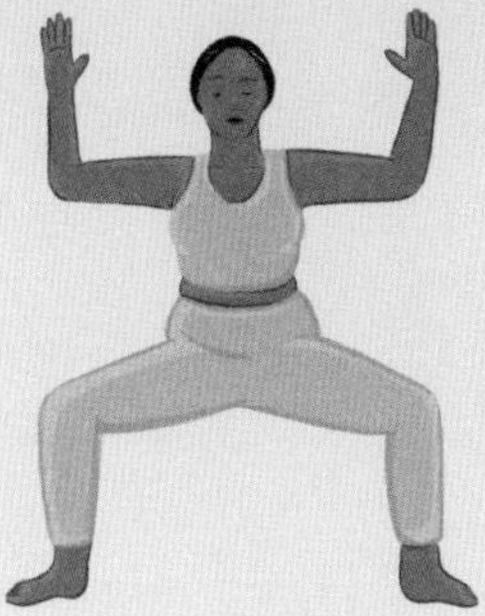

9. GODDESS

Step down and exhale, opening to to goddess. Hold for 5 breaths.

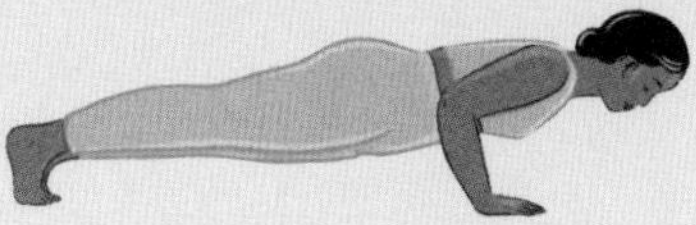

10. YOGA PUSH-UP

Frame the front foot stepping back through plank and exhaling through yoga push-up to your belly.

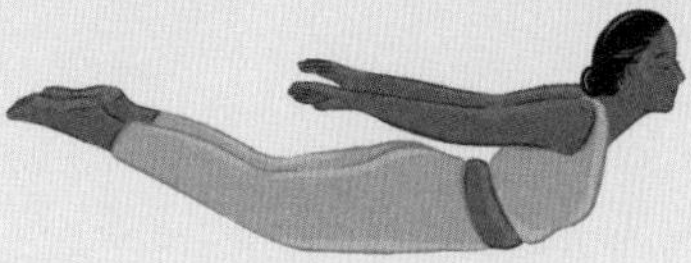

11. LOCUST

Inhale, lifting into locust pose. Hold for 5 breaths. Option to pulse the legs and arms up and down.

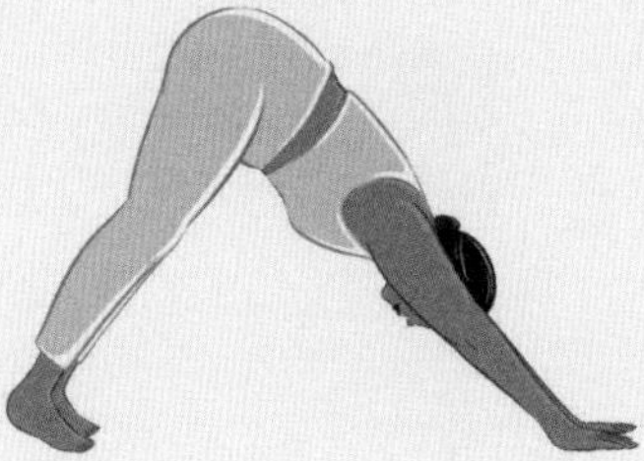

12. DOWNWARD-FACING DOG

Exhale, lifting the hips into downward-facing dog and hold for 3 breaths.

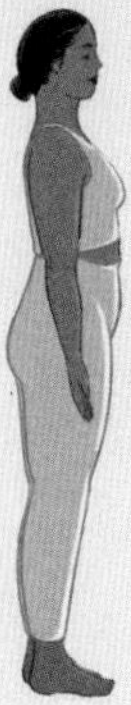

13. MOUNTAIN

Inhale and step the feet forward, lifting up to mountain.

REPEAT ON THE OTHER SIDE

STEPS 5–13

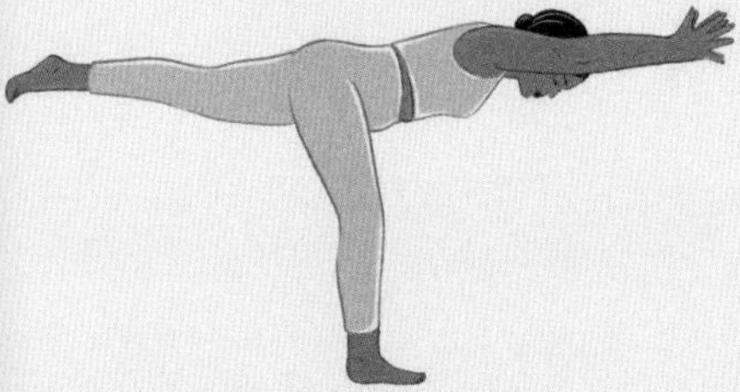

14. WARRIOR III

Exhale as you reach the left leg back into warrior III. Hold for 2 breaths.

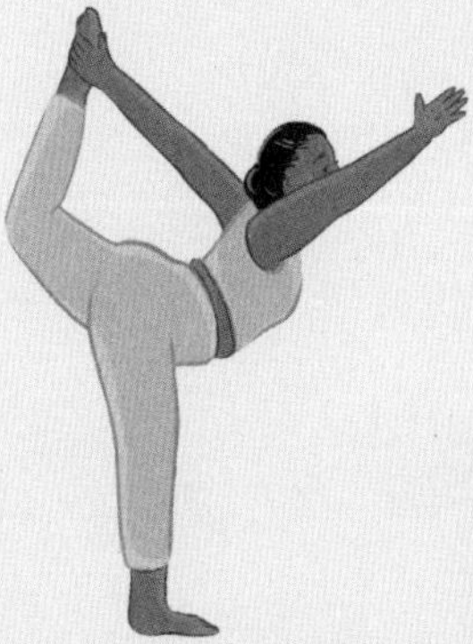

15. DANCER

Inhale to stand, take hold of the left foot behind you with the left hand and exhale to dancer. Hold for 5 breaths.

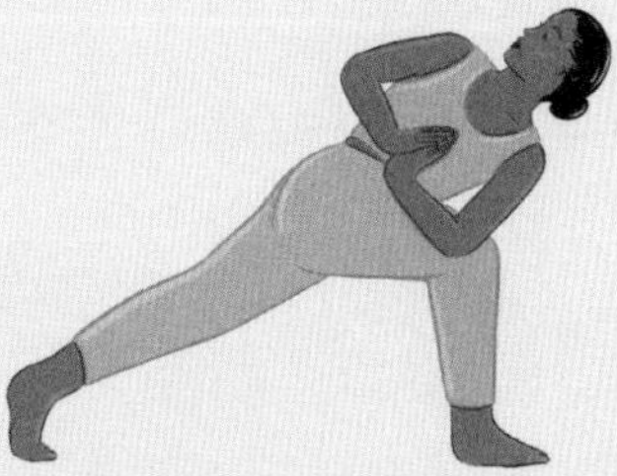

16. TWISTED CRESCENT LUNGE

Release the foot and step back to high lunge, exhale and twist. Hold for 5 breaths.

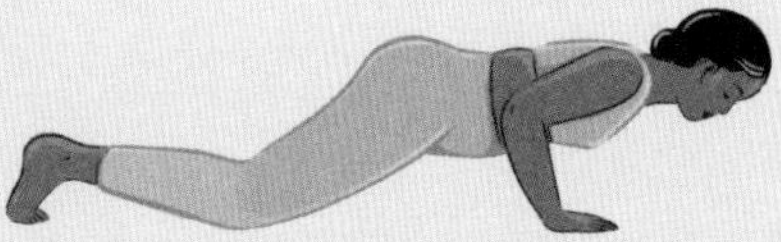

17. YOGA PUSH-UP

Frame the front foot stepping back through plank and exhaling through yoga push-up to your belly.

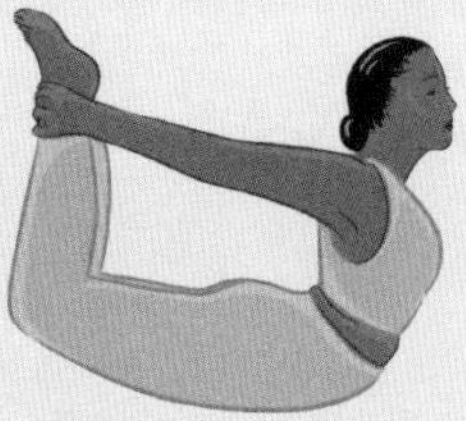

18. BOW POSE

Inhale and lift into bow pose. Hold for 5 breaths.

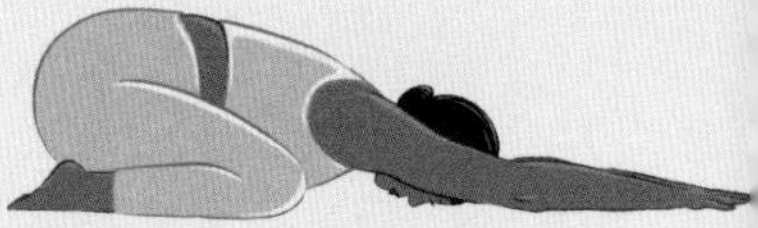

19. CHILD'S POSE

Exhale, sitting the hips to the heels and finding child's pose. Hold for 3 breaths.

REPEAT ON THE OTHER SIDE

STEPS 14–19

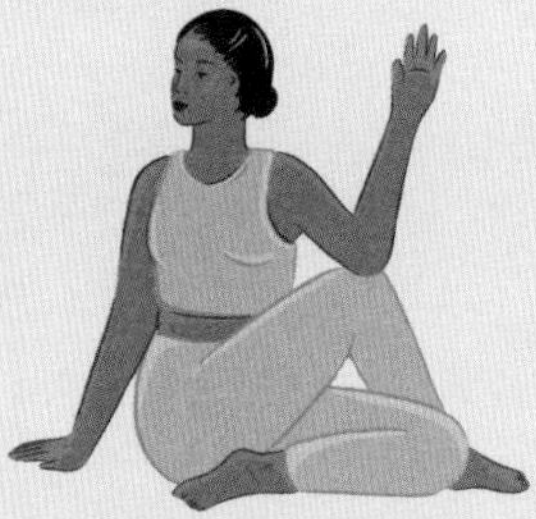

20. HALF LORD OF THE FISHES POSE

Coming to sit on the mat, step the right foot over the left thigh. Inhale to lengthen, exhale to twist. Hold for 5 breaths.

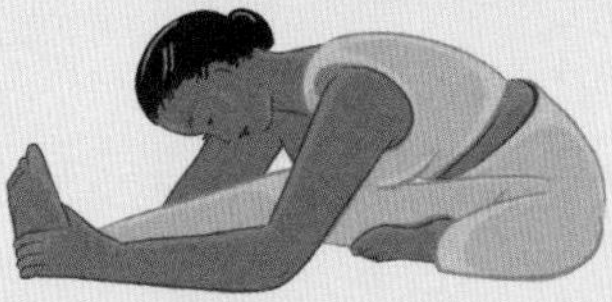

21. HEAD-TO-KNEE FORWARD FOLD

Release the right leg straight, inhale to lengthen, exhale to fold forward. Hold for 5 breaths.

REPEAT ON THE LEFT SIDE

STEPS 20 AND 21

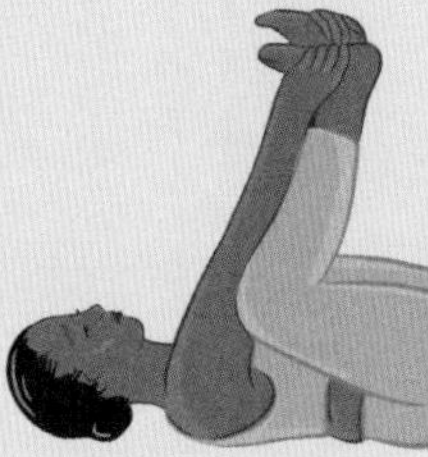

22. HAPPY BABY

Coming onto the back, take hold of both feet and exhale into happy baby. Hold for 5 breaths.

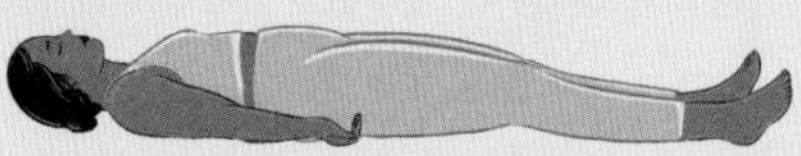

23. SAVASANA

Release softly and melt into savasana for 2 minutes or more.

MEDITATION

WALK AND SMELL THE ROSES

This last meditation is a favourite of mine. It's a walking meditation that channels gratitude and uses the sense of smell as a powerful connection to the present moment. I call it 'walk and smell the roses'. Bring the concept of this meditation into everyday life. Take those pauses, appreciate the beauty around you and remember to stop to smell the roses.

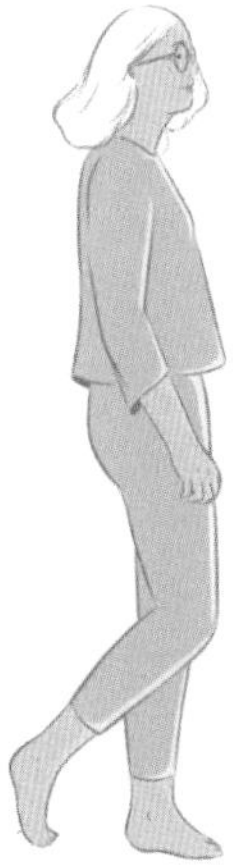

Directions:

1. Set a timer for 10 minutes or more.
2. Take yourself outside to a back garden, park or even a quiet pavement. Choose a place where you are safe, won't be interrupted and where you don't need to make decisions about where you walk.
3. As you walk, bring your full focus into the present moment. Walk at a slightly slower-than-normal pace, observing the world around you.
4. When you see something natural that may have a scent, pause and smell it; it may be a flower, a leaf, a plant or the smell of the ground after the rain.
5. Close your eyes as you smell and bring your full awareness to the aroma.
6. After a few moments, leave the smell and continue walking.
7. When you come across another fragrance, stop and smell it with presence and curiosity. Try to let go of analysis or judgement.
8. Feel free to intentionally move your attention to any sounds, sights or objects, but the key is intention. Intentionally allow the mind to explore and observe them.
9. When you are finished with your walk, try to remember this practice throughout your day, tuning in to any smells that come and go.

JOURNAL PROMPTS

Below I have given you eight self-reflection questions linked to this month's buffalo theme and the *gunas*. Try answering two questions weekly alongside the daily journal prompts set out on pages 8–9.

▸ What practices elevate my mind and spirit towards greater understanding and harmony so that I can cultivate *sattva guna* (see page 180)?

▸ How can I integrate the qualities of a buffalo's connection to the earth into my own life? What positive changes can I make?

▸ In which areas of my life am I driven by restlessness or the need for constant action? Can I find a healthier balance between productivity and personal well-being?

▸ A buffalo has a powerful presence that coexists with its gracefulness. In what ways can I embody both power and grace in my actions?

▸ Which habits or patterns hold me back from growth or positive change?

▸ What challenges am I currently facing? How can the buffalo's resilience in facing the storm inspire me to confront and overcome them?

▸ How can I consciously shift from one *guna* to another when necessary for my well-being?

▸ Buffalos have the ability to adapt to different environments and conditions. What strategies do you use to navigate transitions and shifts in life and remain grounded?

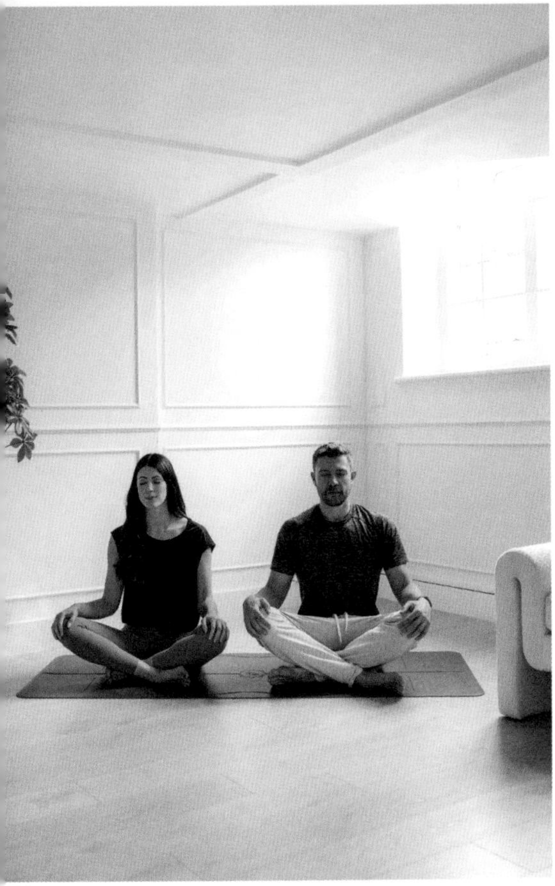
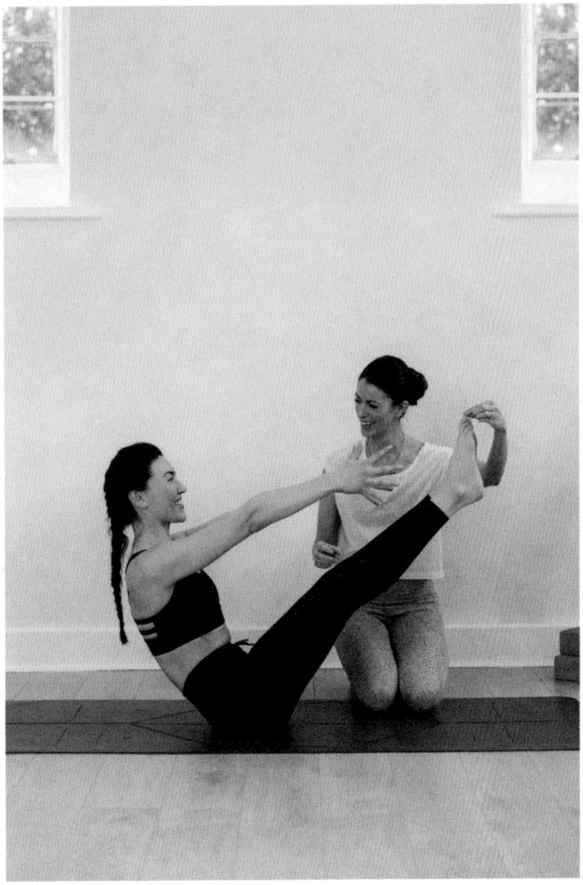
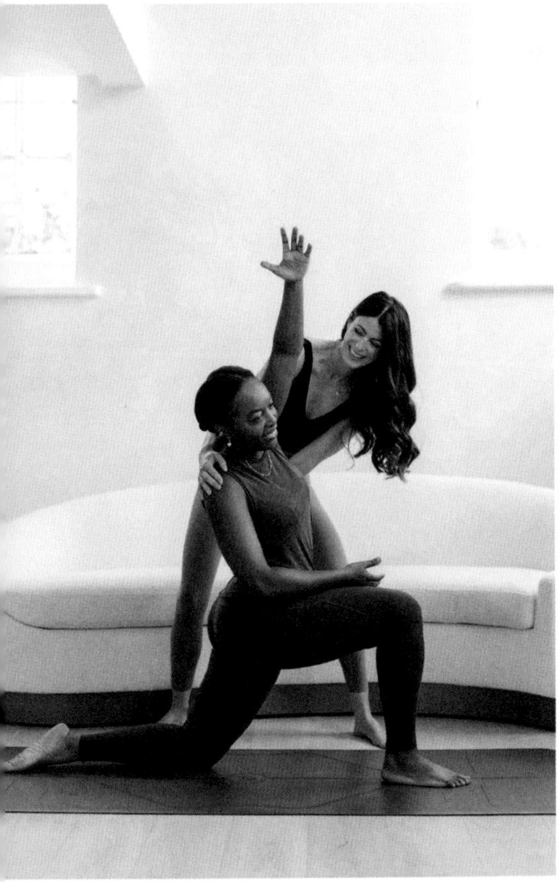
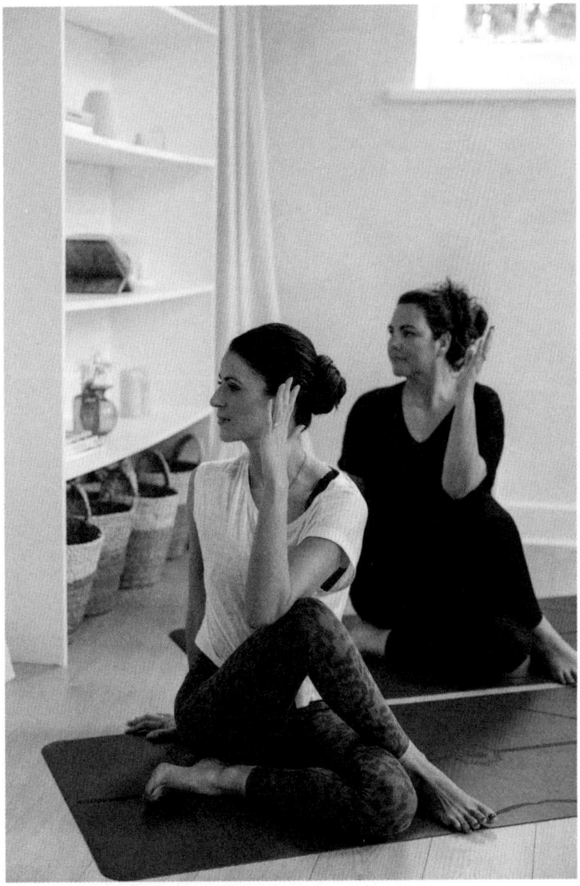

APPENDIX OF POSTURES

‘YOGA ISN’T ABOUT WHAT IT LOOKS LIKE, TUNE IN TO HOW IT FEELS IN YOUR UNIQUE BODY.’

HANNAH BARRETT

BOAT POSE
(Navasana)

Sit on the mat with the knees bent, feet flat on the floor and the spine long.

Exhale as you shift onto the back of the sitting bones, lifting the feet off the floor so that the shins are either parallel to the floor or the legs are straight.

Roll the shoulders back and down, as you imagine a piece of string is pulling the crown of the head away from you to lengthen the spine. Keep the chest lifted and the chin slightly tucked. Hug the inner thighs towards each other and point the toes.

Stretch the arms out parallel to the floor, palms facing one another, fingertips reaching away from the body. Hold for 5 breaths, ensuring the spine stays long and the core strong. Exhale and release the legs to the floor.

Option to modify by holding onto the backs of the thighs or placing one or both feet on the floor.

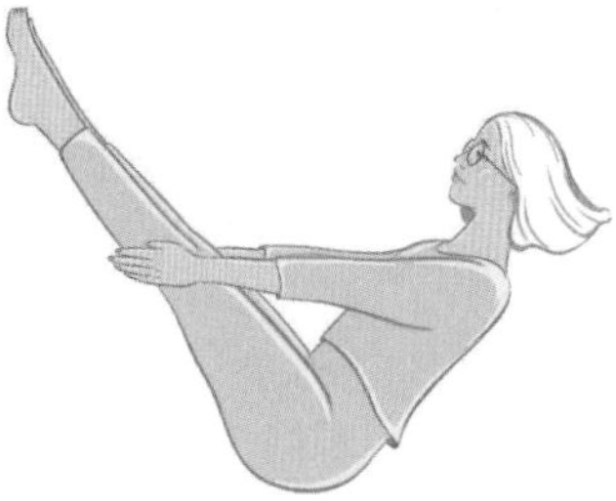

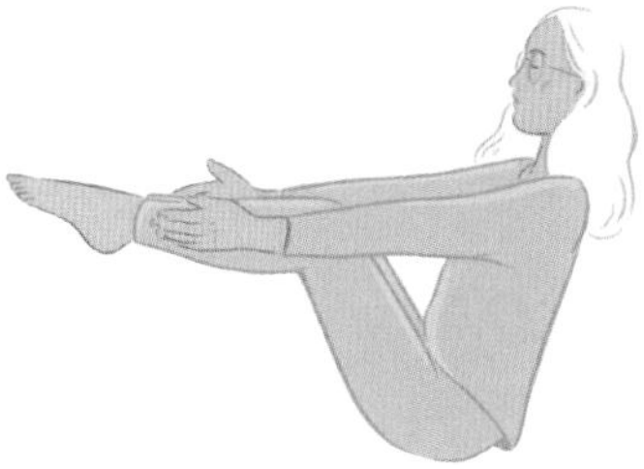

BOW POSE
(Dhanurasana)

Lie on your stomach with your legs extended.

Bend the knees and reach back to grab the ankles, one in each hand. You can hold the ankles from the outside or inside, whichever is most comfortable for you.

Inhale as you press the hands into the feet and kick the feet into the hands to lift the chest and thighs. Squeeze the shoulder blades together and squeeze the glutes to lift the thighs even higher.

Gaze forward or gently lift the head, maintaining a neutral neck. Reach the crown of the head away from the tailbone to keep a long spine.

Push down gently through the pubic bone into the mat to avoid overextending the lower back. Don't let the knees splay to the sides and hug them gently towards the centre keeping them around hip distance apart. Hold for 5 breaths before exhaling and gently releasing.

To modify, if you can't reach the feet you can lift without connecting the hands to the ankles. Alternatively, use a yoga strap around one ankle and keep the other leg straight and grounded.

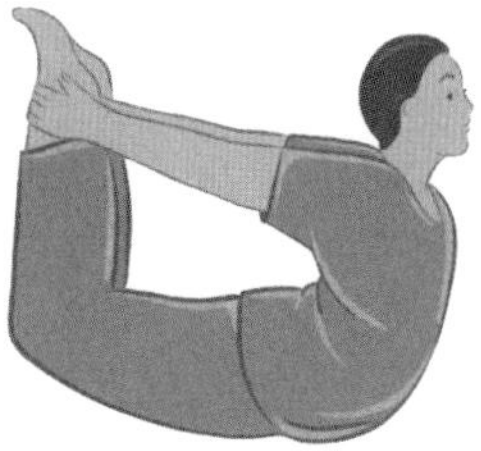

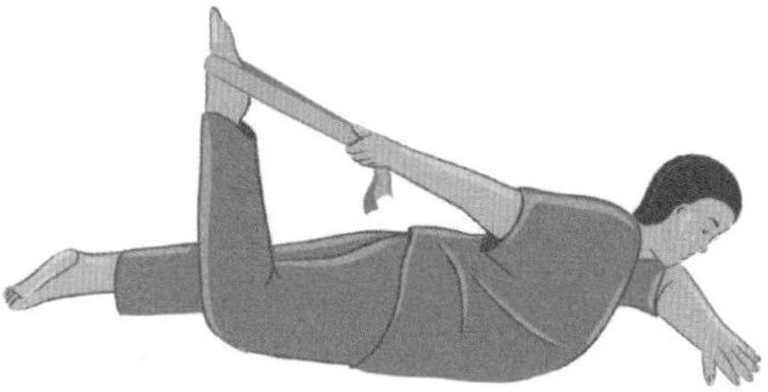

BRIDGE POSE
(Setu bandhasana)

Lie on your back with the knees bent, feet flat and hands by your side. Feet are hip width apart, toes pointing forward and heels about a hand's distance from the buttocks.

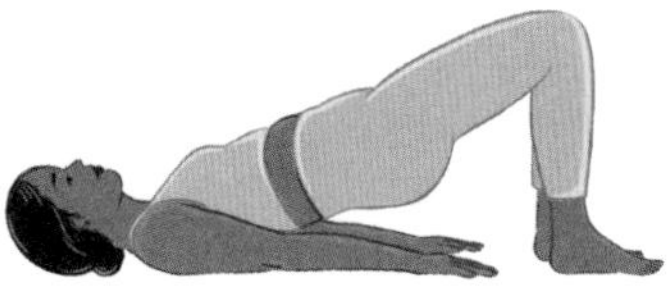

Exhale and press firmly into both feet lifting the hips off the floor, lengthening through the tailbone keeping the spine neutral and neck long.

Imagine a heavy weight is balancing on your hips and resist against it. Hold for 5 breaths.

Inhale and release the hips back towards the floor.

SUPPORTED BRIDGE POSE

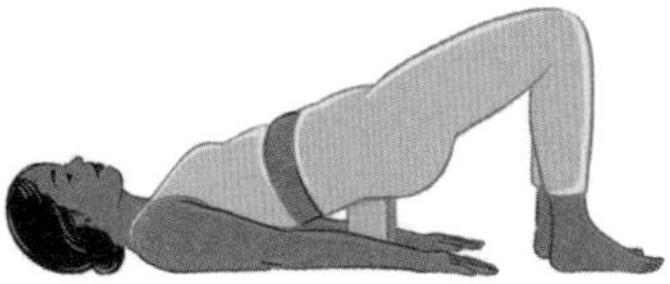

Placing a block or cushion underneath the sacrum can be a really nice restorative version of this posture.

COBBLER'S BRIDGE

Instead of having the feet hip distance apart, bring the soles of the feet together, letting the knees fall to opposite sides and lift the hips from the floor from here.

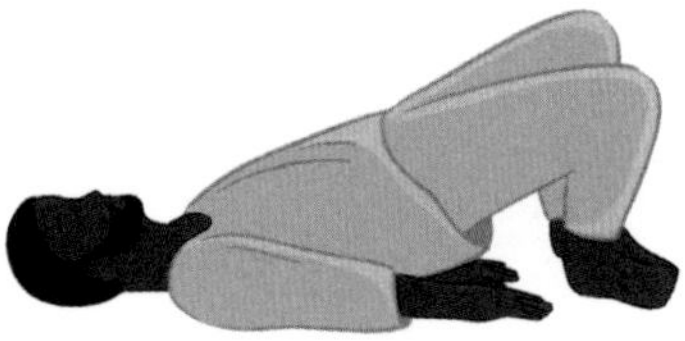

CAMEL POSE
(Ustrasana)

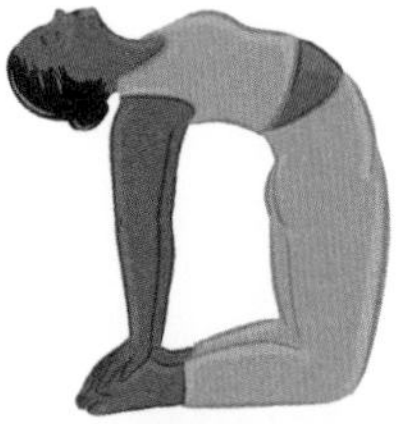

Begin in a kneeling position on your mat, with the knees under your hips and shins parallel to each other. Toes can be tucked or untucked.

Bring your hands onto your sacrum, fingers pointing down, and inhale as you lift the chest toward the ceiling. Gently arch the back and press the hips forward. Option to stay here.

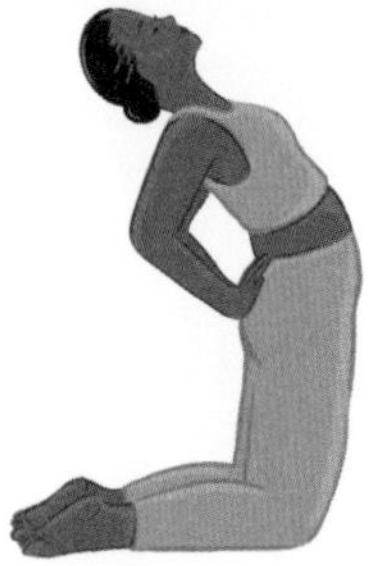

If you want more depth, reach one hand at a time toward the heels or onto secure blocks by your ankles.

Option to tilt your head back, gazing toward the ceiling or keep the chin tucked if that feels better for you.

Imagine there's a piece of string attached to the centre of the chest and it's lifting you upwards as you breathe the chest open. Keep the hips over your knees.

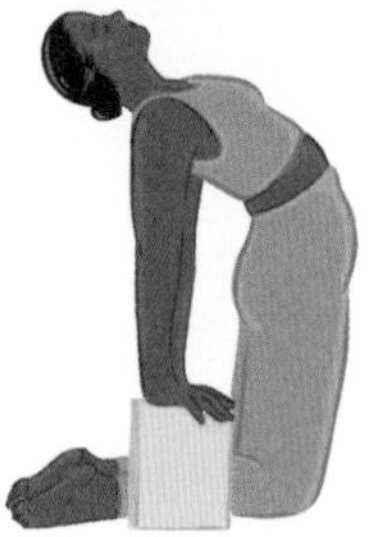

Hold for 5 slow breaths and then release, using your core to gently lift yourself back up. Sit back on your heels with a neutral spine to take a few grounding breaths.

CAT AND COW
(Marjariasana and bitilasana)

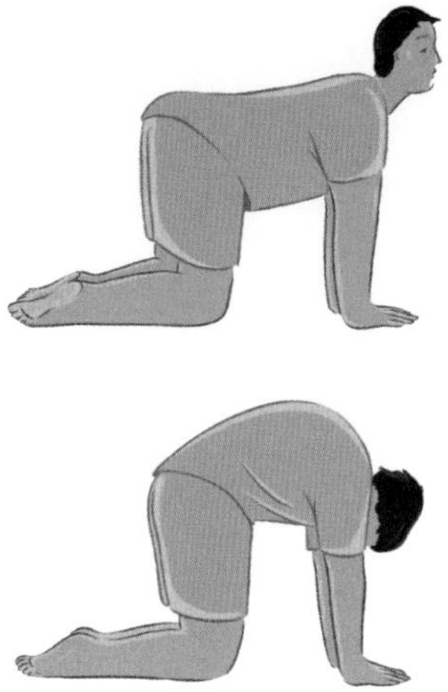

Start on all fours, wrists under shoulders, knees under hips.

Inhale into cow pose lifting the tailbone and arching the spine, having a sensation of pulling the hands backwards to help open the chest. Gaze forwards, keeping the neck long.

Exhale into cat pose drawing the tailbone down and rounding the back, relaxing the head, drawing the navel to spine and pushing the ground away to pull the shoulder blades away from the spine.

Continue moving through cow and cat for 5 full breaths.

CHAIR POSE
(Utkatasana)

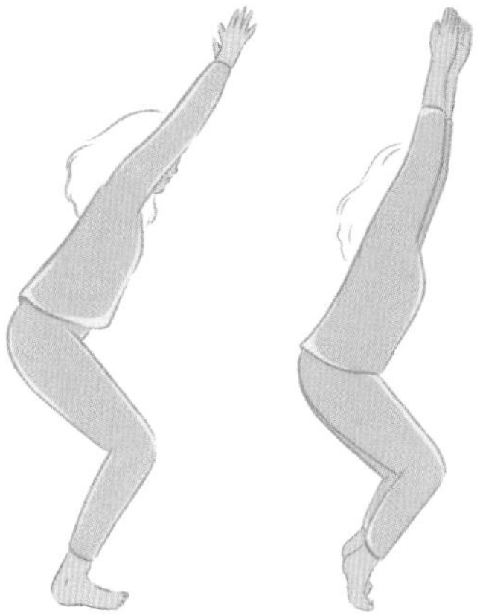

Stand at the top of the mat, toes together, heels slightly apart, or feet hip width apart, if that's more comfortable.

Inhale, raising the arms overhead (palms facing each other), lengthening the spine and bending the knees as if sitting back into a chair. Hug the inner thighs in, feeling the thighs and glutes fully engage.

Gaze forward and keep the chest lifted and spine long and neutral. Gently draw the ribs in to avoid them flaring. Hold the posture for 5 slow breaths.

CHAIR ON TIPTOES

From chair pose, see if you can lift the heels and balance on the toes. The heels may want to splay out, keep drawing them in to keep them parallel.

FIGURE FOUR CHAIR

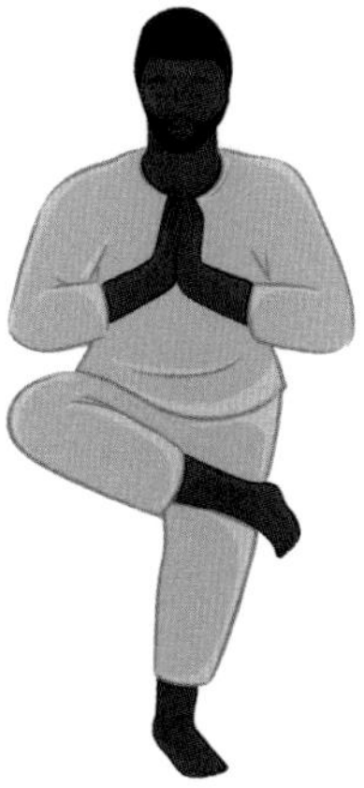

A nice variation of chair pose is to lift the right left and bring the ankle just above the left knee into a figure four position, opening the knee out to the right.

Hold for 5 slow breaths and then repeat on the opposite side.

TWISTED CHAIR
(Parivrtta Utkatasana)

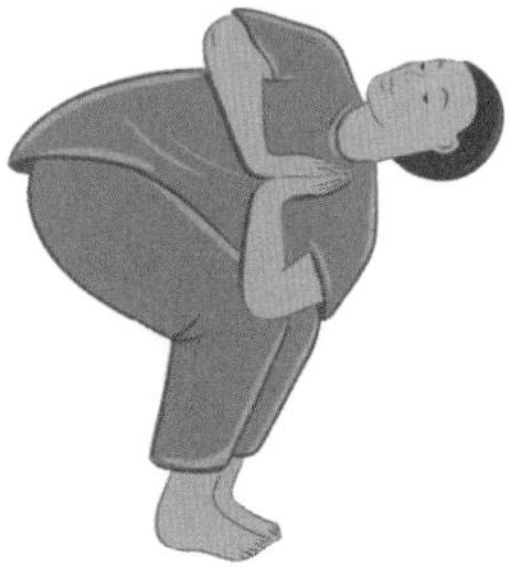

From chair pose, exhale as you bring the hands into prayer at heart centre and inhale to roll the shoulders back and down, opening through the chest. Exhale to rotate the torso to the right (the lower body doesn't move).

Option to hold here or connect the left elbow to the outside of the right thigh or on top of the thigh (keeping the chest open).

The left knee may want to creep forward; draw it back to keep it in line with the right. Roll the right shoulder back to keep the chest open.

Hold for 5 slow breaths before inhaling back to centre and releasing. Repeat on the left side.

CHILD'S POSE
(Balasana)

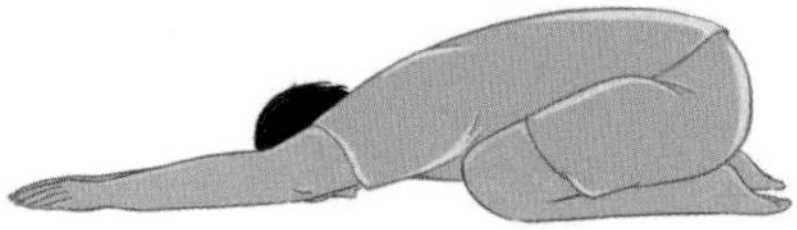

Kneel on the mat with the big toes together and the knees about hip width apart.

Exhale and lay your torso down between the thighs keeping the spine long. Stretch the arms forwards feeling a stretch from the tailbone out through the fingertips.

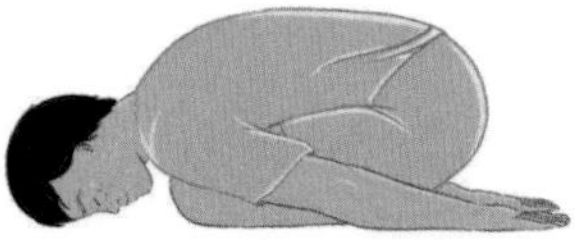

Alternatively, bring the knees together and/or bring the arms back and place the hands on the floor alongside the torso with the palms up, releasing the fronts of the shoulders toward the floor.

Rest here for 5 slow breaths or longer if required.

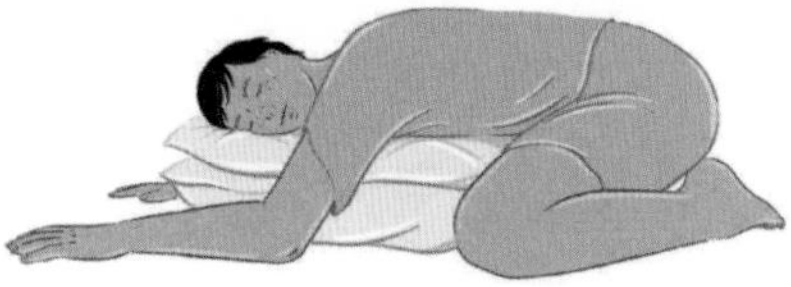

To make this pose really restorative, place a pillow between the thighs and melt the torso over it. You can also place a pillow or block under the hips if more comfortable.

COBBLER'S POSE
(Baddha konasana)

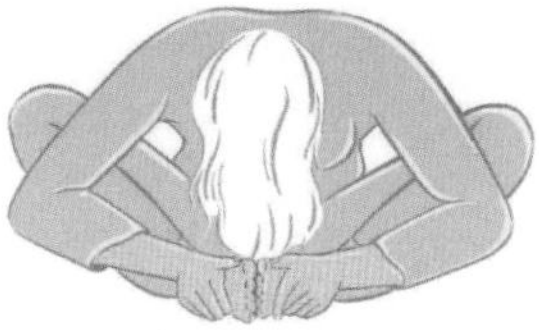

From a seated position, bring the soles of the feet together letting the thighs gently open.

Draw the feet in as close to the body as is comfortable (avoiding any pain in the knees). Gently interlace the fingers around the feet.

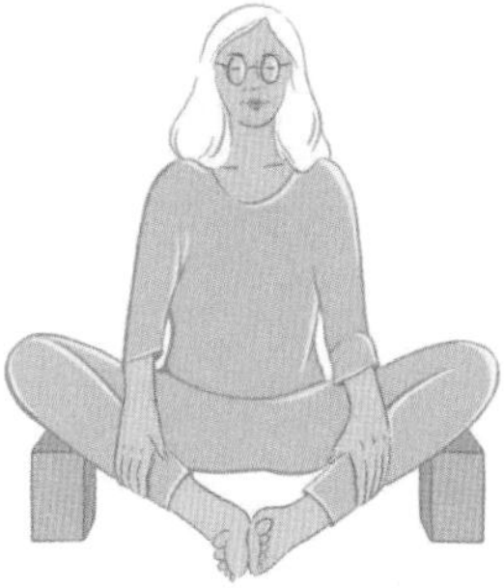

Inhale and find length through the spine, exhale keeping the spine neutral and hinge forward from the hips as far as comfortable. Option to release the head down and round through the back if that feels good.

Hold for 5 slow breaths, then gently inhale back up to centre and release.

If hinging forwards feels too intense, stay upright. You can even use blocks or blankets under the thighs for added support.

RECLINED COBBLER'S POSE
(Supta baddha konasana)

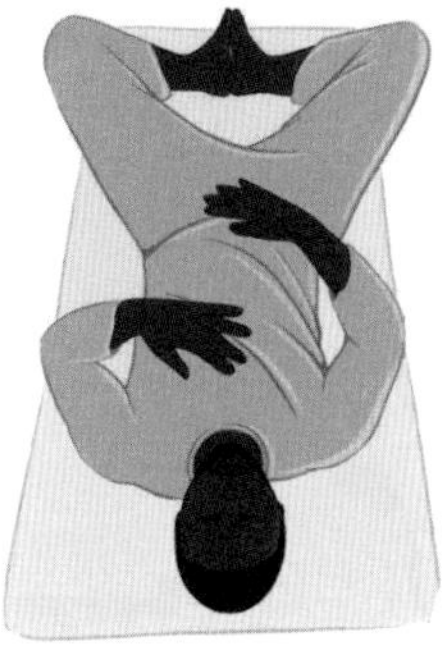

Lying on your back, bring the soles of the feet together letting the thighs gently open. Draw the feet in as close to the body as is comfortable (avoiding any pain in the knees).

Place a blanket or blocks under the knees for support. Use blankets, pillows or bolsters behind the back, head and arms for ultimate relaxation.

Stay for as long as needed, breathing mindfully.

COBRA POSE
(Bhujangasana)

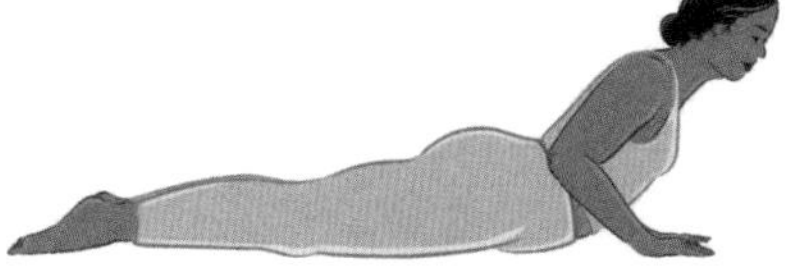

Lying on your belly, gently push down through the tops of the feet and the pubic bone, engaging through the glutes.

Bring the hands underneath the shoulders. Inhale and use your back muscles to lift the upper body off the mat and have the sensation of the hands pulling backwards (without them actually moving) to help lengthen the spine and open the heart. Keep the neck long and gaze slightly forward.

Avoid pushing down through the floor and draw the shoulder blades back and down. Engage the glutes to avoid overextending the lower back.

Hold for 5 slow breaths and then exhale and gently release.

COW FACE
(Gomukhasana)

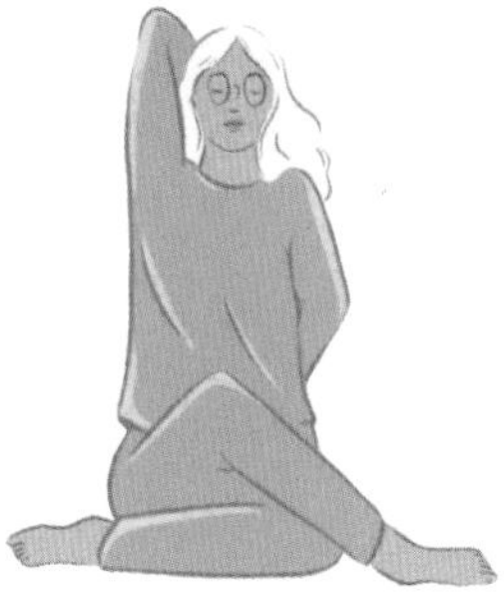

From a seated position with the legs out in front of you, cross the right leg over the left, stacking the right knee on top of the left and bringing the right ankle to the outside of the left hip and left ankle to the outside of the right hip. If this feels too intense, option to keep the left leg straight out in front.

With the knees stacked and centred, press down through your sitting bones and lengthen through the crown of your head as if being pulled upwards by an imaginary piece of string.

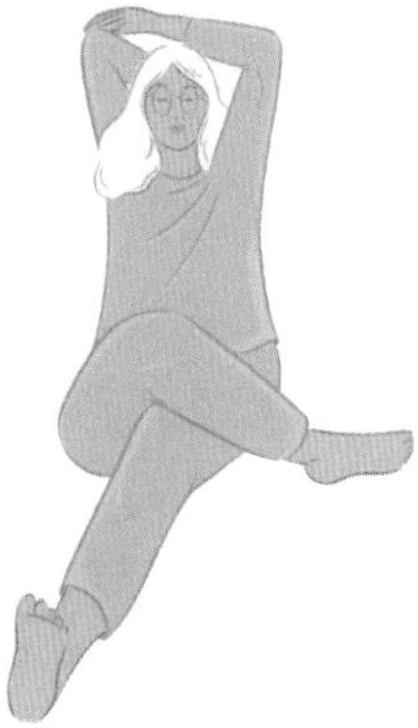

Inhale as you reach your right arm up overhead, bending the elbow up towards the ceiling, and hand down towards your upper back, palm facing your back.

Option to reach the left hand behind the back, palm facing away from the body and fingers clasping the right hand. Alternatively, the left hand can grab hold of the right elbow – press the elbow into the hand and the hand into the elbow. Keep the sensation of lifting up through the right elbow.

Option to fold forward in this posture if it feels good for your body, or simply gaze forward keeping the spine long. Hold for 5 breaths before repeating on the opposite side.

CROW POSE
(Bakasana)

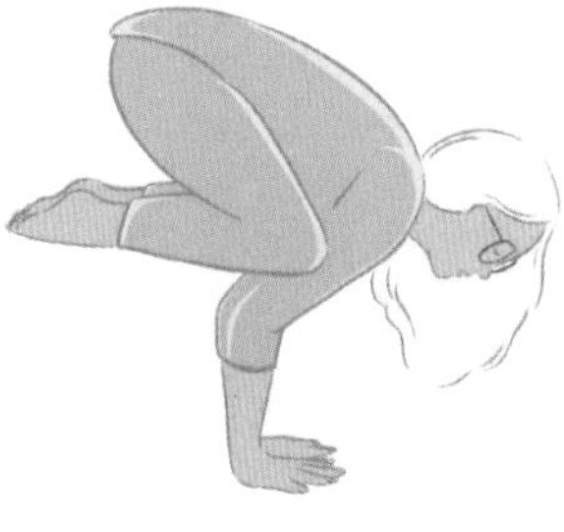

Begin in a squatting position with the feet hip-width apart.

Place the hands on the mat, shoulder-width apart, and spread the fingers. Ground down through your index finger knuckle and thumb and grip the fingers into the mat as they will help you balance in the posture. Push firmly into the mat to stabilise through your shoulders.

Shift your weight forward onto the hands, bending the elbows slightly and lifting the hips high.

Bring the knees to the backs of your upper arms, near the armpits, or balance the elbows on the knees, as you lean the body forwards. Exhale as you slowly lift the feet off the ground, toes pointed and legs strong and hugging inwards. Keep the core strong and have a sense of lift within the pose, lifting up the pelvic floor as you balance on the hands.

Keep the gaze slightly forward to help with balance. Hold the pose for 1–5 breaths and then gently release by lowering your feet back to the mat.

Option just to lift one leg or, to advance the pose, work on straightening the arms.

DANCER POSE
(Natarajasana)

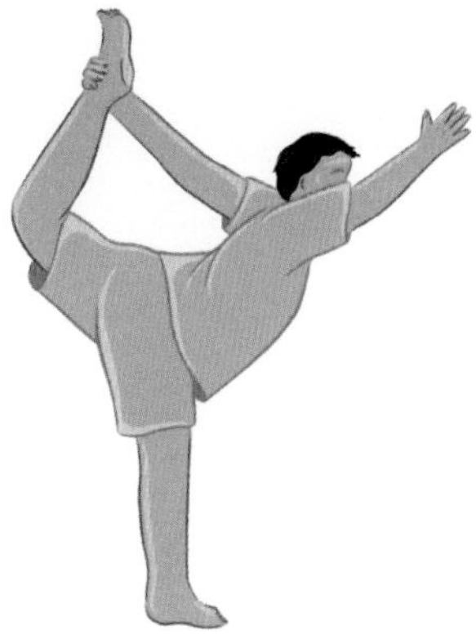

Start at the top of the mat in mountain pose *(tadasana,* see page 207). Shift your weight onto the right foot, pressing it down firmly and firming the muscles of the hip.

Kick the left foot back in towards the body keeping the knees together.

Reach back with the left fingers to grab the outside of the left foot. Option to use a yoga strap if this isn't accessible to you or to grab the inside of the foot if this feels better in your body.

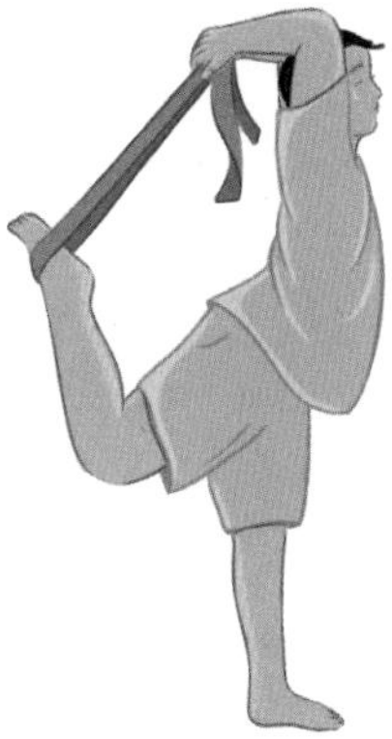

Inhale and reach the right arm to the ceiling as you press the left foot into the left hand and resist the hand into the foot, lifting the left leg back behind you and opening through the chest and shoulders.

Exhale and hinge at the hips, allowing your torso to move forward while keeping your chest open a little like the shape of an archer's bow.

Hold the pose for 5 slow breaths and then gently return to standing. Repeat on the opposite side.

DOLPHIN POSE
(Ardha pincha mayurasana)

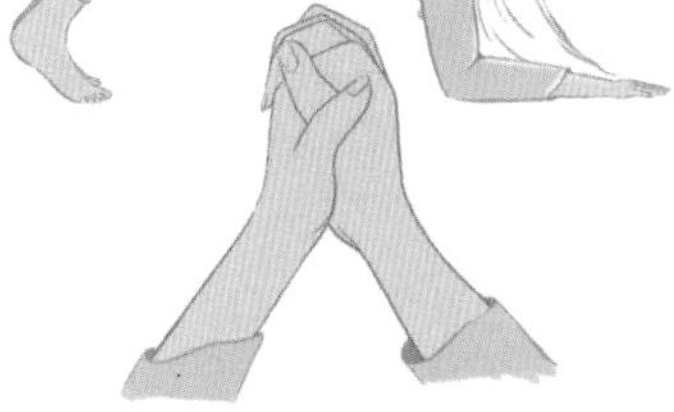

Starting on hands and knees, lower the forearms and palms to the floor shoulder distance apart. If this feels too intense you can clasp the hands together (making a triangle shape with the arms).

Release the head and push down firmly through the forearms drawing the shoulder blades away from your spine.

Exhale and curl the toes under, lifting the knees away from the floor and the hips upwards.

Lift the sitting bones up as you keep the spine long, drawing the heels down (if they don't touch the floor that's okay) and keeping as much of a bend in the knees as needed to keep the spine neutral.

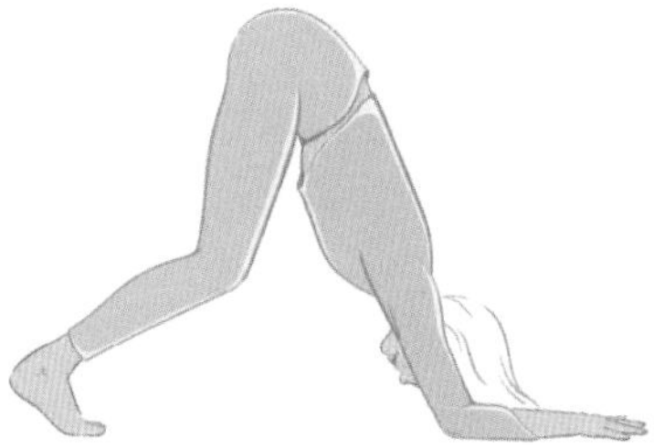

Draw the front ribs gently in towards the back body and hold the head between the upper arms, keeping the neck long.

Hold for 5 slow breaths then exhale and slowly release.

DOWNWARD-FACING DOG
(Adho mukha svanasana)

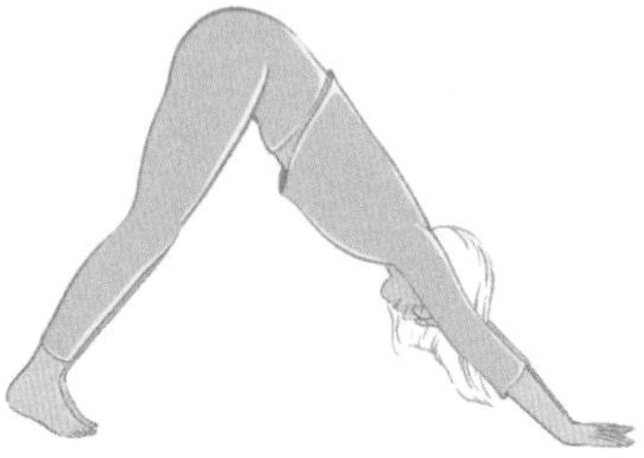

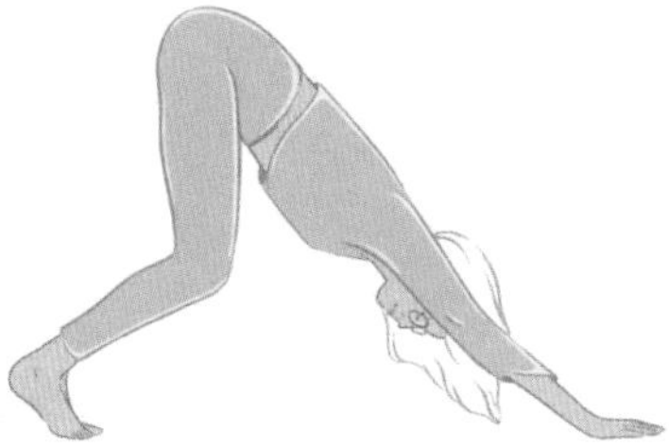

Start on hands and knees with the hands shoulder distance and knees hip distance apart.

Spread the fingers, middle finger facing straight ahead, and press firmly into the mat through the whole hand. Have a sensation of 'dialling' the hands in opposite directions (like screwing jam jar lids) without the hands actually moving. This broadens and stabilises the shoulders.

Exhale, curling the toes under and lifting the hips back and up reaching the sitting bones towards the ceiling. Keep the spine long and neutral as you start to slowly straighten the legs, avoiding any rounding in the lower back. The knees can stay bent. Draw the heels towards the mat but don't worry if they don't reach. Imagine you are shining the backs of the thighs towards the back of the room.

Draw the front ribs gently in towards the back body.

Keep the neck long, between the arms and hold for 5 breaths, then exhale and slowly release.

Option to modify by bending the knees as much as you need to keep the spine long.

DOWNWARD-FACING DOG HIP OPENER

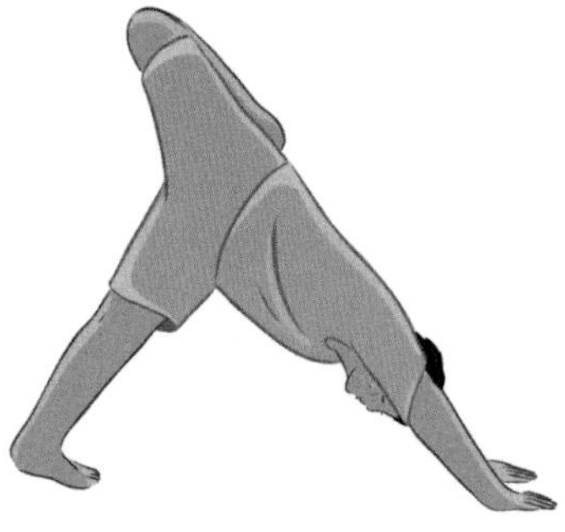

From downward-facing dog, lift the right leg back and up toward the ceiling, then bend the leg to open the hip.

Keep the shoulders square to the mat as you take 5 slow breaths.

Inhale to return to downward-facing dog and repeat on the opposite side.

DOWNWARD-FACING DOG TWISTS

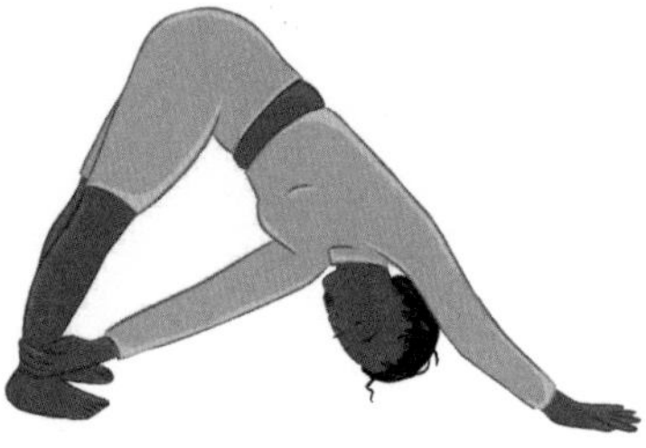

From downward-facing dog, inhale and firmly ground down through the right hand. Exhale to lift the left hand and take a twist underneath grabbing hold of the right thigh, shin or ankle, gazing underneath the right armpit.

Keep the sitting bones lifted towards the ceiling, spine long and heels drawing down.

Hold for 1–5 slow breaths and then inhale back to downward-facing dog and repeat on the opposite side.

EAGLE POSE
(Garudasana)

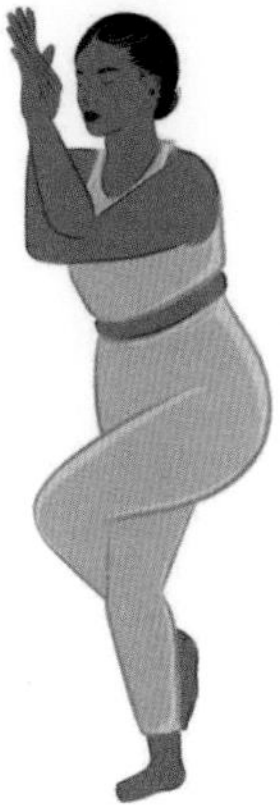

From mountain pose (see page 207), bring your weight to the right foot, grounding down and feeling the muscles of the hip engage.

Inhale as you lift the left foot off the floor, bending the knee and reaching the arms overhead.

Exhale to wrap the left leg around the right (half or full depending on balance and what is comfortable). Bend the right knee as much as needed.

At the same time, wrap the left arm underneath and around the right, bringing the palms or backs of the hands together (whichever is preferred or more comfortable).

Squeeze the inner thighs in towards each other and sit the hips back, feeling strong in the glutes.

Lift the elbows slightly.

Hold for 5 breaths, release and then repeat on the opposite side.

Option to rest the toes gently on the floor for balance.

EXTENDED SIDE ANGLE
(Utthita parsvakonasana)

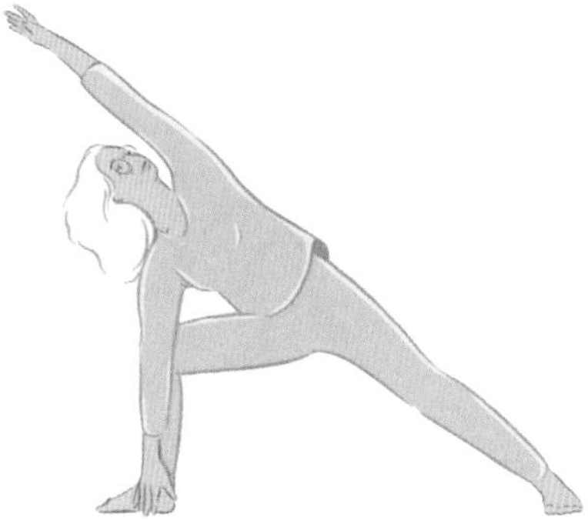

Start from warrior II (see page 219) with your right foot forward.

Exhale as you reach the right hand to the floor or onto a block by the right ankle, or alternatively bring the right forearm lightly onto the right thigh. At the same time, extend the left arm overhead, drawing a straight line from the left heel out through the left fingertips with the palm facing down.

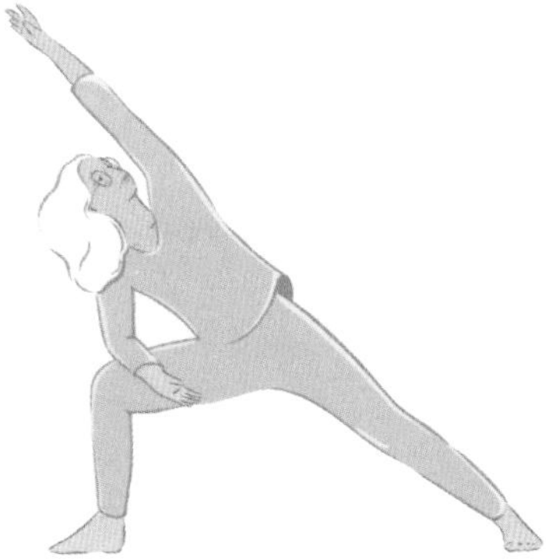

Keep the chest open by rolling the left shoulder back and gaze upward if comfortable or down towards the mat.

Press down firmly through the feet; you can even have a sensation of drawing the feet in opposite directions (as if you're trying to rip the mat apart) to help engage the leg and hip muscles. Keep the spine and torso long.

Take 5 breaths here and then inhale as you return to warrior II slowly, with control, and repeat on the other side.

FOOT AND WRIST SEQUENCE

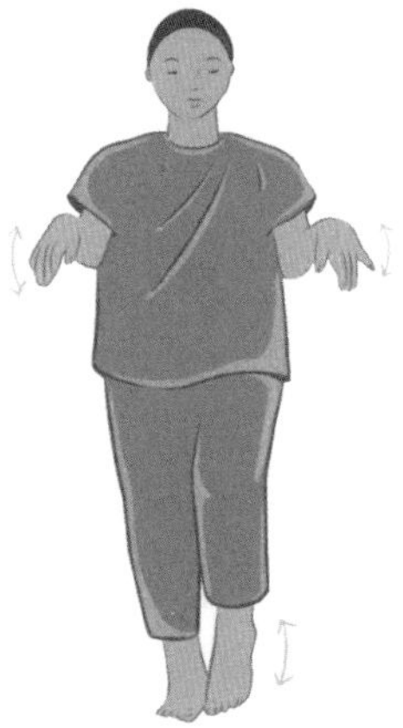

Stand at the top of the yoga mat. Ground down through the right foot, firming the muscles in the hip and inhale as you lift the left foot off the floor, bending the left knee.

Ensure you don't collapse into the right hip by keeping the right foot pushing into the mat.

Start to slowly circle the wrists and left ankle as you slow down the breath and deepen it.

Repeat three times in both directions.

Exhale to slowly release the foot and inhale to repeat on the other side.

This sequence can also be performed seated.

GODDESS POSE
(Utkata konasana)

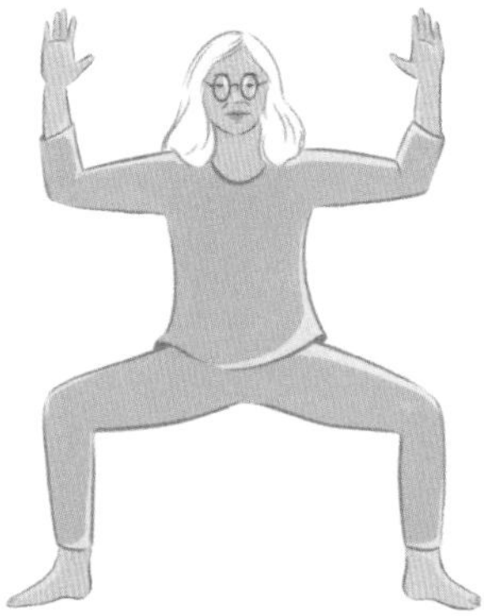

From mountain pose (see page 207), exhale and step the left foot back around 1m (3ft).

Turn the body and feet to face the left side of the mat.

Turn the toes out slightly (about 45 degrees) and inhale to reach the arms overhead.

Exhale to bend the knees, sitting down into the hips and bending the elbows to 90 degrees.

Keep the shoulders strong with the palms facing forward.

Press the feet down and knees gently backwards to engage legs and glutes and to ensure the knees don't collapse in.

Keep the spine long as you take 5 slow breaths here, then inhale as you straighten the legs and step to the front of the mat.

Option to have the feet closer together or to lessen the bend in the knees if more comfortable and to have hands at the heart centre if there is any pain in the shoulders.

HALF LORD OF THE FISHES POSE
(Ardha matsyendrasana)

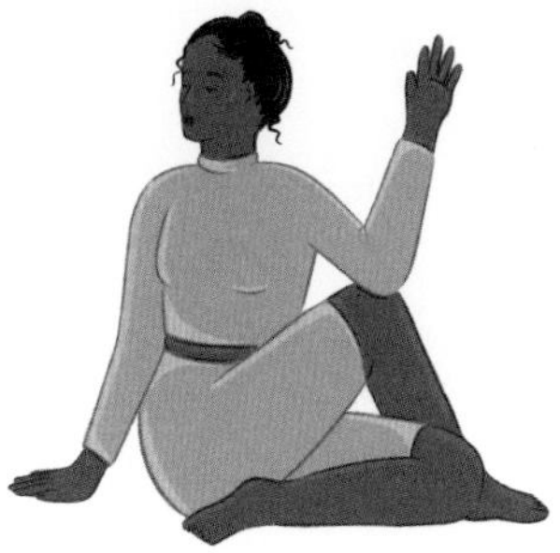

Sit on the mat with your feet flat on the floor and knees bent. Drop your left knee to the floor, tucking the left foot under the right leg, by the right hip. Option to straighten the left leg if this feels too intense.

Place the right fingertips behind you and inhale the left fingertips to the sky as you feel the spine lengthening. Exhale and twist your torso over to the right, imagining you are moving from the chest (avoiding just twisting from the neck).

You can tuck your left elbow on the outside of your right thigh or alternatively, hug the right leg with the left arm.

Hold for 5 slow breaths, growing taller with each inhale and twisting the body a little bit more with each exhale. Inhale slowly to release back to centre and repeat on the opposite side.

HALF MOON
(Ardha chandrasana)

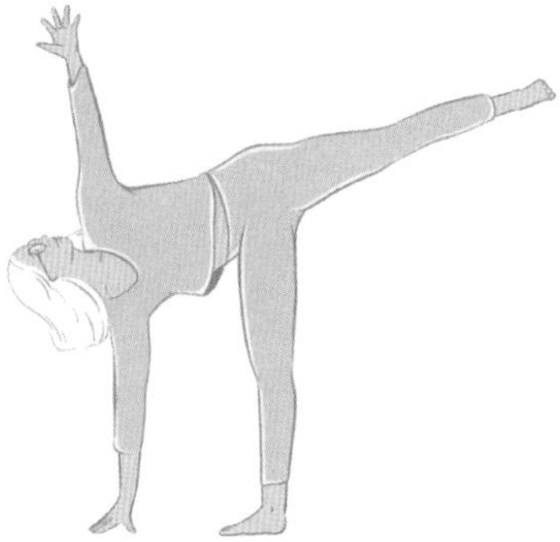

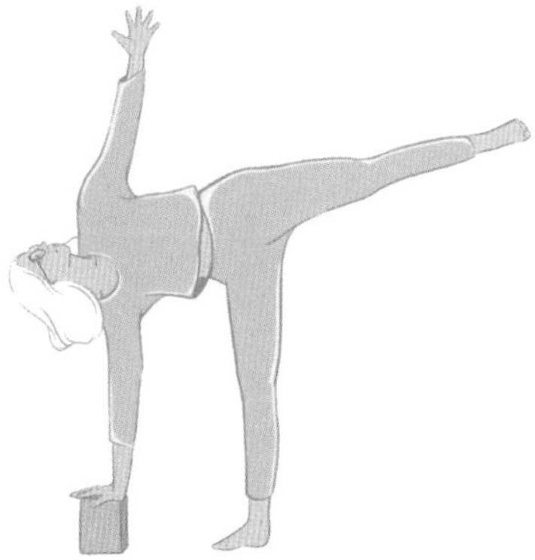

Starting in warrior II (see page 219) with the right foot forward, inhale and slowly hinge the right side of the body forward over the right leg bringing the right hand towards the floor or onto a block in front of the right foot. As you shift the weight forward lift the left leg away from the mat, foot flexed or pointed.

Roll the left hip back opening your body to the left, stacking the hips.

Roll the left shoulder open to stack it over the right shoulder and either keep the left hand on the hip or extend the left arm straight up to the ceiling. Gaze either down at the ground or up at the hand.

Hold for 5 slow breaths.

Exhale and slowly return to warrior II using your core to help control the movement and repeat on the opposite side.

HALF SPLIT
(Ardha hanumanasana)

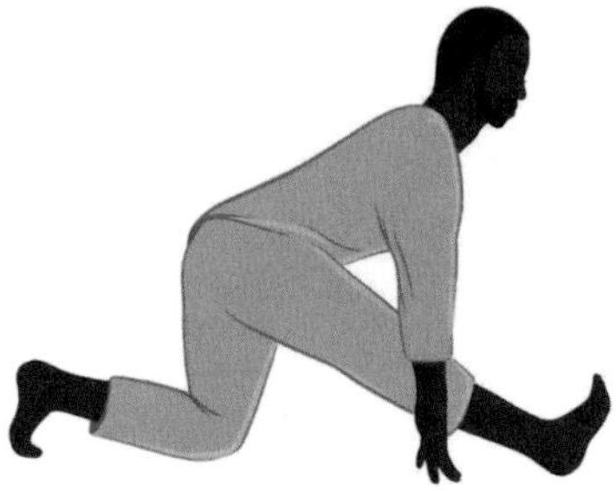

Start in low lunge (see page 206) with the right foot forward, exhale as you slowly start to shift the hips back to stack them over the left knee.

Straighten the right leg (as much as is comfortable) and flex the foot.

Slowly start to fold forward at the hip joint and bring the hands onto the floor (or blocks) to frame the front leg.

Encourage a sensation of pulling the hands back in space, this will help to keep length in the spine.

Only fold as far as you are able to, keeping the spine long and avoiding rounding the lower back.

Push into the heel of the right foot to activate the leg muscles as you take 5 breaths here.

Inhale to slowly release and repeat on the opposite side.

Option to place a blanket or cushion under the back knee or to keep the hands at heart centre.

HAPPY BABY
(Ananda balasana)

Lie on your back, bend the knees and kick the feet up towards the ceiling, flexing the feet.

Take hold of the outer edges of the feet, shins or thighs and gently press the sacrum into the floor.

Take 5 slow breaths here; you might also appreciate finding a gentle rocking sensation side to side.

Inhale to slowly release.

A nice modification can be to do one side at a time.

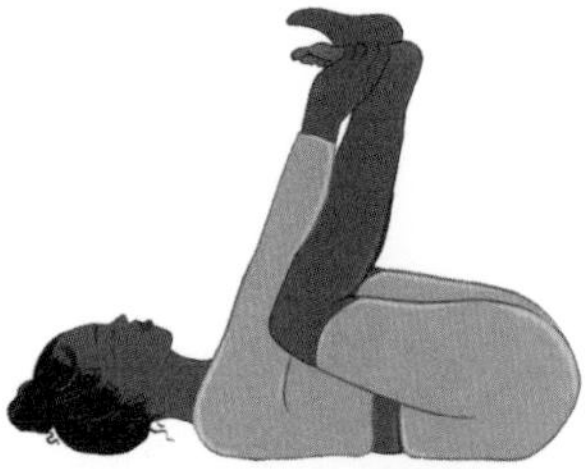

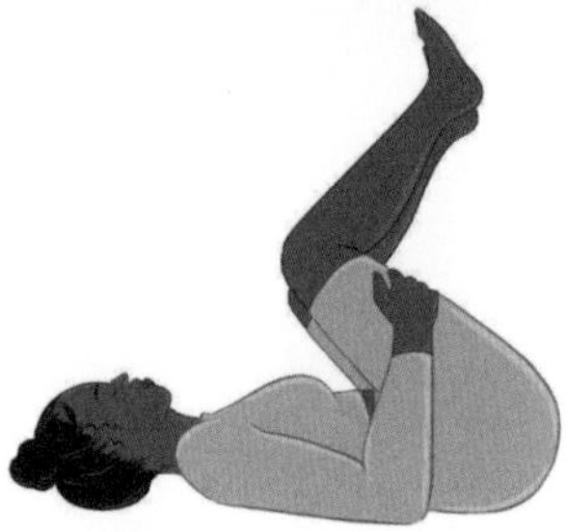

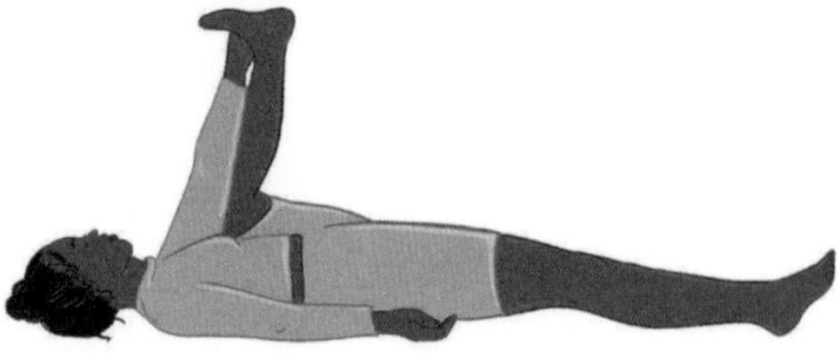

HEAD-TO-KNEE FORWARD FOLD
(Janu sirsasana)

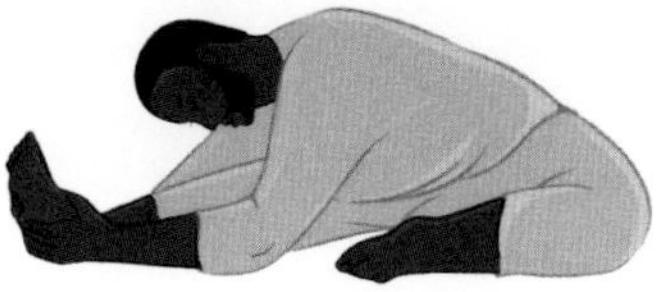

From a seated position, extend the right leg forwards, flexing the foot.

Bend the left knee, placing the sole of the foot on the right inner thigh and relaxing the knee towards the floor.

Turn your torso slightly to face over the extended right leg.

Inhale as you find length in the spine, growing tall through the crown of the head and raising the arms towards the ceiling.

Exhale and fold forward from the hips, draping the body over the thigh and framing the right leg with your fingers. Option to take hold of the ankle or foot or use a strap around the foot.

Keep the spine long and chest open (avoid rounding through the back). Hold for 5 slow breaths.

Inhale to release and then repeat on the opposite side.

Option to place a folded blanket or block under the sitting bones and/or the bent leg thigh.

HIGH LUNGE
(Utthita ashwa sanchalanasana)

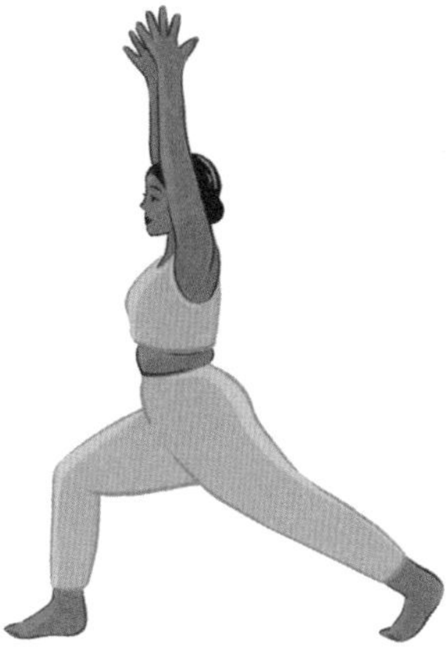

From downward-facing dog (see page 198) exhale and step the right foot between the hands (use your hand to help you if required).

Inhale up to standing, lifting the arms straight up to the ceiling. The hips are facing forward, right knee stacked over ankle. The left knee can have a slight bend to help keep the pelvis and spine neutral.

Press firmly through the feet as you reach up through the crown and fingers tips towards the ceiling.

Hold for 5 slow breaths and then exhale and return to downward-facing dog to repeat on the opposite side.

HIGH LUNGE HEART OPENER

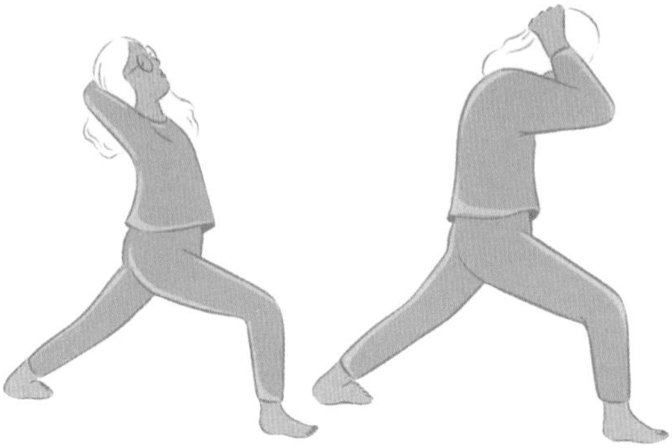

From high lunge, interlace the hands behind the head or bring the fingers to the ears if more comfortable.

Inhale as you open the elbows and chest, breathing up and lifting through the chest bringing a gentle bend into the upper spine.

Exhale and start to round through the back bringing elbow to elbow as you draw navel to spine, round the back and tuck the chin.

Repeat 5 times before gently releasing and repeating on the opposite side.

HINGED HIGH LUNGE

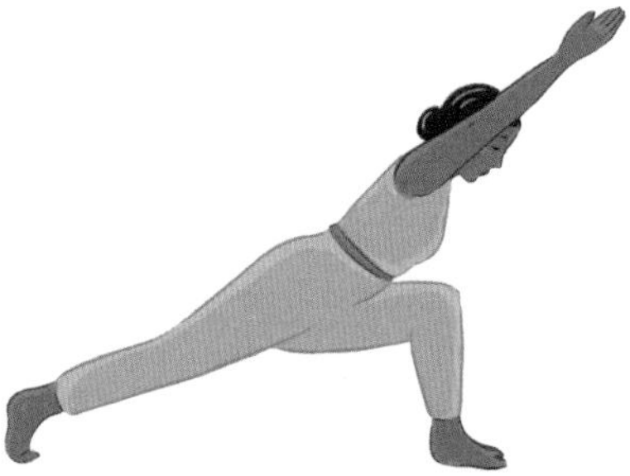

Starting in high lunge, exhale as you hinge from the hips and bring the torso closer to the front thigh. Keep the spine long and legs strong.

Hold for 5 slow breaths, then repeat on the opposite side.

LEGS UP THE WALL
(Viparita karani)

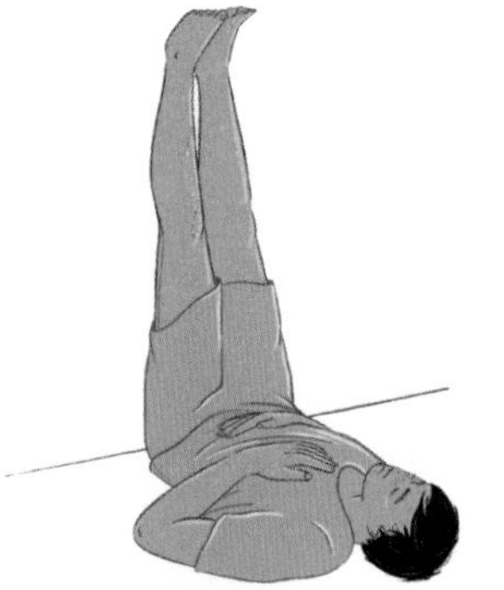

Lying on a mat, bring the hips to the wall, with the upper body flat and sitting bones as close to the wall as is comfortable.

Gently raise the legs straight up, resting them against the wall.

Option to place a pillow or blanket under your sacrum to ease any discomfort in the lower back and help to hinge at the hips.

If you have time, stay here for 5–15 minutes (or longer).

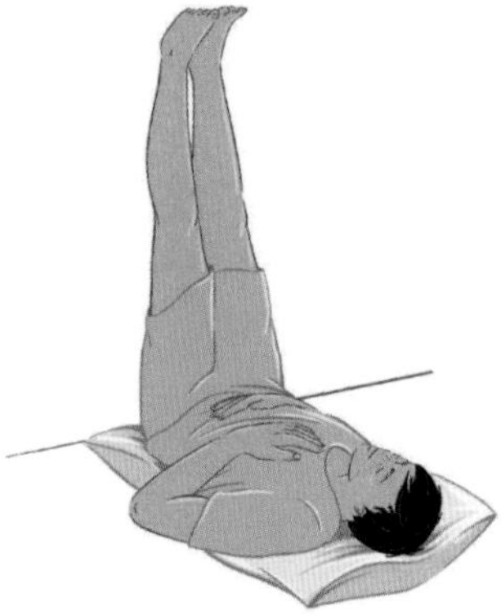

LIZARD POSE
(Utthan pristhasana)

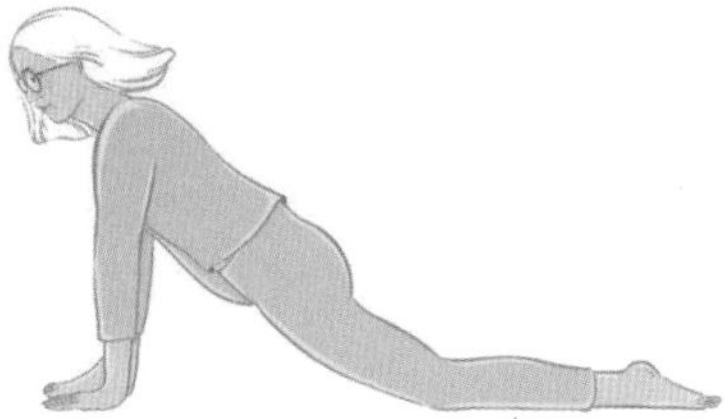

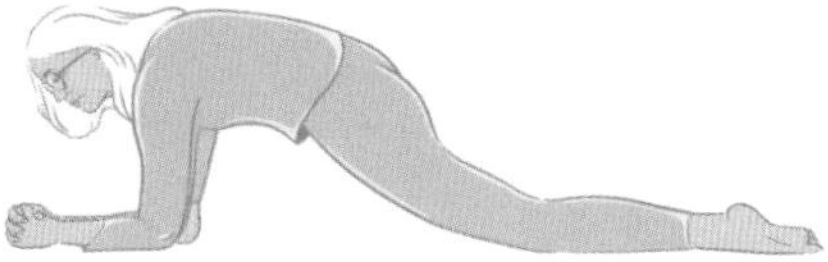

From downward-facing dog (see page 198), exhale and step the right foot forward to the outside of the right hand (use your hand to help you if required) then come down onto the left knee. The further the knee is from the hands, the more intense the stretch in the hip flexor and quadricep (front of the thigh).

Inhale as you find the sensation of pulling back in space with the hands (without moving them) to keep the spine long and the chest open.

Option to deepen the pose by either tucking the toes and lifting the back knee or coming down onto the forearms (ensuring that the spine stays long).

Hold for five slow breaths.

On the next exhale slowly release and repeat on the left side.

Option to place a blanket under the back knee if the knees are sensitive.

LOCUST POSE
(Salabhasana)

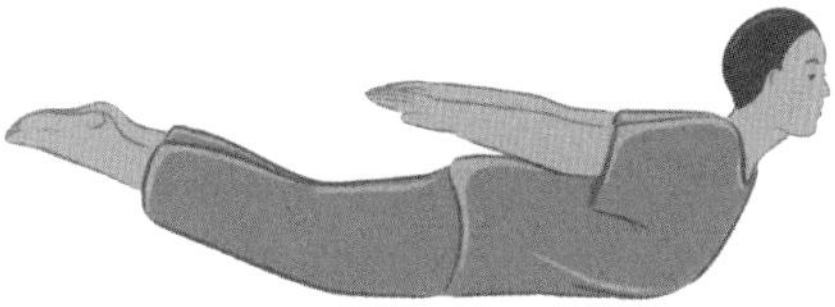

Lie on your stomach with the legs extended hip distance apart.

Reach the arms behind the back, elbows slightly bent and interlace the fingers into a fist. Squeeze the shoulders blades into centre and gently straighten the arms as you reach the fist away from you (the arms don't need to be fully straight). Option to grab a strap instead or to reach the arms back in space alongside the body without interlacing them.

Inhale as you press down through the public bone and lift the lower and upper body off the floor. Keep squeezing the shoulder blades together and squeeze the glutes to lift the thighs even higher.

Reach the toes in the opposite direction to the crown of the head to keep the spine long and the chest open. The gaze is forward and the chin is slightly tucked to keep the neck long.

Hold for 5 slow breaths, then exhale and gently release to the mat.

LOW LUNGE
(Anjaneyasana)

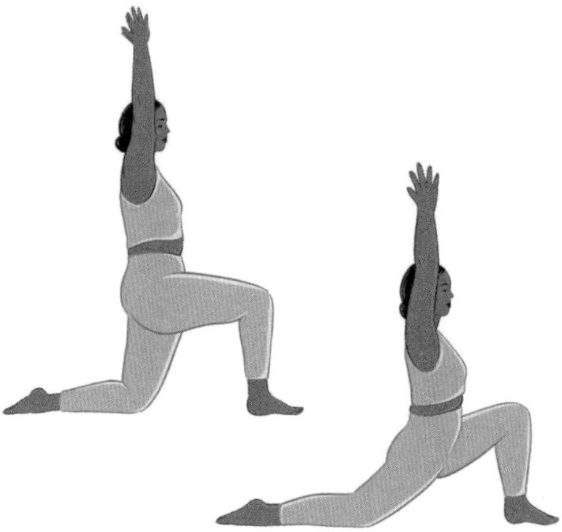

From downward-facing dog (see page 198), exhale and step the right foot forward between the hands (use your hand to help you if required) coming down onto the left knee. Stack the right knee over the right ankle and the left hip over your left knee, engaging the glute to help open the front of the hip.

Inhale and reach the fingers and crown of the head high to the sky, lengthening through the side body and drawing the ribs in gently to avoid them flaring.

Hold for 5 slow breaths then repeat on the other side.

Option to step the right foot forward further to focus the stretch on the front of the thigh, keeping the pelvis in a neutral position.

Option to turn this into a backbend keeping the glutes strong and lifting the chest upwards gently opening through the upper spine.

Place a blanket or cushion under the back knee if needed.

LOW LUNGE SIDE STRETCH
(Parsva anjaneyasana)

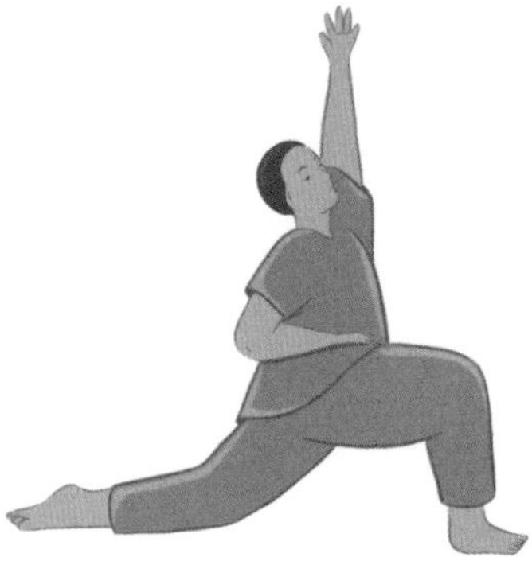

From low lunge with the right foot forward, inhale as you lift the left fingers to the sky and bring the right hand onto the right hip or place it over the belly

Exhale as you take a side stretch over to the right, lengthening through the left side body and keeping the spine long.

Hold for 5 slow breaths, then slowly release and repeat on the opposite side.

LOW LUNGE TWIST
(Parivrtta anjaneyasana)

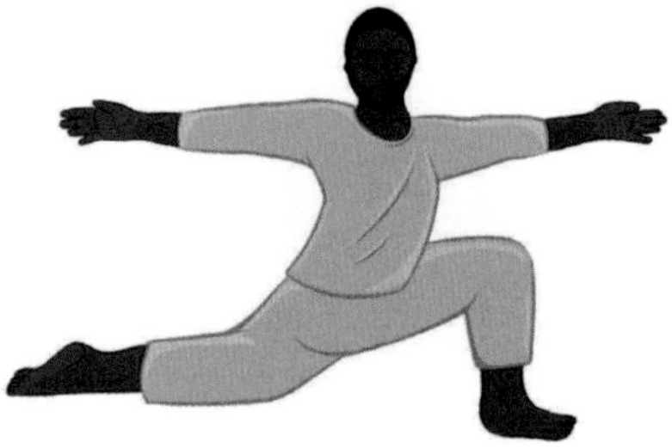

From low lunge with the right foot forward, inhale as you reach the arms to the sky.

Exhale as you reach the right arm backwards and left arm forwards so they are parallel with the floor, fingers reaching away from each other and palms down. At the same time, twist the torso to the right, rotating the chest towards the back of the room.

Keep the hips facing forward, spine long and feel the twist through the whole spine avoiding just rotating from the neck.

Hold for 5 slow breaths, then slowly release and repeat on the opposite side.

LOW LUNGE QUAD STRETCH

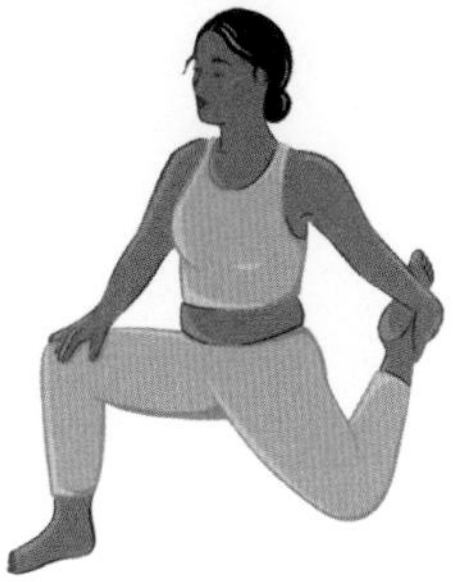

From low lunge with the right foot forward, kick the left foot in towards you and reach back with the left hand to grab hold of the foot (you can use a yoga strap here too). Place the right hand on the right thigh for balance or reach it into the air for an extra challenge.

Take 5 slow breaths as you gently pull the left foot in towards you. Reach tall through the crown of the head to keep the spine long and lengthen the tailbone downwards to increase the stretch sensation on the front of the left thigh and hip.

Exhale to gently release the left foot and repeat on the opposite side.

MOUNTAIN
(Tadasana)

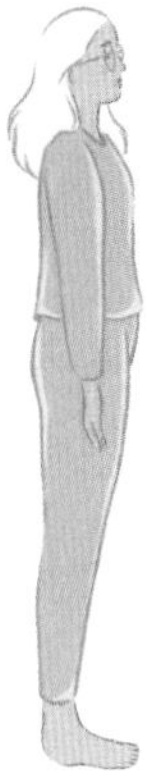

Stand at the top of the yoga mat with the feet facing forward, hip distance apart.

Lift and spread the toes, gently placing them back down on the mat and balancing the weight evenly through the feet.

Ground down through both feet and lengthen through the crown of the head, finding the natural curve of the spine and growing tall. Feel the energy drawing up through the floor into the legs and core.

Energise the arms by the torso, palms facing forward. Aim to stack your ears over the shoulders, the hips, the knees and the ankles. Hold for 5 slow breaths, then gently release.

Option to stand with the big toes touching and heels slightly apart.

PIGEON POSE
(Kapotasana)

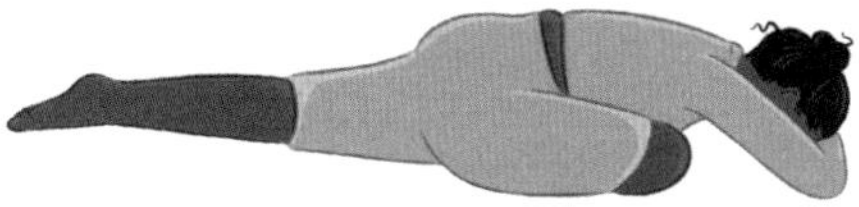

Starting in downward-facing dog (see page 198), bring the right knee to the right wrist and the right foot towards the left wrist, flexing the foot. Place the shin down onto the mat with the left leg stretching straight back behind you.

Lower the hips down towards the mat, squaring them forwards with the option of placing a cushion or block under the right hip.

Place the fingertips down slightly in front of the body and inhale to lengthen the spine as you press down gently through the legs. Exhale, slowly walk the hands forward to lower your torso to the floor, resting on the forearms or extending the arms forward.

Take 5–10 breaths here before gently walking yourself back up and out of the pose and repeating on the opposite side.

If this pose causes knee pain try reclined pigeon instead.

RECLINED PIGEON POSE
(Supta kapotasana)

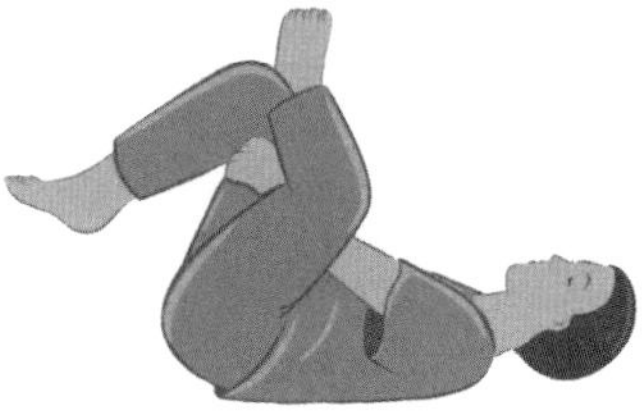

Lie on your back and bend the right leg, keeping the foot on the floor.

Place the left ankle over the right thigh just below the knee, keeping the left foot flexed.

Take the hands around the right shin or thigh and reach the left knee away as you gently pull the right leg towards your chest.

Hold for 5 slow breaths, then inhale to release.

Repeat on the opposite side.

PLANK
(Phalakasana)

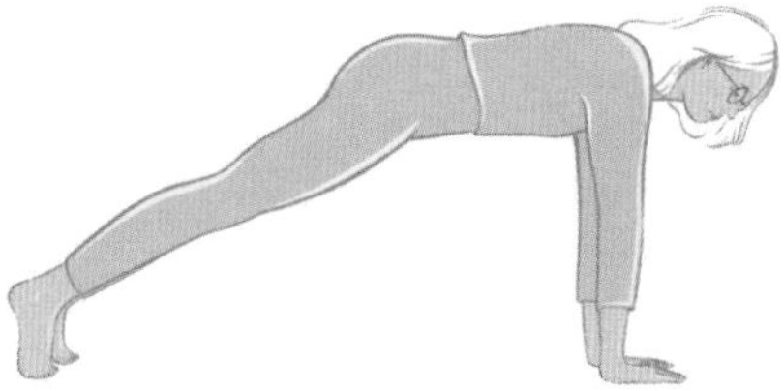

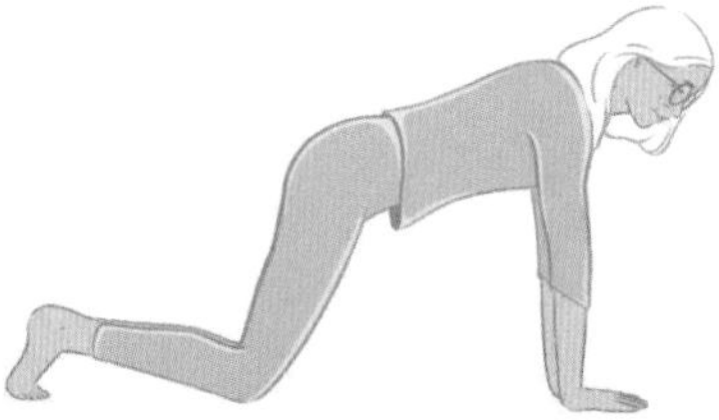

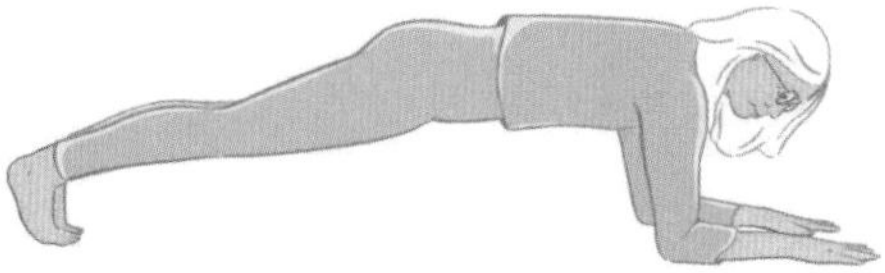

Come onto your hands and knees with the wrists under the shoulders.

Step the feet back, tucking the toes and lifting the knees from the floor. The legs and glutes should be engaged.

Bring the hips in line with the shoulders and keep a neutral spine with the neck long and gaze slightly forward. Avoid the lower back overarching or head dropping and draw the ribs in.

Keep the arms strong and have a sensation of 'dialling' the hands in opposite directions (like screwing jam jar lids) and set the shoulder blades into a neutral position.

Hold for 5 slow breaths then release.

Option to modify this pose by dropping the knees – the closer the knees are to the hands the less intense the pose will be.

Option to come onto the forearms with the knees down or lifted.

PYRAMID POSE
(Parsvottanasana)

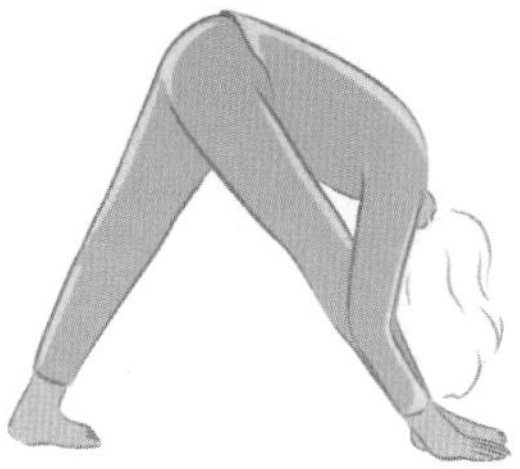

From mountain pose (see page 207), step the left foot back about 1–1.3m (3–4ft), keeping both legs straight and grounding both feet down to engage the muscles of the legs and hips.

The front foot is pointing forward and the back foot turned slightly outwards (around 45 degrees). The hips are square to the front as you inhale and lengthen your spine.

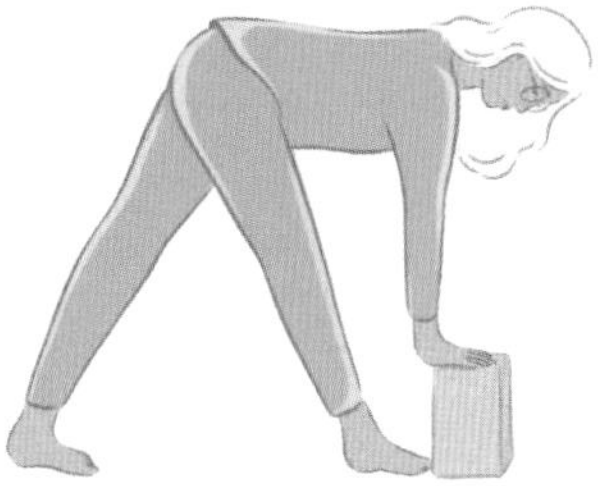

Exhale as you hinge at the hips, bringing your torso forward over the front leg and feeling a stretch on the hamstrings (back of the legs). Keep the spine neutral and long and avoid rounding in the back.

Place your hands on the floor on either side of your front foot. Option to use blocks if needed. Alternatively, bring your hands into prayer at heart centre.

Hold for 5 slow breaths, then inhale to slowly release and repeat on the other side.

RESTORATIVE FISH
(Matsyasana)

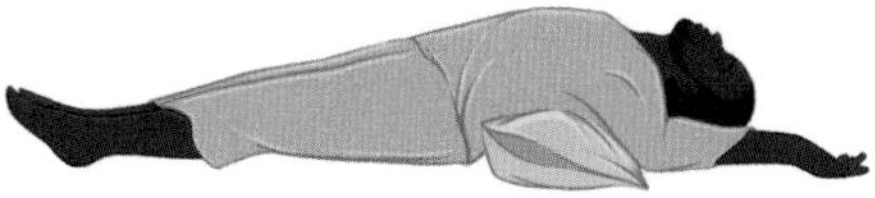

Place a pillow or block parallel to the short edge of your mat about 30–50cm (1½ft) away from the back of the mat.

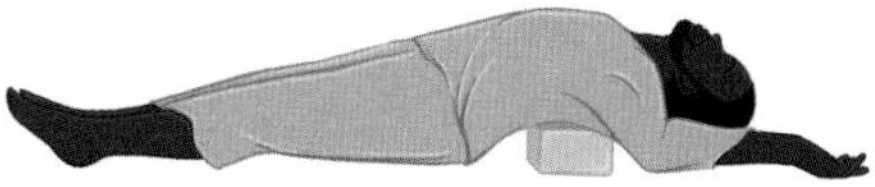

Option to place another pillow or block for your head at the back of the mat. Gently lie back over the prop(s) bringing the bottom edge just below the tips of the shoulder blades and the other under your head (if desired).

Melt the body over the prop(s) and place the arms to the side or overhead – whatever is most comfortable. Stay for 1–2 minutes or more. When exiting the pose gently roll to one side and remove the prop(s).

Option to clasp the hands behind the head, opening the shoulders as much as is comfortable. You can take a gentle side to side movement with the upper back.

RESTORATIVE FISH, CAT AND COW

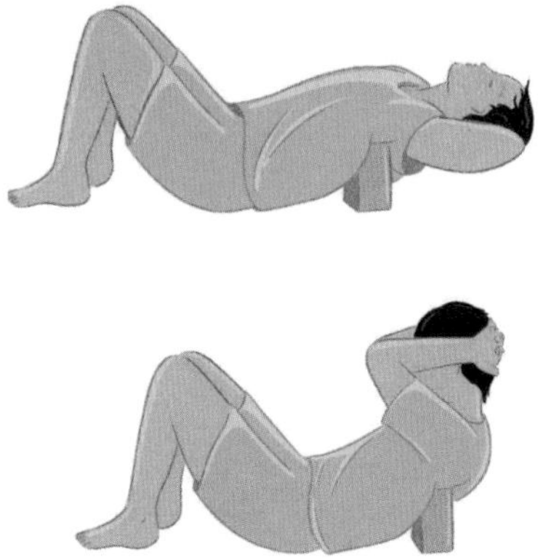

From restorative fish (see page 209), bend the knees and place the feet flat on the ground.

Interlace the hands behind the head, letting the elbows open to the sides.

Inhale gently pushing the skull into the hands and opening through the chest. Exhale to gently round the back, tucking the chin and bringing elbow to elbow.

Repeat for 5 breaths, then gently release the posture.

REVOLVED HEAD-TO-KNEE
(Parivrtta janu sirsasana)

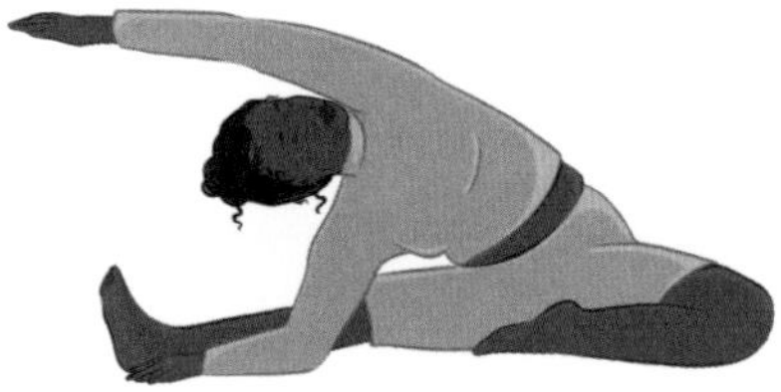

From a seated position, extend the right leg out wide, flexing the foot.

Bend the left knee, placing the sole of the foot on the right inner thigh and relaxing the knee towards the floor.

Place the right arm alongside the right leg and inhale as you find length in the spine and grow tall through the crown of the head.

Exhale to gently open through the left shoulder, twisting the upper body slightly to the left and reaching the left arm overhead as you take a side bend over to the right, stretching the fingertips away from you.

Lift the chest, keeping the left shoulder open, the neck long and chin slightly tucked. Hold for 5 slow breaths.

Inhale to release the posture and repeat on the other side.

Option to place a folded blanket or block under the sitting bones and/or bent leg thigh or to slightly bend the extended leg.

SAVASANA

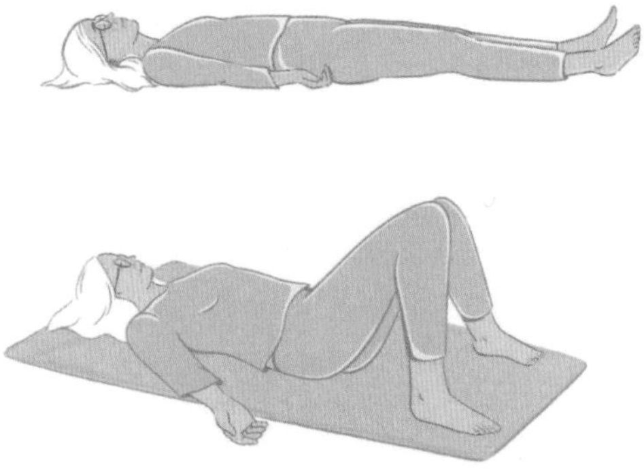

Lie on your back with the feet mat distance apart and let the feet drop open. If there is any pain in the lower back, bend the knees, bringing the feet flat on the floor and let the knees drop in towards each other.

Lay your arms by your sides away from the body, turn the palms to face the ceiling and let the fingers curl in naturally. Relax the shoulder blades evenly on the mat and lengthen through the back of the neck.

Close the eyes and allow the whole body to become soft and heavy, melting into the floor.

Stay here for 5 deep breaths or as long as desired.

SCALE POSE
(Tolasana)

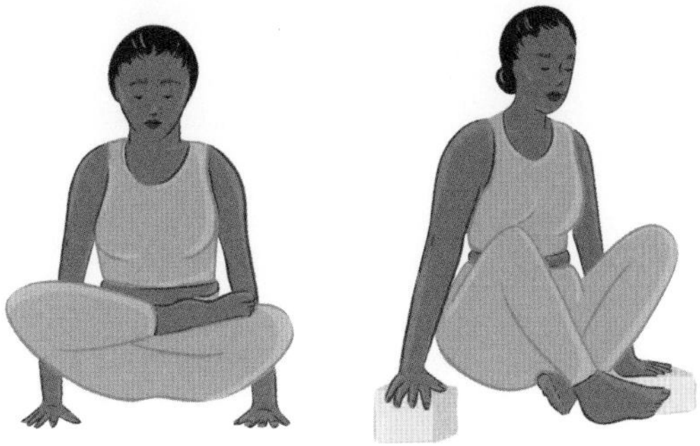

Start from easy pose (see page 211) or alternatively, lotus or half lotus pose, if either is in your practice.

Place the hands on the mat beside your hips, fingers pointing forward (they can be on blocks if required).

On an exhale, gaze forward and press firmly into the ground or blocks, feeling the core engage to help lift your lower body off the ground. Imagine a sensation of suctioning your legs into their sockets to help you find that lift.

Hold for 1–5 breaths, then slowly release back to the ground.

SEAL POSE
(Bhujangasana)

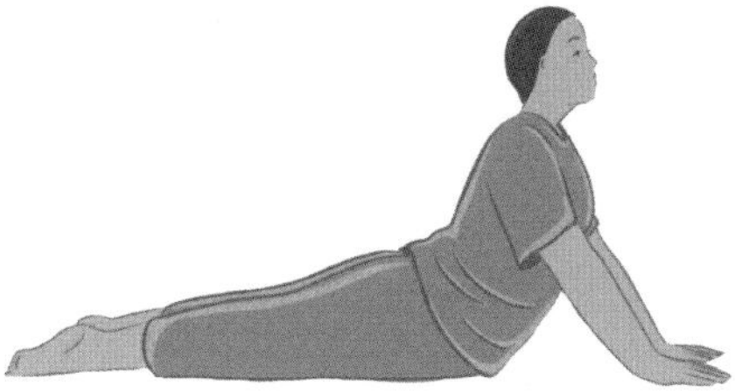

Starting from sphinx (see page 213), push the top of the feet and the pubic bone into the mat as you squeeze the shoulder blades together and push firmly into the hands to straighten the arms (they don't need to straighten fully).

Reach the crown of the head away from the toes to keep the spine long. Keep the chest open and gently squeeze the glutes to help avoid overextending the lower back.

Have a sensation of pulling the hands back in space (they don't actually move) and use the back muscles to help hold the posture rather than just relying on the strength of the arms.

Hold for 5 slow breaths, then slowly release to the mat.

SEATED POSTURES

EASY POSE
(Sukhasana)

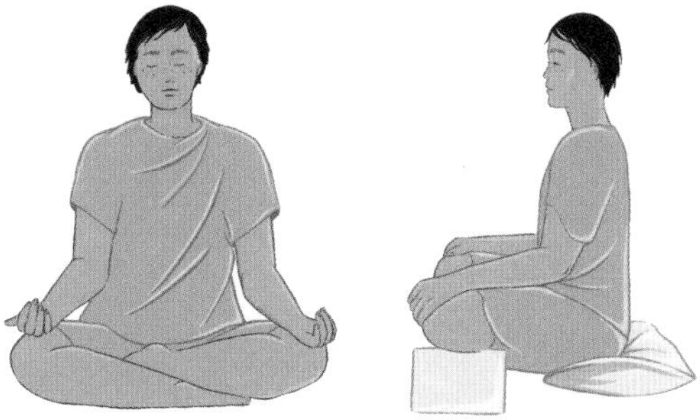

Come onto the floor, crossing one leg in front of the other, resting the hands on the knees or lap. Feel the sitting bones in contact with the ground as if rooting down and find length in the spine.

If this is uncomfortable (as it is for many), you can sit on a block or pillow to allow gradual release in the hips and help you find length in the spine. You can also do this for any seated posture that follows. Option to also place pillows under the thighs.

Hold for 5 slow breaths or more.

SEATED HEART OPENER

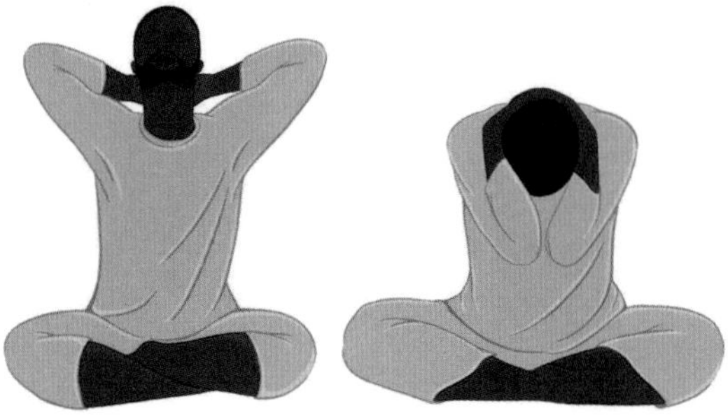

From a seated position, interlace the fingers behind the head or bring the fingers to the ears if more comfortable.

Inhale as you open the elbows and chest, breathing up and lifting through the chest bringing a gentle bend into the upper spine.

Exhale and start to round through the back bringing elbow to elbow as you draw navel to spine, round the back and tuck the chin.

Repeat 5 times.

SEATED FOLD

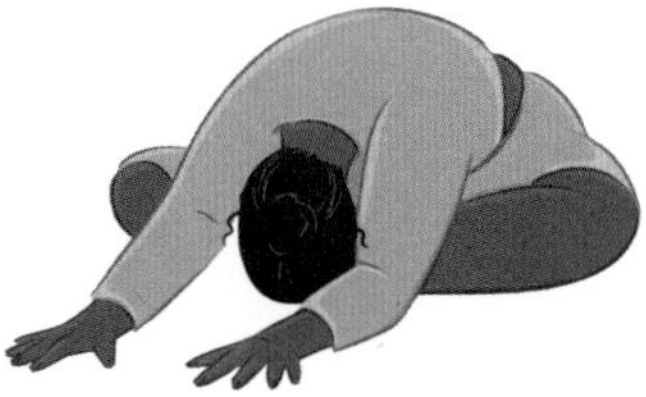

From a seated position, bring the fingertips slightly in front of the body.

Inhale as you roll the shoulders back and lengthen the spine, exhale to gently fold the body forward keeping the spine long. If you only fold a small distance that is okay. With each inhale, feel your spine growing a little longer, with each exhale, perhaps fold a tiny bit more.

Option to rest the head on a block or pillow.

Hold for 5 slow breaths and then inhale to gently walk yourself back to a seated position.

SEATED NECK STRETCH

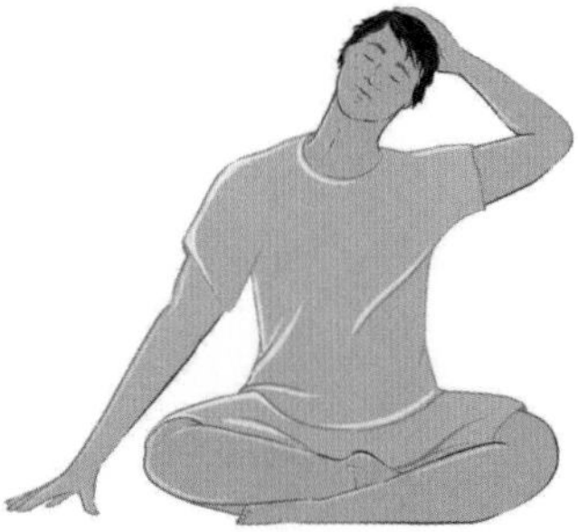

From a seated position, gently rest the right fingertips on the ground beside the right hip.

Take a breath in as you bring the left hand to the crown of the head, and as you breathe out slowly bring the left ear towards the left shoulder using the hand as a gentle guide.

Take 5 breaths here and then inhale, release and repeat on the other side.

SEATED SIDE STRETCH

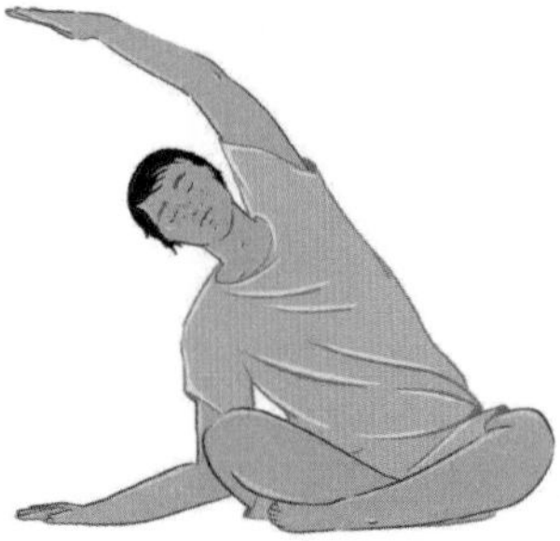

From a seated position, gently inhale, lifting the left arm up towards the sky finding length in the side body. As you exhale take a side bend over to the right-hand side keeping the sit bones grounded.

Inhale brings you up through centre then repeat on the other side.

Repeat 5 times.

SEATED TWIST

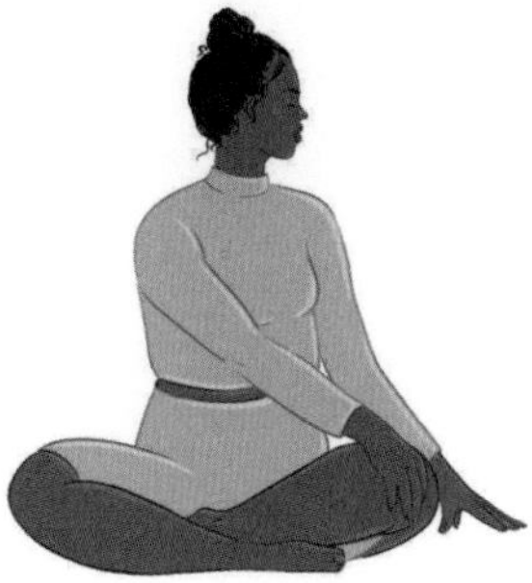

From a seated position, bring the right hand to the left knee and the left fingertips behind you.

Inhale to find length through the spine, growing tall through the crown of the head. As you exhale take a gentle twist gazing over your left shoulder. Imagine the twist going all the way up the spine, avoiding just twisting the cervical spine (the neck).

Hold this posture for 3–5 breaths and then slowly release before repeating on the opposite side.

SIDE PLANK
(Utthita vasisthasana)

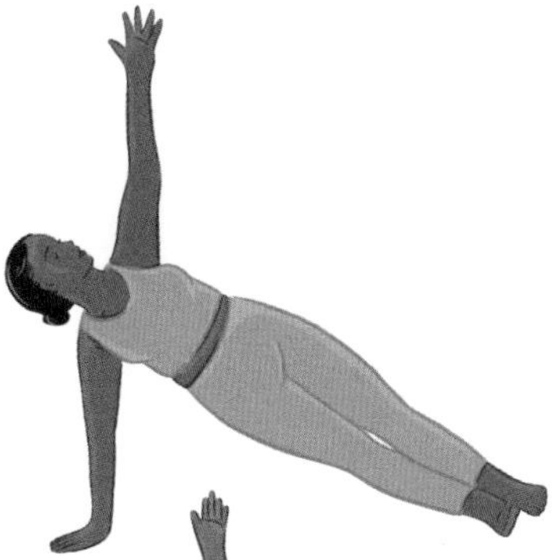

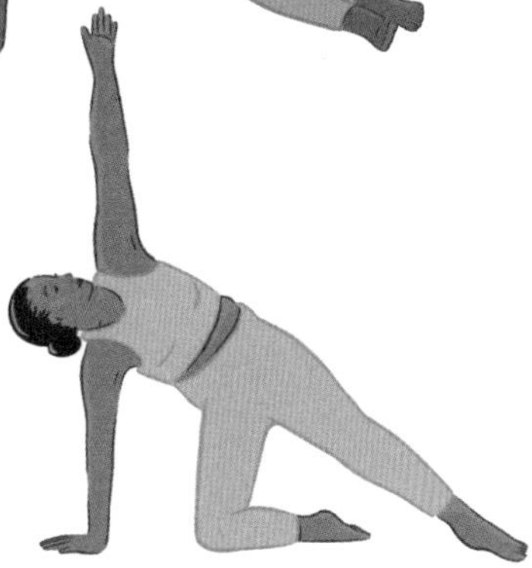

Starting in plank pose (see page 208), inhale as you shift the weight onto the right hand and the edge of the right foot. Stack the shoulders, feet and hips on top of each other and reach the left fingers straight up towards the ceiling.

Create a straight line from the crown of your head through to your heels.

Firmly press the right hand down and imagine suctioning the shoulder blade onto the back ribs for stability. The gaze can be up, straight ahead or down, depending on preference.

Keep the bottom hip pressing upwards and feel strength in the core while doing so.

Hold for 5 slow breaths and slowly return to plank before repeating on the opposite side.

Option to modify by keeping the bottom knee grounded.

SPHINX
(Salamba bhujangasana)

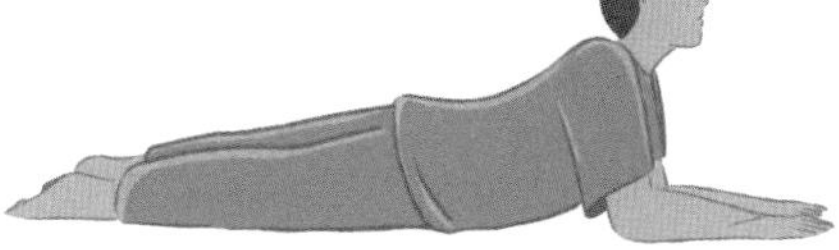

Begin by lying on your stomach with the legs extended, hip distance apart and your elbows placed directly beneath your shoulders, forearms flat on the mat.

As you inhale, press your forearms into the mat and lift your chest, imagining there's a piece of string lifting the centre of your chest forward and up. Have a feeling of pulling backwards with the forearms (they don't move).

Gaze forward and relax your shoulders away from your ears as the spine stays long.

To make this pose more restorative, you can release the head by dropping it down.

STANDING FORWARD BEND
(Uttanasana)

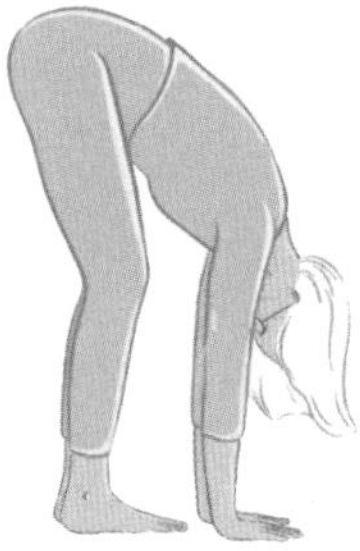

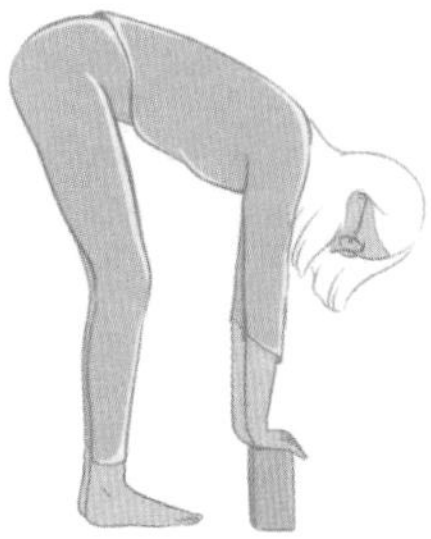

Stand at the top of the mat, feet hip distance apart, spine long and with a small bend in the knees.

Exhale, pressing the feet into the mat, and slowly hinge forward at the hips melting the torso towards the thighs, keeping the spine long. Imagine you have a heavy backpack on your back and you're resisting the weight as you move. Feel the engagement in the body as you do this.

Bring the hands to the floor, to your shins or onto blocks placed on the mat in line with the shoulders (wherever is comfortable). Bend the knees as much as you need to keep length in the spine.

Take 5 slow breaths here, then slowly return back to the upright position.

STANDING FORWARD BEND WITH LOCK

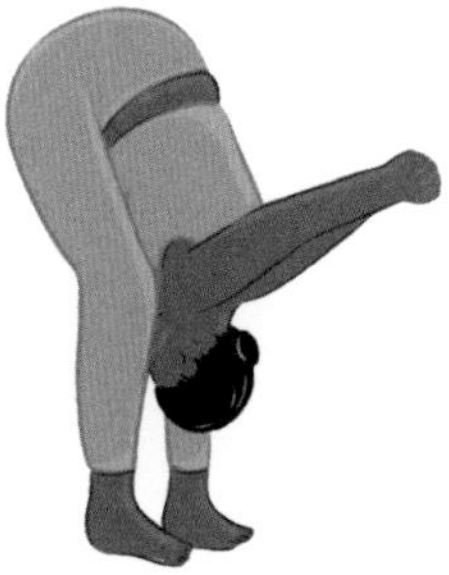

A nice variation of this pose is to interlace the hands behind the back (or grab a yoga strap or belt) and reach the fists away from you as you draw the arms overhead, keeping the arms fairly straight. Move slowly and mindfully, paying attention to both balance and sensation.

STANDING HALF FORWARD BEND
(Ardha Uttanasana)

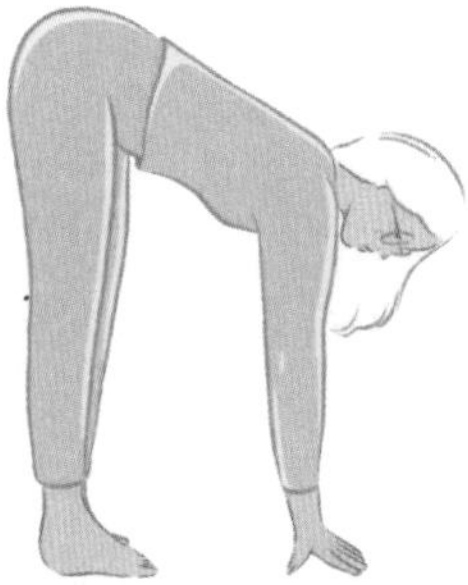

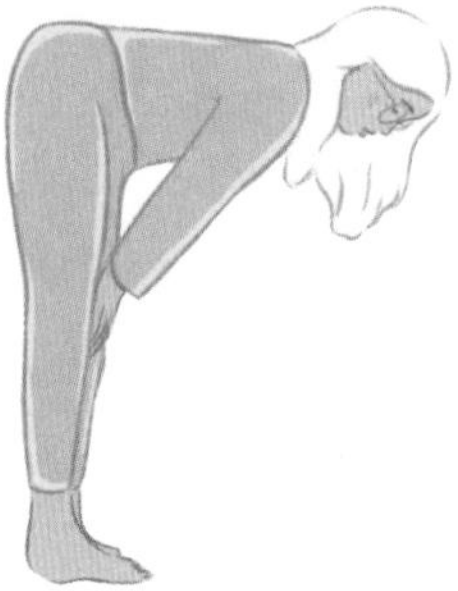

From standing forward bend (see above), ground through the feet as you inhale and use the back and core muscles to lift the upper body to come into a long and neutral spine.

The fingertips can be down on the mat if flexibility allows, or on a block or resting lightly on the shins or thighs.

Keep the chin tucked and imagine a piece of string is drawing the crown of the head forward helping you find even more length in the spine.

As you exhale, slowly release back to forward fold. Option to hold for multiple breaths too.

STANDING SIDE STRETCH

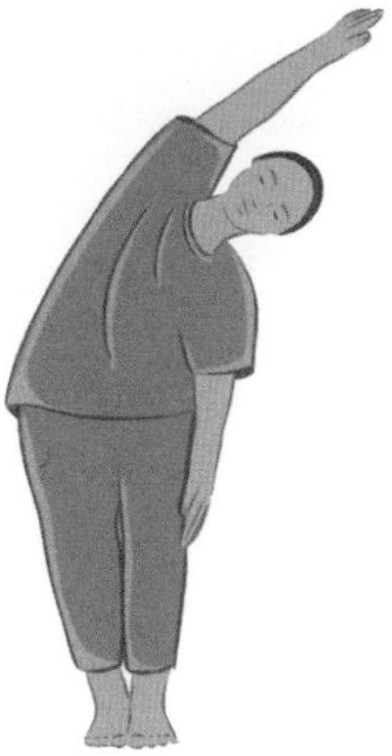

From mountain pose (see page 207), ground down through the feet and inhale, lifting the right fingertips to the sky.

Exhale to take a side bend over to the left-hand side, gently pressing the hips to the right to counterbalance the movement. Keep the spine long and the legs and glutes engaged.

Inhale back to centre and repeat on the other side.

Repeat 5 times.

STANDING HEART OPENER

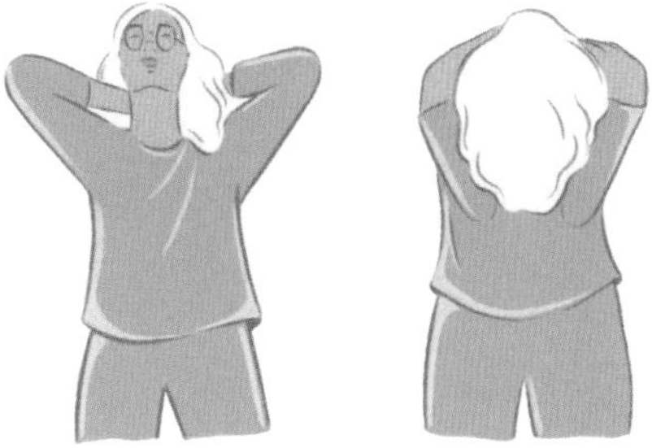

From mountain pose (see page 207), interlace the fingers behind the head or bring the fingers to the ears if more comfortable.

Inhale as you open the elbows and chest, breathing up and lifting through the chest bringing a gentle bend into the upper spine.

Exhale and start to round through the back bringing elbow to elbow as you draw navel to spine, round the back and tuck the chin.

Repeat 5 times.

SUPINE TWIST
(Supta matsyendrasana)

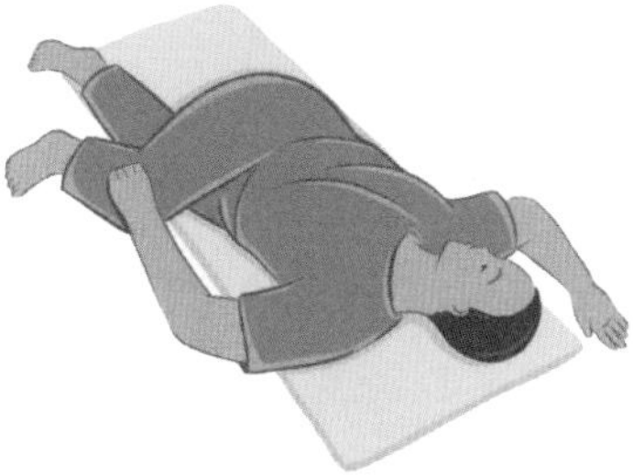

Starting on your back, hug the right knee into your chest and gently start to rotate it over to the left-hand side, bringing the gaze to the right and stretching the right arm in line with the shoulder, or with a bend in the elbow.

The left hand can come onto the knee to intensify the stretch. Try and keep the shoulders grounded, but if the knee doesn't touch the floor, that's okay. Hold for 5 breaths and repeat on the other side.

Option to either extend the bent leg or bring both knees in and twist.

THREAD THE NEEDLE
(Urdhva mukha pasasana)

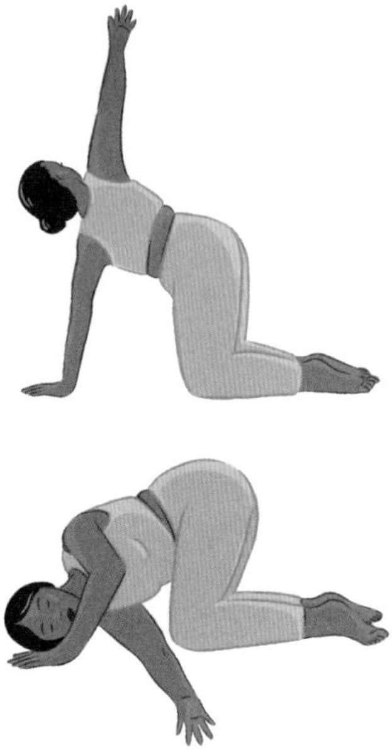

Start in tabletop with the wrists underneath the shoulders and knees underneath the hips.

Inhale and reach the right fingertips up towards the ceiling, opening the body to the right.

Exhale and mindfully thread the right arm through and underneath the body, bringing the right shoulder and right cheek down towards the ground (they don't need to touch).

Inhale, reaching the arm back up and repeating the movement.

Repeat 5 times, then repeat on the opposite side.

TREE POSE
(Vrikshasana)

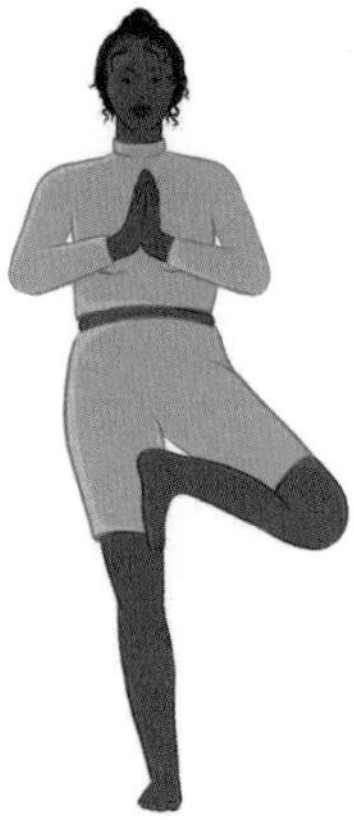

From mountain pose (see page 207), bring the weight into your right foot, grounding down and feeling the muscles of the hip engage.

Inhale and lift the left knee, taking hold of the foot.

Guide the foot to the right inner thigh, shin or ankle letting the knee open to the left. Keep the hips and shoulders facing forward.

Lift through the crown of the head, keeping the spine long and neutral. Avoid collapsing into the right hip; stand tall.

The hands can come into prayer at the heart centre or you can lift them into a 'V' towards the sky.

Hold for 5 breaths, then release and repeat on the opposite side.

TRIANGLE POSE
(Trikonasana)

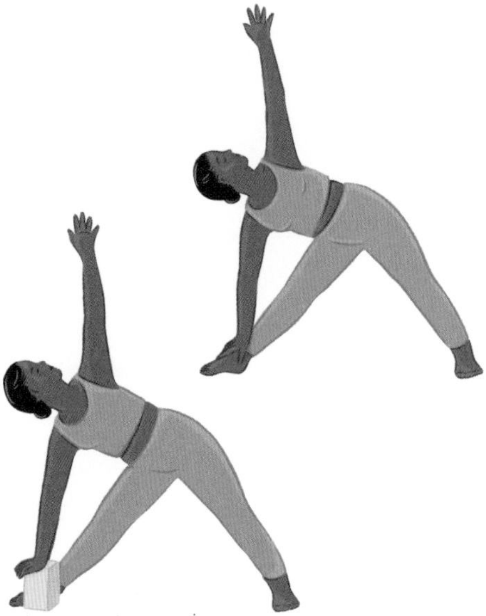

Start in warrior II (see page 219) with the right foot forward. Straighten both legs and step the left foot in a little so the feet are around 1m (3ft) apart.

The front toes point forward, the back foot is parallel to the end of the mat with the heels in line. Ground down through the feet, energising the legs as you raise the arms parallel to the floor with the palms facing down and fingers reaching away from each other.

Inhale as you reach towards the front of the mat keeping the lower body still and finding length in the side body.

Exhale as you extend the right hand towards the ground, taking hold of the big toe or resting it on the shin or a block and reach the left hand towards the ceiling.

Keep the upper body in line with the right leg as the left hip and torso rotate open, with the spine long.

The gaze can follow the left hand or be down towards the floor if more comfortable. Stay here for 5 slow breaths. Exhale to release and then repeat on the opposite side.

TWISTED CRESCENT LUNGE

(Parivrtta anjaneyasana)

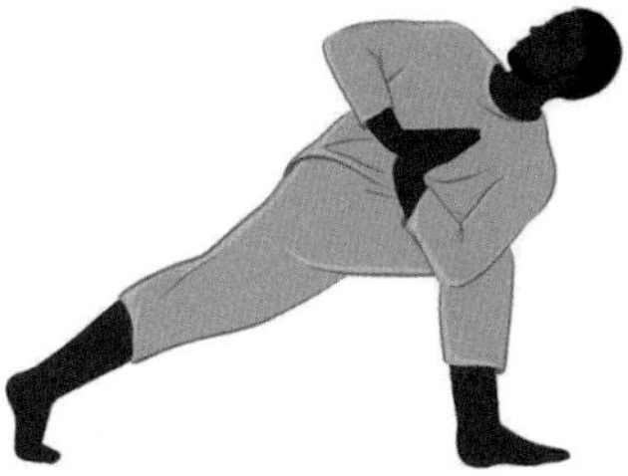

From low lunge, right foot forward, exhale as you bring the hands into prayer at heart centre and inhale to roll the shoulders back and down, opening through the chest. Exhale to rotate the torso to the right (the lower body doesn't move).

Option to hold here, connect the left elbow to the outside of the right thigh, or place the elbow on top of the thigh (keeping the chest open).

Option to intensify the pose by lifting the back knee and straightening the back leg.

Lengthen the spine, creating a line from the crown of the head to your left heel. Take 5 breaths here then inhale to come back to the centre and step to the front of the mat. Repeat on the other side.

UPWARD-FACING DOG

(Urdhva mukha svanasana)

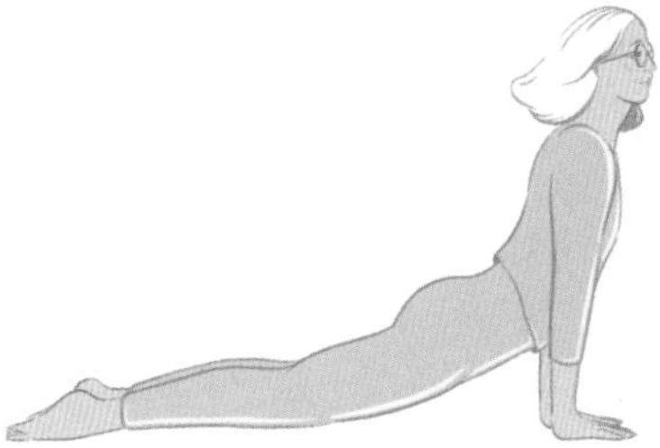

Starting in plank (see page 208), exhale as you slowly lower through yoga push-up (see page 222) and inhale coming onto the tops of the feet as you straighten the arms.

There can be a gentle bend in the elbows to help open the chest. Roll the shoulders back and down, opening through the heart space. Imagine a piece of string attached to the centre of your chest pulling you forward and up. Create a feeling of dragging the hands backwards and press down into the mat to help draw the chest through the arms.

Activate the front of your thighs by pushing the tops of the feet into the floor, keeping the knees lifted off the floor. The glutes should be engaged to keep the pelvis neutral and avoid overextending the lower back.

Gaze forwards, keep the neck long and grow tall through the crown of the head. Hold for 5 slow breaths and then slowly on an exhale lift the hips up and back to downward- facing dog (see page 198).

Option for cobra pose instead (see page 195) if that feels better for your body.

UPWARD SALUTE
(Urdhva hastasana)

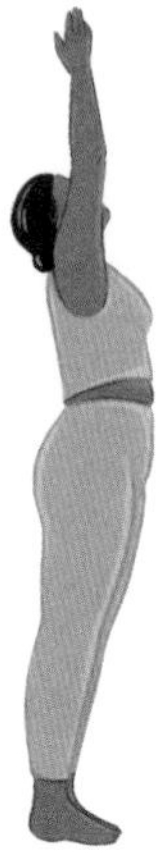

From mountain pose (see page 207), ground down through the feet as you inhale the arms to the sky, reaching tall through the crown of the head and lifting the fingertips high to the sky.

The hands can come together or be shoulder-distance apart.

A gentle squeeze of the glutes and hug in of the ribs will help you keep the spine neutral.

Exhale and return to mountain pose (see page 207) or fold into standing forward bend (see page 214).

WARRIOR I
(Virabhadrasana I)

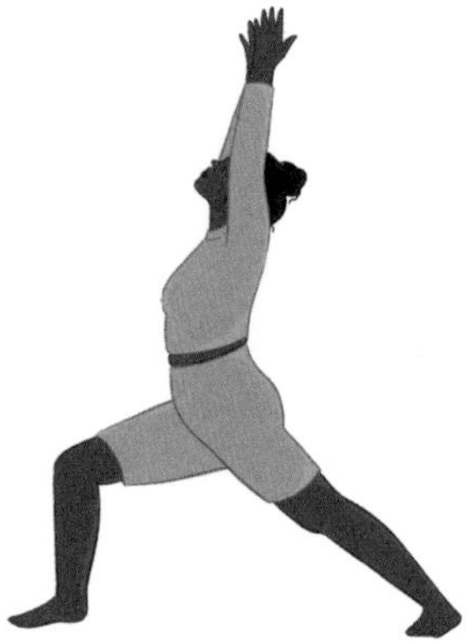

From mountain pose (see page 207), exhale and step the left foot back around 1m (3ft).

Bend the right knee and stack it over the ankle, turning your left toes out (around 45 degrees).

Keep the heels hip distance apart to help to square the hips forward. Press evenly into both feet to lift the arches and engage the front glute to avoid the knee collapsing in.

Inhale, raising the arms overhead, reaching the fingers up towards the sky, lengthening the torso, opening through the heart and gently hugging the front ribs in.

Option to bring the hands together or have them slightly apart if more comfortable.

The gaze can be up towards the hands or forward, if preferred.

Take 5 breaths here, then inhale as you step the left foot to the front of the mat and repeat on the other side.

Option to have the feet closer together if more comfortable and the hands at the heart centre if there is any pain in the shoulders.

WARRIOR II
(Virabhadrasana II)

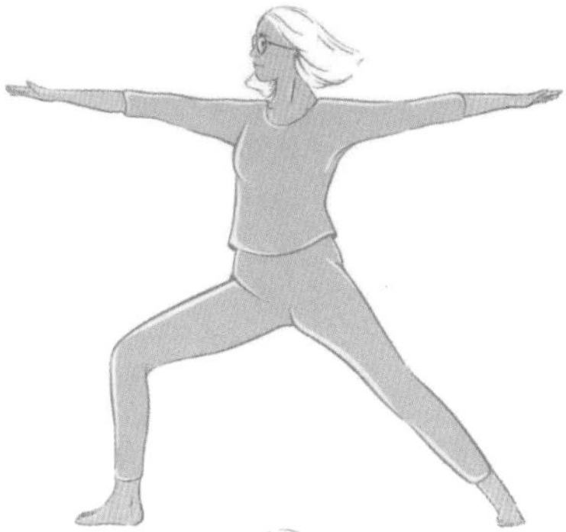

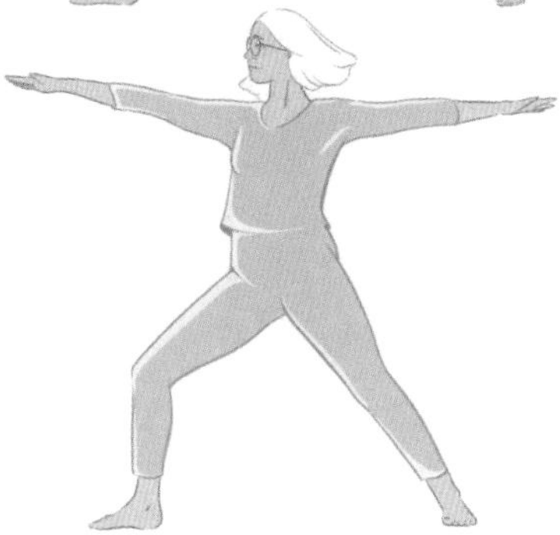

From mountain pose (see page 207), exhale and step the left foot back around 1m (3ft).

Bend the right knee so it is stacked over the ankle and come onto the sole of the left foot. The outer edge of the left foot should be parallel with the back of the mat. The right heel can be in line with the arch or heel of the left foot. The torso is facing the left side of the mat.

Press evenly into both feet to lift the arches and engage the front glute to avoid the knee collapsing in.

Raise the arms so they are parallel to the floor, palms facing down, and lengthen them in opposite directions. Keep the torso long, spine neutral and shoulders strong.

Check that the shoulders are away from the ears and gaze at the middle fingertip of the right hand.

Take 5 breaths here and then inhale as you step the left foot to the front of the mat and repeat on the other side.

Option to have the feet closer together if more comfortable and the hands at the heart centre if there is any pain in the shoulders.

WARRIOR III
(Virabhadrasana III)

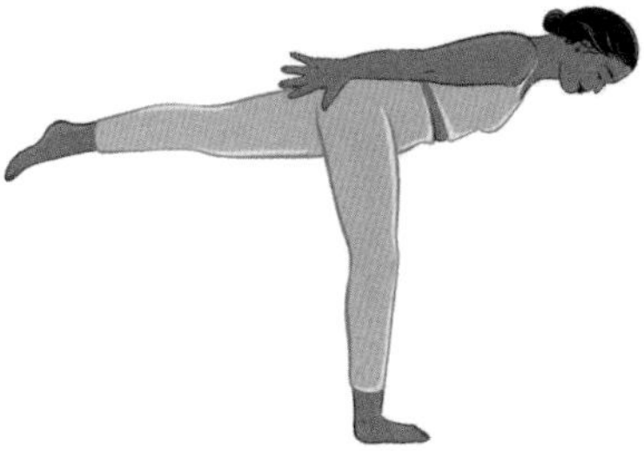

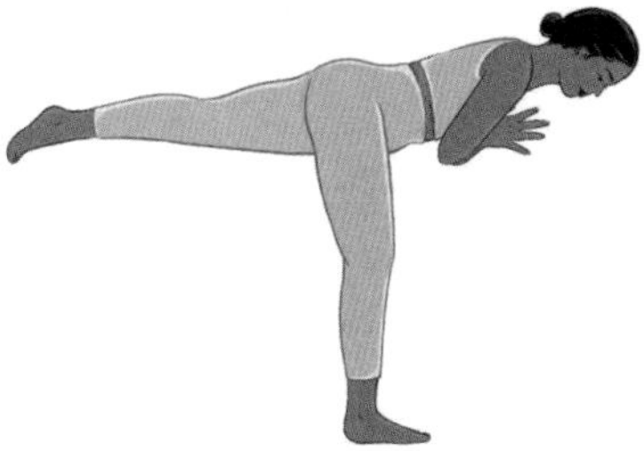

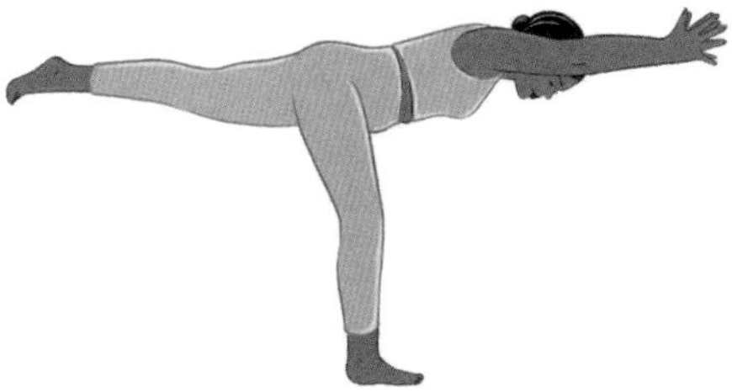

From high lunge (see page 203), exhale slowly, shifting the weight forwards, hinging from the hips and bringing the left leg back up behind you, pointing the toes and squeezing the glutes.

Push firmly through the grounded foot and big toe mound to activate the stabilising muscles in the hip. The left hip will want to lift up; try to square it in line with the right (placing the hands on the hips can be helpful).

The spine stays long, creating a long line from the crown of your head to your left toes. The hands can come to the hips, heart centre, behind or reach out in front.

Hold for 5 slow breaths. Inhale to return to high lunge and repeat on the opposite side.

WIDE-ANGLE SEATED FORWARD BEND
(Upavistha konasana)

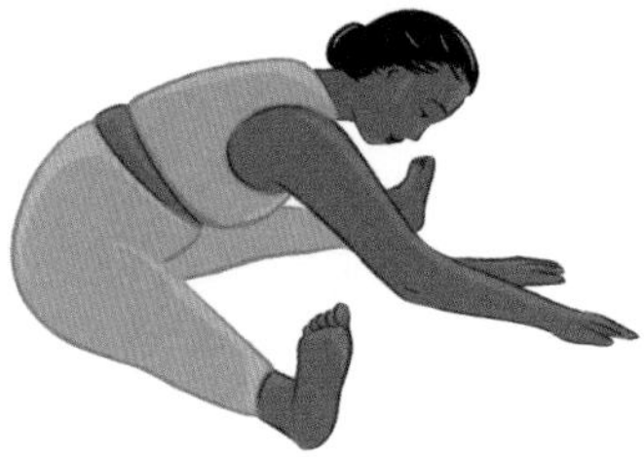

Sitting on your mat, extend the legs into a 'V' shape with the feet flexed.

You want a long, neutral spine; if this is difficult, sitting on a block or rolled up blanket can be helpful.

Bring the fingertips between the legs as you inhale, lifting through the crown of the head and lengthening the spine.

Exhale to slowly start to walk the hands forward, hinging from the hips and folding down between the legs. The spine stays long, the chest open and legs active.

Each inhale find length through the spine, each exhale maybe reach a little bit deeper.

Hold for 5 slow breaths, then release back to sitting.

WILD THING
(Camatkarasana)

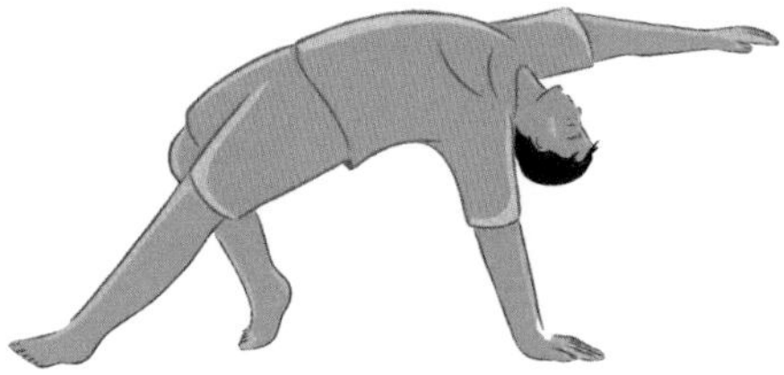

From downward-facing dog hip opener (see page 198), right side, exhale to softly place the right toes on the floor behind you with the knee partially bent and the heel can be lifted or flat to the floor, firm the left shoulder blade onto the back ribs.

Inhale to sweep your right arm overhead, arching through the upper back and lifting the hips, activating through the glutes.

Imagine there's a piece of string attached to the centre of your chest, drawing you upwards and opening the heart.

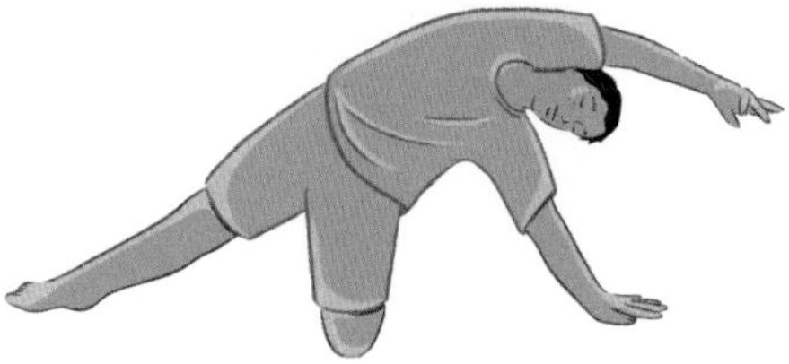

Hold for 5 slow breaths, then slowly return to downward-facing dog (see page 198) before repeating on the opposite side.

Option to start from kneeling plank, keep the left knee grounded and the right leg straight.

WRIST WARM-UP SEQUENCE

This sequence can be used to warm up and strengthen the wrists whenever you need it.

FISTS AND STARS

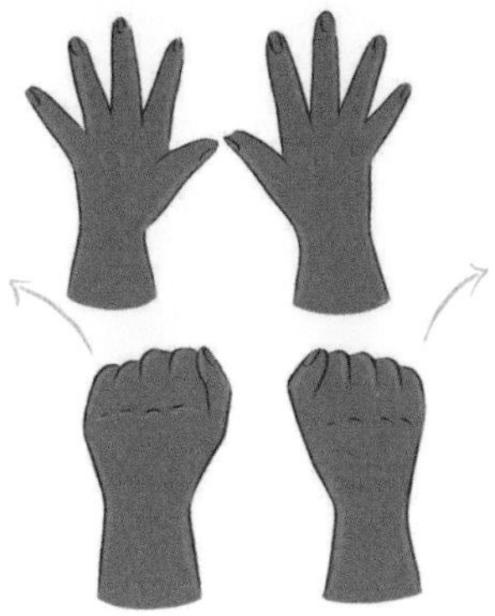

From a seated or standing position, reach the arms straight out in front of you parallel to the floor.

Make a strong fist with both hands, then stretch out the fingers as wide as you can to make a shape a little like a star.

Repeat the fist and star movement as quickly as you can for 30–60 seconds, being mindful with both movements.

TABLETOP CIRCLES

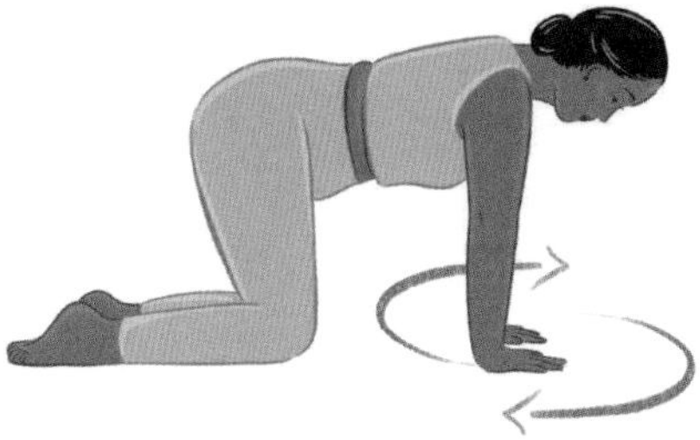

From tabletop, gently start to circle the body, inhaling forward, circling the shoulders over the wrists as far as is comfortable and exhaling, circling back bringing the hips towards the heels.

Repeat 5 times and then switch direction.

TABLETOP ROUND THE CLOCK

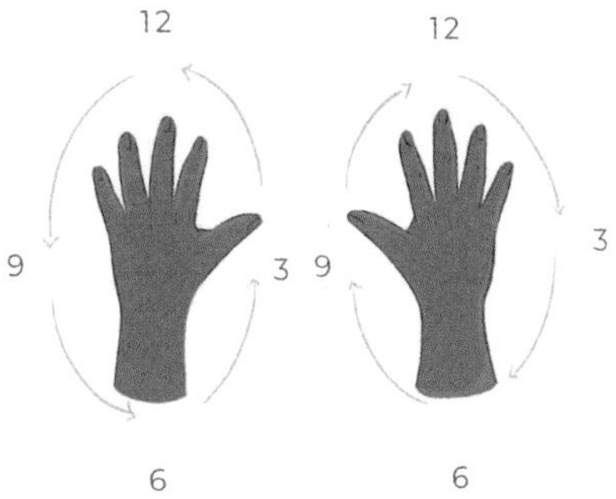

From tabletop pose, gently pad the left hand to face 9 o'clock and the right hand to face 3 o'clock.

Hold for a moment then continue moving them round so they both point to 6 o'clock.

Bring them back to 9 o'clock and 3 o'clock, then back to 12 o'clock and then the left hand to 3 o'clock and the right hand to 9 o'clock.

Repeat 5 times.

YOGA PUSH-UP
(Chaturanga)

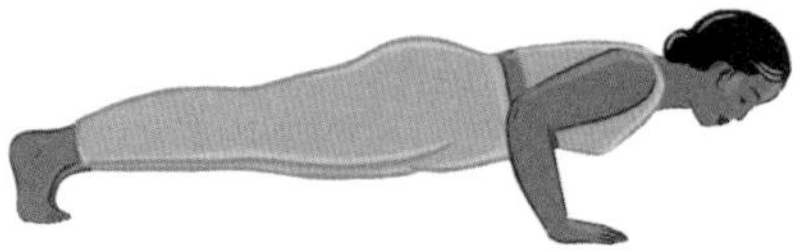

Start in plank (see page 208) with the spine neutral, the legs active, glutes activated, core engaged and ribs drawing in. Imagine there's a heavy weight on your back and you're resisting against it.

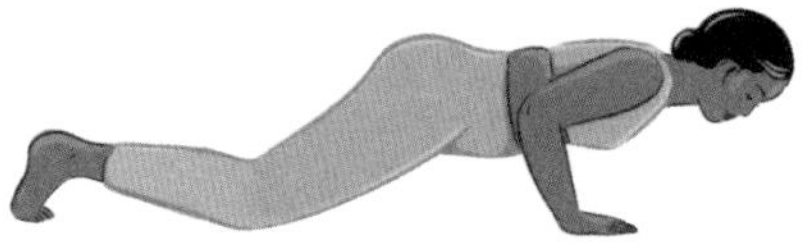

Exhale as you start to lower the body in one straight line, elbows pointing backwards. Have a sensation of 'dialling' the hands in opposite directions (like screwing jam jar lids) and pulling back with the hands to keep the shoulder tips lifted (the hands don't actually move).

Lower as much as you can control or until the upper arms make a 90-degree angle with the floor; avoid the head and shoulders dipping down.

Hold for 1–5 breaths. Either inhale and lift into upward-facing dog (see page 217), or exhale and push back up to plank.

Option to lower the intensity by dropping the knees – this is a challenging posture so tune in and be mindful of your body.

YOGI SQUAT
(Malasana)

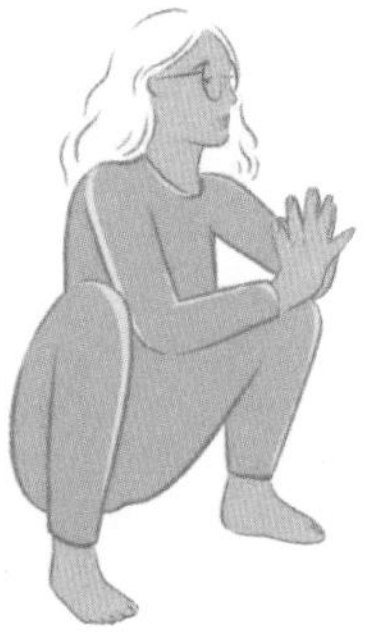

Begin standing at the top of the mat, feet slightly wider than hip distance and toes turned slightly outwards.

Exhale as you squat down and lower the hips down close to the ground.

Bring the hands into prayer at heart centre, using the elbows to gently push the knees outwards.

Inhale, growing tall through the crown of the head, lifting the chest and lengthening through the spine as your feet push firmly into the mat engaging through the legs and hip muscles.

Hold for 5 slow breaths before inhaling back up to standing.

If your heels don't reach the ground, you can place a rolled-up mat or a blanket under them for support. You can also place a block under your sit bones.

INDEX

ACKNOWLEDGEMENTS

It takes a village to make a book dream a reality and I feel beyond grateful to have so many incredible people in my life that support me every step of the way.

Giles, the biggest thank you as you truly never stop believing in me and making life more fun. Your calm strength inspires me more than you know and I love that you could be part of this book.

Jack and Amelie, you teach me presence and how to be a better person and I love you with all my heart. Jack, I love how you have learnt to use my meditations to help you fall asleep. Amelie, I adore how you join me on the mat, from flowing with me to just being with me playing 'the floor is lava' with all the yoga props.

Thank you to all my family – the Gillinsons and the Barretts. You put up with me lugging my yoga mat to any and every destination and never fail to support me in everything I do. I love you all and thank you for being there for me. And James, I miss you every day.

A huge thank you to my literary agent Jenny. I trust and value you so much. Thanks for continuing to be a sounding board and for always believing in me.

Imogen, you are so wonderful and talented and I was delighted to be back working with you. Your continued patience and valuable insight is appreciated always.

To the whole team at Quadrille, thank you for making this vision a reality. In particular, Gemma, Sophie and Ore – thank you for creating such a beautiful book, the little touches of thoughtfulness do not go unnoticed.

Eleanor, our magical illustrator. Yet again you have blown us away with your talent. This book wouldn't be the same without you.

Cecilia, Mike and Grace, my lovely photographer and videographers. You know I come back to using you time and time again because the passion, care and dedication you put into your work is astounding. Thank you for being part of this project.

My beam of sunshine Celest, the past few years creating Alba Yoga Academy have been incredible. You have taught me so much and lots of that has fed into this book. Thank you for making working so darn fun and for all the belly laughs along the way.

Elspeth, you were one of the first people to read *The Yoga Happy Year* and I was beyond nervous. I value your opinion so greatly and was thrilled when you loved it. Thank you always for your insight and honesty and for all the walks and pep talks on the range.

To my Yoga Happy Khala. You've been part of my community from the very start, grateful for your friendship and so happy you could be part of this book. Thank you also to my other models, Maria and Geri – you are both wonderful. And to Ami, I was so grateful to receive your philosophy insight, thank you.

A huge thank you to all my students, teachers, the other special people I have in my life and for everyone who has picked up this book. You all teach me so much and inspire me each and every day to do my best and to share my passion. I wouldn't be the same without you all.

And to Juliet and Nicky, life can be cruel and it isn't the same without you. You both spread ripples of joy and positive change with everything you did. You inspired me in so many ways and I promise to 'go grab life' and find joy in the big and small parts.